AF556765

Monogenic Hyperinsulinemic Hypoglycemia Disorders

Frontiers in Diabetes

Vol. 21

Series Editors

M. Porta Turin
F.M. Matschinsky Philadelphia, Pa.

Monogenic Hyperinsulinemic Hypoglycemia Disorders

Volume Editors

Charles A. Stanley Philadelphia, Pa.

Diva D. De León Philadelphia, Pa.

54 figures, 10 in color, and 20 tables, 2012

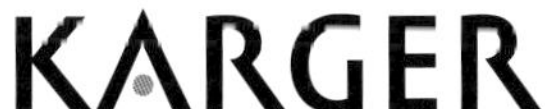

Basel · Freiburg · Paris · London · New York · New Delhi · Bangkok · Beijing · Tokyo · Kuala Lumpur · Singapore · Sydney

Frontiers in Diabetes
Founded 1981 by F. Belfiore, Catania

Charles A. Stanley, MD
Division of Endocrinology/Diabetes
The Children's Hospital of Philadelphia and
Department of Pediatrics
Perelman School of Medicine
University of Pennsylvania
Philadelphia, Pa., USA

Diva D. De León, MD
Division of Endocrinology/Diabetes
The Children's Hospital of Philadelphia and
Department of Pediatrics
Perelman School of Medicine
University of Pennsylvania
Philadelphia, Pa., USA

Library of Congress Cataloging-in-Publication Data

Monogenic hyperinsulinemic hypoglycemia disorders / volume editors, Charles A. Stanley, Diva D. De León.
p.; cm. -- (Frontiers in diabetes, ISSN 0251-5342 ; v. 21)
Includes bibliographical references and indexes.
ISBN 978-3-8055-9943-6 (hard cover: alk. paper) -- ISBN 978-3-8055-9944-3 (electronic version)
I. Stanley, Charles A. II. De León, Diva D. III. Series: Frontiers in diabetes; v. 21. 0251-5342
[DNLM: 1. Hyperinsulinism. 2. Hypoglycemia. 3. Insulin--metabolism. 4. Pancreatic Diseases.
W1 FR945X v.21 2012 / WK 880]
616.4'66--dc23

2011048792

Bibliographic Indices. This publication is listed in bibliographic services.

www.karger.com
Printed in Germany on acid-free and non-aging paper (ISO 9706) by Kraft Druck GmbH, Ettlingen
ISSN 0251–5342
e-ISSN 1662–2995
ISBN 978–3–8055–9943–6
e-ISBN 978–3–8055–9944–3

Contents

Preface

This volume of *Frontiers in Diabetes* is devoted to genetic defects associated with hyperinsulinemic hypoglycemia. Although hypoglycemia disorders might seem a peculiar topic for a series on diabetes mellitus, these diseases provide unique perspectives on basic mechanisms regulating insulin secretion in both normals and diabetics. The contributors to this monograph represent many centers around the world that have been responsible for the rapid advances in this field over the past two decades (although we confess to not being able to include other significant investigators for lack of space).

This volume is the third in a series devoted to discussing broadly the molecular basis of monogenic disease of glucose homeostasis (see vol. 15 and 16). We hope that it will be recognized as the third guidepost for an investigative strategy which continues to elucidate the biochemistry of rare molecular genetic 'experiments of nature' in fuel metabolism, many yet to be discovered, thereby increasing the understanding of the enormous complexities of blood glucose regulation in health and disease, and facilitating the development of new therapies that would benefit the patients suffering from diabetes mellitus, hyperinsulinemic hypoglycemia, and related disorders.

The Editors wish to thank Dr. Franz M. Matschinsky, series editor for *Frontiers in Diabetes*, for suggesting this volume and for his encouragement.

Charles A. Stanley, Philadelphia, Pa.
Diva D. De León, Philadelphia, Pa.

Stanley CA, De León DD (eds): Monogenic Hyperinsulinemic Hypoglycemia Disorders.
Front Diabetes. Basel, Karger, 2012, vol 21, pp 1–6

Historical Perspective on the Genetic Forms of Congenital Hyperinsulinism

Charles A. Stanley[a] · Franz M. Matschinsky[b]

[a]Division of Endocrinology/Diabetes, The Children's Hospital of Philadelphia and [b]Institute for Diabetes, Obesity and Metabolism, University of Pennsylvania School of Medicine, Philadelphia, Pa., USA

Abstract

Since 1995, a total of 8 genetic defects in the pathways of beta-cell insulin secretion have been identified that cause congenital hyperinsulinism. These advances parallel the discovery of 10 different monogenic diabetes disorders. Together these disorders of islet regulation provide important insight into the mechanisms controlling beta-cell insulin secretion not only in patients, but also in normal humans.

As shown in the table 1, the major historical landmarks in congenital hyperinsulinism (HI) in children roughly parallel the discoveries of monogenic forms of diabetes mellitus [maturity-onset diabetes of the young (MODY)]. Recognition of HI actually predates MODY by two decades, beginning with Irvine McQuarrie [1] in 1954, who devoted his presidential address to the American Pediatric Society to a description of 'idiopathic hypoglycemia of infancy'. He was among the first to recognize that endogenous hypoglycemia, as opposed to hypoglycemia from iatrogenic insulin overdose, could occur in children. He emphasized that delays in diagnosis and inadequate early therapy of this idiopathic disorder all too frequently result in 'irremediable brain injury'. Shortly thereafter, in 1956, Cochrane et al. [2] described children with a form of hypoglycemia that was not improved, but aggravated by a high-protein diet. He found that leucine was the most potent amino acid inducing hypoglycemia, leading to the term 'leucine sensitivity'. Both Dr. McQuarrie and Dr. Cochrane described familial cases in their series, implying that genetic factors might be involved in 'idiopathic hypoglycemia'. In contrast, MODY was first recognized in 1975 by Tattersall and Fajans [3].

In 1960, one of the first important applications of the insulin radioimmunoassay of Rosalind Yalow and Solomon Berson was to prove that 'leucine-sensitive

Table 1. Historical landmarks in the genetics of hyperinsulinism and monogenic diabetes

Hyperinsulinism	Monogenic diabetes
1950s	
Description of 'idiopathic hypoglycemia of infancy' [1]	
Description of 'leucine-sensitive hypoglycemia' [2]	
1960s	
Insulin radioimmunoassay of Yalow and Berson [4]	
Diazoxide Rx of 'leucine-sensitive hypoglycemia' [5]	
1970s	
'Nesidioblastosis' [6]	Description of MODY [3]
1980s	
Diffuse vs. focal hyperinsulinism defined [7]	
1990s	
Recessive inheritance of hyperinsulinism [8]	
Dominant inheritance of hyperinsulinism [9]	
	MODY2 (glucokinase) [11]
SUR1 mutations (recessive) [12]	MODY3 (HNF1A) [13]
Kir6.2 mutations (recessive) [14]	MODY1 (HNF4A) [15]
Glucokinase mutations (dominant) [16]	MODY4 (PDX1) [17]
GDH mutations (dominant) [18]	MODY5 (HNF1B) [19]
	DIDMOAD (WFS) [20]
	MODY6 (NEUROD1) [21]
2000s	
SUR1 mutations (dominant) [22]	PNDM (Kir6.2) [23]
SCHAD mutations (recessive) [24]	CEL diabetes [25]
Kir6.2 mutations (dominant) [26]	PNDM (SUR1) [27]
MCT1 mutations (dominant, exercise HI) [28]	INS [29]
HNF4A mutations (dominant, transient HI) [10]	
UCP2 mutations (dominant) [30]	

hypoglycemia' was, in fact, due to insulin, thus highlighting the importance of amino acids, as well as glucose, as regulators of insulin secretion [4]. As discussed in the chapters by Kelly et al. [pp. 100–111] and Li et al. [pp. 112–124], recent studies of children with HI show that protein and leucine sensitivity are not necessarily synonymous and are not found in all genetic forms of the disorder. In 1965, Drash and Wolf [5] at Pittsburgh Children's Hospital first reported the use of diazoxide, an antihypertensive drug with the unfortunate side effect of suppressing insulin secretion, to successfully control hypoglycemia in some cases of idiopathic hypoglycemia. To this day, diazoxide continues to be the mainstay for treating HI, although it is ineffective in a large proportion of the most severely affected cases with mutations at the site for diazoxide action (fig. 1).

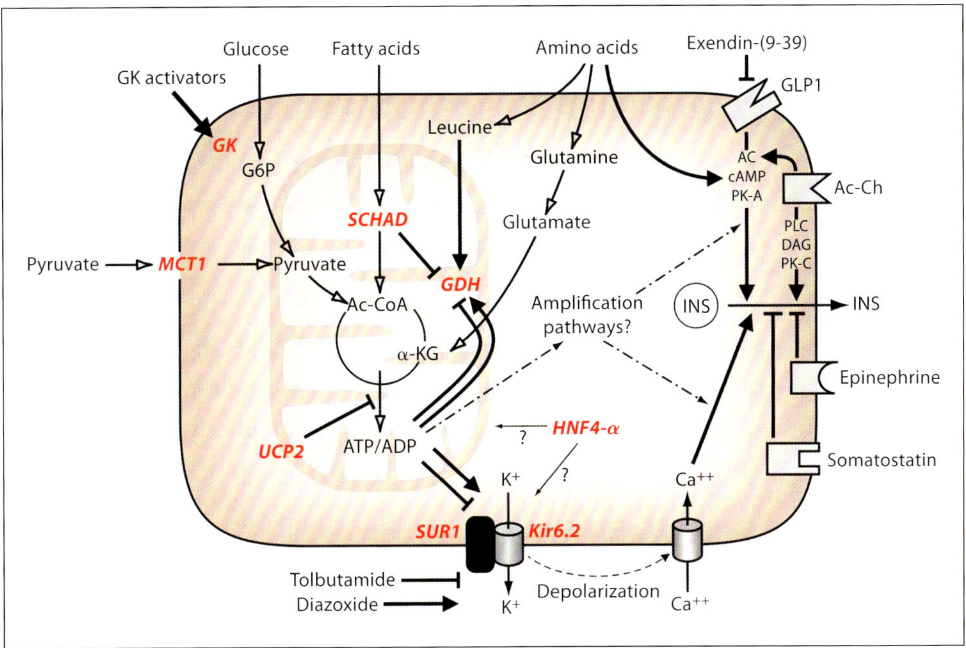

Fig. 1. Sites of genetic defects causing hyperinsulinism. For this introductory perspective, this diagram provides a minimalist consensus view, leaving the discussion of further details and controversial views to the individual chapters. Shown are the pancreatic beta-cell signaling pathways of fuel-mediated insulin secretion and their modifications by the neuroendocrine system and relevant drugs. Open arrowheads indicate directionality of metabolite flux and solid arrowheads the presence of stimulatory signaling, whereas terminal crossbars denote inhibitory effects. Glucose and amino acids, but not fatty acids, are the major fuel signals. The eight known gene defects are shown in bold italics in red. Five are inactivating mutations: SUR1 (sulfonylurea receptor), Kir6.2 (potassium channel), UCP2 (uncoupling protein 2), HNF4-alpha (hepatic nuclear transcription factor 4-alpha, a transcription factor with the biochemical effects of a genetic defect still unknown), SCHAD (short-chain 3-OH acyl-CoA dehydrogenase functioning as inhibitor of GDH through direct protein/protein interaction). Three are activating mutations: GK (glucokinase), GDH (glutamate dehydrogenase), MCT1 (monocarboxylate transporter 1). Note that all of the known defects affect the 'triggering' pathway of insulin secretion in which increased production of ATP in mitochondria associated with a lowering of ADP levels leads to inhibition of plasma membrane ATP-dependent potassium channels. Adenine nucleotides, or other mitochondrial derived signals and cell membrane receptors (such as the GLP-1-R and the acetylcholine receptor), also promote insulin release by 'amplification' pathways (some of them poorly defined but usually in the presence of elevated cytosolic calcium). G6P = Glucose-6-phosphate; Ac-CoA = acetyl-CoA; α-KG = alpha-ketoglutarate; INS = insulin; GLP-1-R = glucagon-like-peptide 1 receptor; Ac-Ch = acetylcholine; cAMP = cyclic adenosine monophosphate; PK-A = protein kinase A; PK-C = protein kinase C; DAG = diacylglycerol; PLC = phospholipase C.

In the 1970s, increasing recognition of the central role of insulin led to the introduction of 'nesidioblastosis' to replace 'idiopathic hypoglycemia of infancy' [6]. While the term, unfortunately, continues to have currency in adult diabetology, pediatricians abandoned it long ago after pathologists pointed out that 'nesidioblastosis' is a normal feature of the pancreas in neonates and young infants [7].

In the early 1990s, the possibility of a genetic basis for HI was rediscovered through reports of families showing autosomal recessive or autosomal dominant modes of inheritance [8, 9]. Using new technologies of positional cloning and mutation analysis, it became feasible to associate HI (and MODY) with specific genetic loci by analysis of multiplex families or candidate gene approaches. The past two decades have generated 8 genes for HI and 10 for MODY. Note that several genes contribute to both disorders: glucokinase, SUR1, Kir6.2, and the transcription factor HNF4A.

As shown in figure 1, nearly all the disease-causing HI mutations involve metabolic steps in beta-cell fuel-mediated insulin secretion: the so-called 'triggering' pathway of insulin release which links substrate oxidation through plasma membrane depolarization to trigger a rise in cytosolic calcium and subsequent release of insulin from storage granules. Interestingly, steps downstream of cytosolic calcium remain as potential candidate disease loci, including receptor signaling via glucagon-like peptide-1 and acetylcholine on the one hand, and somatostatin and epinephrine on the other (fig. 1). In contrast with HI disorders, most of the MODY defects cannot be easily diagrammed because they involve gene transcription factors whose complex effect(s) on beta-cells are still being elucidated. For this reason, figure 1 does not identify a specific mechanism for HI due to mutations of the HNF4A transcription factor, which was recently shown to cause a transient form of neonatal hyperinsulinism that resolves within several months or years after birth (Kapoor et al. [this vol., pp. 182–190]) [10].

This monograph explores the pathophysiologic consequences for each of the large number of genetic disorders of HI in detail. As indicated by table 1, this is a rapidly expanding field with interesting and exciting implications for understanding the central mechanisms of beta-cell regulation. Glucokinase-HI has already provided insights on the development of glucokinase activator drugs for diabetes. Several of the chapters touch on new approaches to diagnosis (e.g. ^{18}F-DOPA PET scans for preoperative localization of focal hyperinsulinism – States and Adzick [this vol., pp. 71–78]) and potential new treatments (e.g. green tea polyphenols for GDH-HI and GLP-receptor antagonists for SUR1 and Kir6.2-HI – Smith [this vol., pp. 87–99] and De León [this vol., pp. 79–86]).

Acknowledgements

This work was supported in part by grants from the NIH: RO1-DK-22122 (F.M.M.), R37-DK056268 (C.A.S.), R01-DK053012 (C.A.S.), DK-19525, and UL1-RR024134.

References

1 McQuarrie I: Idiopathic spontaneously occurring hypoglycemia in infants: clinical significance of problem and treatment. AMA Am J Dis Child 1954;87:399–428.

2 Cochrane WA, Payne WW, Simpkiss MJ, Woolf LI: Familial hypoglycemia precipitated by amino acids. J Clin Invest 1956;35:411–422.

3 Tattersall RB, Fajans SS: A difference between the inheritance of classical juvenile-onset and maturity-onset type diabetes of young people. Diabetes 1975;24:44–53.
4 Yalow RS, Berson SA: Immunoassay of endogenous plasma insulin in man. J Clin Invest 1960;39:1157–1175.
5 Drash A, Wolff F: Drug therapy in leucine-sensitive hypoglycemia. Metabolism: clinical and experimental. Metabolism 1964;13:487.
6 Yakovak WC, Baker L, Hummeler K: Beta cell nesidioblastosis in idiopathic hypoglycemia of infancy. J Pediatr 1971;79:226–231.
7 Rahier J: Relevance of endocrine pancreas nesidioblastosis to hyperinsulinemic hypoglycemia. Diabetes Care 1989;12:164–166.
8 Thornton PS, Sumner AE, Ruchelli ED, Spielman RS, Baker L, Stanley CA: Familial and sporadic hyperinsulinism: histopathologic findings and segregation analysis support a single autosomal recessive disorder (see comments). J Pediatr 1991;119:721–724.
9 Thornton PM, Glaser B, Herold K, Chiu KC, Satin-Smith MS, Permutt MA, et al. (eds): Familial Hyperinsulinism Inherited in an Autosomal Dominant Form Differs Clinically and Genetically from the More Common Autosomal Recessive Form (abstract No. 587 presented orally). San Diego, Society for Pediatric Research, 1995.
10 Kapoor RR, Locke J, Colclough K, Wales J, Conn JJ, Hattersley AT, et al: Persistent hyperinsulinemic hypoglycemia and maturity-onset diabetes of the young due to heterozygous HNF4A mutations. Diabetes 2008;57:1659–1663.
11 Froguel P, Aouali H, Vionnet N, Velho G, Vaxillaire M, Sun F, et al: Familial hyperglycemia due to mutations in glucokinase: definition of a subtype of diabetes mellitus. N Engl J Med 1994;328:697–702.
12 Nestorowicz A, Wilson BA, Schoor KP, Inoue H, Glaser B, Landau H, et al: Mutations in the sulonylurea receptor gene are associated with familial hyperinsulinism in Ashkenazi Jews. Hum Mol Genet 1996;5:1813–1822.
13 Yamagata K, Oda N, Kaisaki PJ, Menzel S, Furuta H, Vaxillaire M, et al: Mutations in the hepatocyte nuclear factor-1alpha gene in maturity-onset diabetes of the young (MODY3). Nature 1996;384:455–458.
14 Nestorowicz A, Inagaki N, Gonoi T, Schoor KP, Wilson BA, Glaser B, et al: A nonsense mutation in the inward rectifier potassium channel gene, Kir6.2, is associated with familial hyperinsulinism. Diabetes 1997;46:1743–1748.
15 Yamagata K, Furuta H, Oda N, Kaisaki PJ, Menzel S, Cox NJ, et al: Mutations in the hepatocyte nuclear factor-4alpha gene in maturity-onset diabetes of the young (MODY1). Nature 1996;384:458–460.
16 Glaser B, Kesavan P, Heyman M, Davis E, Cuesta A, Buchs A, et al: Familial hyperinsulinism caused by an activating glucokinase mutation. N Engl J Med 1998;338:226–230.
17 Stoffers DA, Ferrer J, Clarke WL, Habener JF: Early-onset type-II diabetes mellitus (MODY4) linked to IPF1. Nat Genet 1997;17:138–139.
18 Stanley CA, Lieu YK, Hsu BY, Burlina AB, Greenberg CR, Hopwood NJ, et al: Hyperinsulinism and hyperammonemia in infants with regulatory mutations of the glutamate dehydrogenase gene. N Engl J Med 1998;338:1352–1357.
19 Horikawa Y, Iwasaki N, Hara M, Furuta H, Hinokio Y, Cockburn BN, et al: Mutation in hepatocyte nuclear factor-1 beta gene (TCF2) associated with MODY. Nat Genet 1997;17:384–385.
20 Inoue H, Tanizawa Y, Wasson J, Behn P, Kalidas K, Bernal-Mizrachi E, et al: A gene encoding a transmembrane protein is mutated in patients with diabetes mellitus and optic atrophy (Wolfram syndrome). Nat Genet 1998;20:143–148.
21 Malecki MT, Jhala US, Antonellis A, Fields L, Doria A, Orban T, et al: Mutations in NEUROD1 are associated with the development of type 2 diabetes mellitus. Nat Genet 1999;23:323–328.
22 Huopio H, Reimann F, Ashfield R, Komulainen J, Lenko HL, Rahier J, et al: Dominantly inherited hyperinsulinism caused by a mutation in the sulfonylurea receptor type 1. J Clin Invest 2000;106:897–906.
23 Gloyn AL, Pearson ER, Antcliff JF, Proks P, Bruining GJ, Slingerland AS, et al: Activating mutations in the gene encoding the ATP-sensitive potassium-channel subunit Kir6.2 and permanent neonatal diabetes. N Engl J Med 2004;350:1838–1849.
24 Clayton PT, Eaton S, Aynsley-Green A, Edginton M, Hussain K, Krywawych S, et al: Hyperinsulinism in short-chain L-3-hydroxyacyl-CoA dehydrogenase deficiency reveals the importance of beta-oxidation in insulin secretion. J Clin Invest 2001;108:457–465.
25 Raeder H, Johansson S, Holm PI, Haldorsen IS, Mas E, Sbarra V, et al: Mutations in the CEL VNTR cause a syndrome of diabetes and pancreatic exocrine dysfunction. Nat Genet 2006;38:54–62.
26 Pinney SE, MacMullen C, Becker S, Lin YW, Hanna C, Thornton P, et al: Clinical characteristics and biochemical mechanisms of congenital hyperinsulinism associated with dominant KATP channel mutations. J Clin Invest 2008;118:2877–2886.

27 Proks P, Arnold AL, Bruining J, Girard C, Flanagan SE, Larkin B, et al: A heterozygous activating mutation in the sulphonylurea receptor SUR1 (ABCC8) causes neonatal diabetes. Hum Mol Genet 2006;15:1793–1800.
28 Otonkoski T, Jiao H, Kaminen-Ahola N, Tapia-Paez I, Ullah MS, Parton LE, et al: Physical exercise-induced hypoglycemia caused by failed silencing of monocarboxylate transporter 1 in pancreatic beta cells. Am J Hum Genet 2007;81:467–474.
29 Stoy J, Edghill EL, Flanagan SE, Ye H, Paz VP, Pluzhnikov A, et al: Insulin gene mutations as a cause of permanent neonatal diabetes. Proc Natl Acad Sci USA 2007;104:15040–15044.
30 Gonzalez-Barroso MM, Giurgea I, Bouillaud F, Anedda A, Bellanne-Chantelot C, Hubert L, et al: Mutations in UCP2 in congenital hyperinsulinism reveal a role for regulation of insulin secretion. PLoS One 2008;3:e3850.

Charles A. Stanley, MD
Division of Endocrinology/Diabetes
The Children's Hospital of Philadelphia
34th Street and Civic Center Boulevard
Philadelphia, PA 19104 (USA)
Tel. +1 215 590 3420, E-Mail stanleyc@email.chop.edu

Stanley CA, De León DD (eds): Monogenic Hyperinsulinemic Hypoglycemia Disorders.
Front Diabetes. Basel, Karger, 2012, vol 21, pp 7–17

Biochemistry and Physiology of the ATP-Sensitive Potassium Channel

Maria S. Remedi · Colin G. Nichols

Department of Cell Biology and Physiology, Washington University School of Medicine, St. Louis, Mo., USA

Abstract

ATP-sensitive potassium (K_{ATP}) channels are present in the surface membranes of many organs and cell types. In the pancreatic beta-cell, they play a critical role in coupling glucose metabolism to insulin secretion, and over the last few years, significant advances have been made in understanding the molecular basis of K_{ATP} channel activity, as well as the role of these channels in physiology and disease. K_{ATP} channels are generated from coassembly of Kir6.2 pore-forming subunits with sulfonylurea receptor 1 (SUR1) regulatory subunits. They are inhibited by intracellular ATP, and activated by ADP, so that glucose oxidation in beta-cells leads to a rise in [ATP]:[ADP] ratio, which reduces K_{ATP} channel activity and causes membrane depolarization. This leads to the opening of voltage-dependent Ca^{2+} channels, elevated intracellular [Ca^{2+}], and insulin exocytosis. Sulfonylureas, hypoglycemic agents used in the treatment of type 2 diabetes, act by binding to the regulatory SUR1 subunit and directly inhibiting the K_{ATP} current, bypassing metabolism to trigger insulin secretion. Conversely, K_{ATP}-specific channel openers (diazoxide) suppress insulin release by activating K_{ATP} and preventing a depolarization-dependent rise in intracellular [Ca^{2+}]. Loss-of-function mutations in the genes (*KCNJ11, ABCC8*) that encode the two subunits (Kir6.2 and SUR1, respectively) of the K_{ATP} channel underlie hyperinsulinism that can in some cases be treated by potassium channel openers. This chapter will focus on advances in K_{ATP} channel biochemistry and physiology, and consider implications for future understanding of the mechanisms of control of insulin secretion in normal and diseased states.

Molecular Basis of the ATP-Sensitive Potassium Channel

ATP-sensitive K^+ (K_{ATP}) channels are present in the membranes of many organs and cell types, and play a critical role in linking metabolism to the electrical activity of the cell [1]. The pancreatic K_{ATP} channel is a hetero-octameric complex of two separate proteins: the sulfonylurea receptor (SUR) subunit and the pore-forming (Kir6.x) subunit (fig. 1a). Kir6.1 *(KCNJ8)* or Kir6.2 *(KCNJ11)* are members of the inwardly rectifying potassium channel family. The regulatory subunits, SUR1 *(ABCC8)* and SUR2 *(ABCC9)*, belong to the ATP-binding cassette (ABC) superfamily of membrane proteins

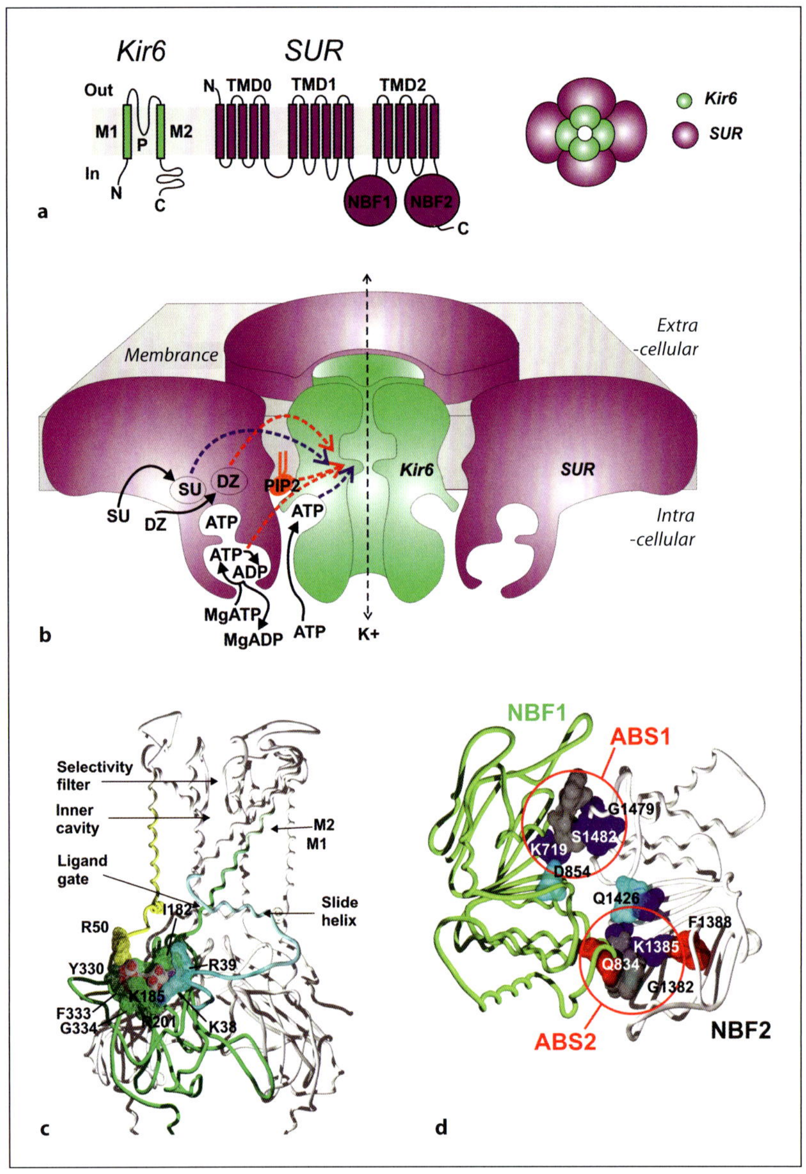

Fig. 1. Biochemical control of K_{ATP} channel activity. **a** Kir6 subunits generate the channel pore and SUR subunits serve the regulatory role, with each channel being a functional octamer of four Kir6 subunits and four SUR subunits. **b** The metabolically controlled gate of the channel is located at the cytoplasmic end of the inner cavity. ATP binds to Kir6 subunits and this provides the energetic push to channel closure. MgATP binds to the ATP-binding sites (ABS) formed at the NBF1-NBF2 interface on SUR subunits. ATP hydrolysis results in a conformational 'activated' state that is transduced to 'override' ATP inhibition. The 'activated state' persists through ADP dissociation and can be maintained by ADP rebinding. In addition, PIP_2 interaction at a site near the ATP inhibitory site also provides an energetic pull to open channels, and sulfonylureas (SU) or diazoxide (DZ), interacting with the SUR subunit within the membrane, respectively, cause channel closure or opening. **c** Three subunits of Kir6.2 are shown with the rear-most subunit removed. Specific regions of the channel are indicated, as well as ATP and one ATP-binding site in the space-filling model. The subunit positioned to the front provides the bulk of one ATP-binding site in its green C-terminal cytoplasmic domain. (continued on p. 9)

[1]. In recombinant expression, functional channels can be generated by C-terminally truncated Kir6.x subunits without SUR subunits [2], but in this case, C-terminal truncation removes a sequence (Arg-Lys-Arg) that normally causes a retention signal in the endoplasmic reticulum in the absence of SUR. SUR, which contains a similar endoplasmic reticulum-retention sequence, is also not efficiently trafficked to the surface membrane in the absence of Kir6.x. Thus, association of one subunit with the other is normally required for efficient trafficking of each to the plasma membrane [3].

Architecture of the ATP-Sensitive Potassium Channel

Crystallographic studies of bacterial and eukaryotic Kir channels [4, 5] demonstrate a conserved architecture of Kir channels consisting of two transmembrane helices (M1, M2) bridged by an extracellular loop that generates the narrow portion of the pore and controls ion selectivity. This structure (fig. 1c) is likely to be present in all major cation channel family members, including the Kir6.x family. Based on such structures, consensus models of Kir6.x agree in regards to the inhibitory ATP-binding site [1] (fig. 1c). As with other ABCC family members, SURs contain two six-helix transmembrane domains, TMD1 and TMD2, but SURs also have an additional N-terminal TMD0 domain consisting of five transmembrane helices (fig. 1a), critical for Kir6.x trafficking and gating [6]. SURs also contain one nucleotide-binding fold (NBF1) between TMD1 and TMD2, and a second (NBF2) after TMD2 in the cytoplasmic loops (fig. 1a). NBFs from bacterial ABC proteins crystallize as 'head-to-tail' dimers, and this is likely the functional arrangement between NBF1 and NBF2 in SUR (fig. 1d) [1]. How the Kir6 and SUR subunits are physically connected remains unknown, but electron micrography of complete K_{ATP} complexes suggest an intimate packing of four SUR and four Kir6.x subunits [7] (fig. 1a).

Biochemical Regulation of ATP-Sensitive Potassium Channel Activity

Nucleotide Gating of the Channel

Nucleotide regulation of K_{ATP} channels is unique among K channels: the channel is rapidly and reversibly inhibited by binding of cytoplasmic adenosine nucleotides, and exhibits complex activation by nucleotide tri- and diphosphates [1, 8] (fig. 1b).

(fig. 1 continued from p. 8) The N-terminal domain of this subunit provides the blue 'slide-helix' overlying the binding site to the right and then curves back to close the binding pocket around the adenine ring. Beyond the slide helix, residue R50 from the subunit to the left (yellow) is predicted to close the binding pocket at the gamma-phosphate of ATP. **d** Heterodimeric structure of SUR1 NBFs, highlighting ATP-binding sites (red circles) formed at the dimer interface. ATP is rendered in gray in ABS1 and ABS2. Mutation of residues in dark and light blue cause reduced or slowed MgADP activation of channel activity, respectively. Mutation of residues in red causes enhanced MgADP activation.

Inhibition by nucleotides requires at least one phosphate, with potency increasing from AMP ($K_{1/2[AMP]}$ approx. 10 mM; $K_{1/2}$ = nucleotide concentration causing half-maximal inhibition), to ADP ($K_{1/2[ADP]}$ approx. 250 μM), to ATP ($K_{1/2[ATP]}$ approx. 10–25 μM) in native K_{ATP} channels [9]. Thus, the free ATP concentration that causes half-maximal channel inhibition is in the micromolar range. It is important to note that cytosolic ATP concentration is in the millimolar range (1–5 mM), and changes little with metabolism. Thus [ATP] is probably always sufficient to almost fully inhibit channel activity. Channel activation then arises from the activating effects of Mg-nucleotides on the SUR subunit [10] as discussed below. Even though this MgADP activation is essential for the physiological opening of K_{ATP}, ATP-sensitivity of the channel is still critical in determining the magnitude of K_{ATP} current; therefore, a decrease in sensitivity to inhibitory ATP will enhance absolute currents at any given [MgADP] and thereby decrease excitability.

Nucleotide Binding to the Kir6.2 Subunit

ATP-inhibition of the K_{ATP} channel results from ATP binding to the Kir6.x subunit [1] (fig. 1b, c). GTP and pyrimidine triphosphates have essentially no inhibitory effects, thus the adenosine moiety seems to be critical for inhibition. Truncations of 10–30 amino acids from the Kir6.2 N-terminus and point mutations throughout the N- and C-terminal regions of Kir6.2 all significantly decrease ATP sensitivity. Most of these mutations seem to affect ATP-sensitivity allosterically by altering the intrinsic stability of the open state, but other mutations directly affect the ATP-binding site. Residues R50, I182, K185, R201, and G334, located at very different positions in the primary sequence, were all identified as controlling ATP affinity (fig. 1c). Satisfyingly, they are all predicted to be extremely close in models based on Kir crystal structures [11], which predict an ATP-binding site located at each of the interfaces between the four subunits in the tetramer (fig. 1c).

Nucleotide-Binding Domains in Sulfonylurea Receptor 1 Subunits

The SUR subunit determines the activating effects of Mg-nucleotides [10], as well as sensitivity of the channel to pharmacological channel openers and blockers [10, 12, 13]. Sulfonylureas, such as tolbutamide and glibenclamide (glyburide), bind directly to the SUR1 subunit (fig. 1b), leading to inhibition of K_{ATP} channel activity, membrane depolarization, and triggering of insulin secretion. These drugs are widely used to treat type 2 diabetes because of their ability to secrete insulin independently of the metabolic state of the beta-cell. Conversely, K_{ATP} channel openers such as diazoxide bind directly to the SUR1 subunit and activate K_{ATP} channels, thereby inhibiting insulin secretion [1].

As with all other ABC proteins, SURs contain NBFs that typically dimerize to form two ATP-binding sites at the dimer interface. The first clue to the role of the SUR subunit in K_{ATP} channel gating was demonstrated by a mutation (G1479R) in NBF2 that caused human hyperinsulinism [10] (fig. 1d). This mutation, and other disease-causing NBF2 mutations selectively abolished MgADP- and diazoxide-mediated stimulation of channel activity, with no effect on ATP inhibition [1]. Mutation of the conserved lysine residues in the Walker A motifs of either NBF1 (mutation K719A) or NBF2 (mutation K1384M), predicted to reduce ATP hydrolytic activity, also block the stimulatory effect of MgADP [13] (fig. 1d).

Electrophysiological and biochemical studies have suggested that both NBFs are involved in channel stimulation by MgADP and by channel opening drugs such as diazoxide. They have also shown that while ATP binds to NBF1 in a Mg^{2+}-independent manner, ATP and ADP binding to NBF2 require Mg^{2+} [14]. Furthermore, nucleotide binding to NBF2 stabilizes ATP binding to NBF1, either as a result of binding to NBF2 or by hydrolysis of bound MgATP [15], and mutations in the nucleotide-binding motifs of NBF2 (K1385M and D1506N) abolish this cooperative binding of nucleotides to the two NBFs (fig. 1d).

Other Modulators of ATP-Sensitive Potassium Channel Activity

K_{ATP} channels are also modulated by cytoplasmic factors and by the lipid composition of the membrane, especially by negatively charged phospholipids. The application of PIP_2 to inside-out patches causes an increase in channel open probability and a decrease in sensitivity to ATP; PIP_2 interacting residues (i.e. R54, R176, R177, R206) are also on the top surface of the domain (fig. 1b, c). Thus, the overlapping nature of the ATP-binding sites and the PIP_2 interacting sites is very consistent with the proposed negative interaction of these two groups in channel regulation. There is also evidence that protein kinase A and protein kinase C mediate phosphorylation of Kir6.2, increasing channel open probability and decreasing ATP sensitivity [16]. Neurotransmitters that couple to adenylate cyclase, and therefore protein kinase A, are also likely to affect Kir6.2 phosphorylation and hence channel activity.

ATP-Sensitive Potassium Channels and Insulin Secretion

The unique dependence of K_{ATP} activity on nucleotides provides the pancreatic beta-cell with a mechanism to couple cellular metabolism to electrical activity, and thus to insulin release [17]. During the fed state, when glucose metabolism is increased, beta-cell K_{ATP} channels become inhibited due to the elevated intracellular [ATP]/[ADP] ratio. This causes membrane depolarization, leading to Ca^{2+} entry through voltage-dependent Ca^{2+} channels, and calcium influx. The resultant rise in intracellular calcium concentration ($[Ca^{2+}]_i$) triggers insulin secretion in two phases: an early transient first phase and a sustained secondary phase (fig. 2a). A rise in circulating insulin then leads to increased glucose uptake in the peripheral tissues, and a compensatory drop in blood glucose. Conversely, a fall in the intracellular [ATP]/[ADP] ratio during the fasting state relieves inhibition of K_{ATP} channels, resulting in membrane hyperpolarization and cessation of insulin release (fig. 2a). However, this straightforward scenario does not account for the entire picture

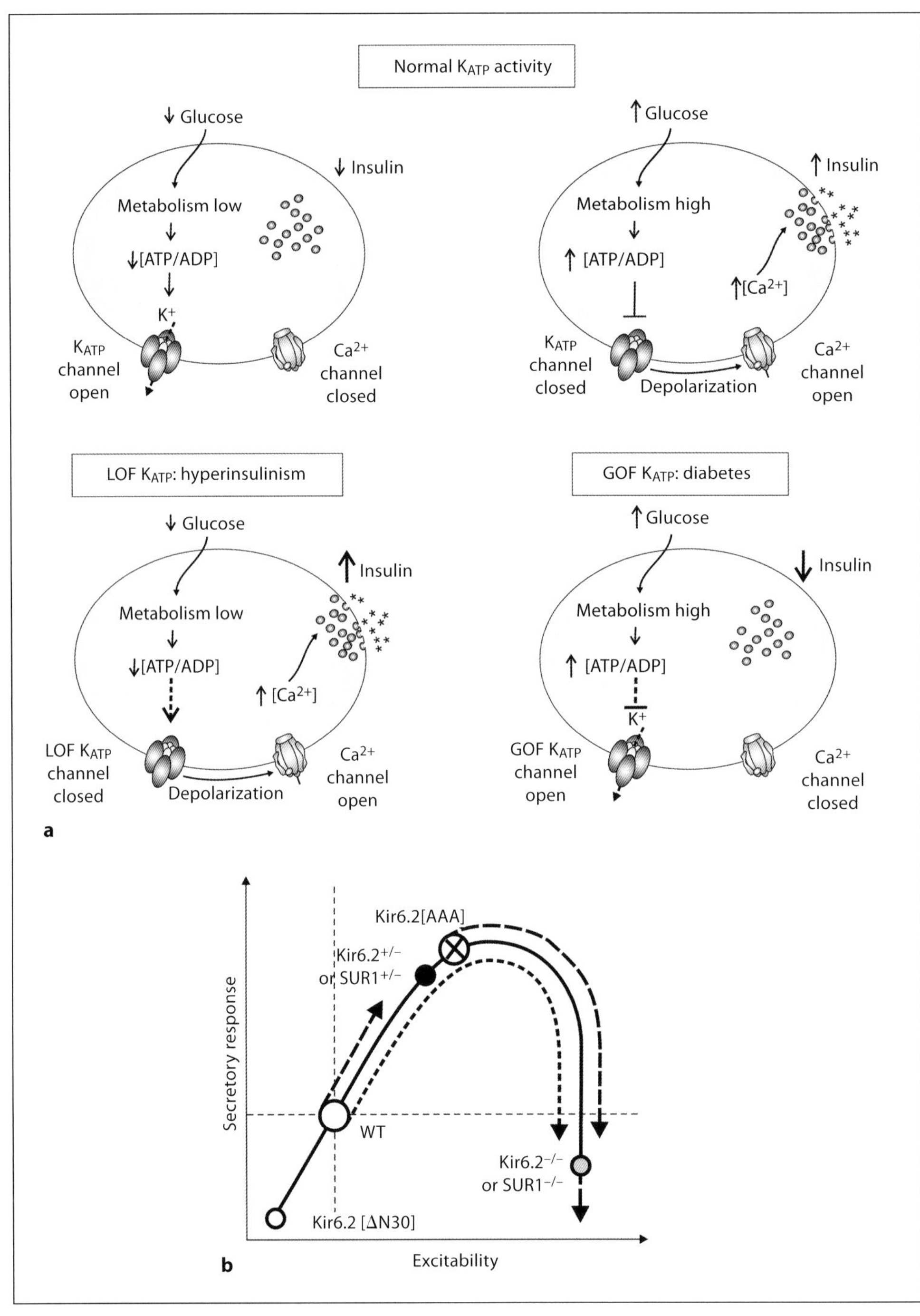

Fig. 2. Physiologic control of K_{ATP} activity and failure in disease. **a** When glucose is low in the pancreatic beta-cell, metabolism is inhibited, lowering the [ATP]/[ADP] ratio. This normally causes K_{ATP} channels to open, hyperpolarizing the cell, inhibiting voltage-dependent Ca^{2+} channels, and inhibiting insulin secretion. Conversely, when glucose rises, metabolism is stimulated, raising the [ATP]/[ADP] ratio. This normally closes K_{ATP} channels, depolarizing the cell, opening Ca^{2+} channels, causing Ca^{2+} to rise, and triggering insulin secretion. The consequences of mutant K_{ATP} channel activity in the (continued on p. 13)

of insulin secretion. Under conditions in which K_{ATP} channels are maximally activated by diazoxide, a glucose-dependence of insulin secretion can still be detected in isolated islets. Thus, even though a K_{ATP}-dependent increase in $[Ca^{2+}]_i$ is the primary trigger of insulin release, so-called K_{ATP}-independent mechanisms modulate release.

Congenital Hyperinsulinemia

The K_{ATP} channel is clearly a key controller of insulin secretion and inappropriate control of excitability resulting from changes in channel activity result in human diseases [1] (fig. 2a; see Shyng et al. [this vol., pp. 30–42]). Reduced or absent K_{ATP} channel activity will result in enhanced or constitutive membrane depolarization, elevated $[Ca^{2+}]_i$, and insulin hypersecretion (fig. 2a). This could result from enhanced metabolism (see Kelly et al. [this vol., pp. 100–111]), enhanced sensitivity of the K_{ATP} channel to metabolic inhibition, or reduction of the number of active K_{ATP} channels (see the chapters by Shyng et al. [pp. 30–42] and Li et al. [pp. 112–124]). Congenital hyperinsulinemia (see De León and Stanley [this vol., pp. 18–29]), is the most common cause of hypoglycemia in infancy and more than 50 loss-of-function hyperinsulinemia mutations have now been recognized in K_{ATP} genes [18] (see Shyng et al. [this vol., pp. 30–42]). While some mutations are in the Kir6.2 subunit, the majority are in SUR1 (see Shyng et al. [this vol., pp. 30–42]). Most of them cause defects in the biosynthesis or trafficking of the subunits which leads to absent or reduced surface expression of K_{ATP}, or loss of MgADP activation of the channel. In either case, beta-cells remain depolarized and persistently secrete insulin.

Neonatal and Type 2 Diabetes

K_{ATP} channels are now also known to be involved causally in both type 2 diabetes and monogenic forms of diabetes [19]. Neonatal diabetes mellitus (NDM) is typically diagnosed by presentation of hyperglycemia within the first 6 months of life, and multiple gain-of-function mutations in the genes encoding for Kir6.2 and SUR1 subunits

(fig. 2 continued from p. 12) beta-cell highlights the role of this channel as a critical regulator of cell function in response to metabolic status. Loss-of-function (LOF) K_{ATP} mutants that reduce channel activity cause beta-cells to become hyperexcitable and persistently hypersecreting insulin (hyperinsulinemia). Conversely, gain-of-function (GOF) K_{ATP} mutants that increase channel activity cause underexcitability of the beta-cell and failure to secrete insulin. **b** Proposed 'inverse-U' model for response to beta-cell hyperexcitability. Wild-type (WT) islets show a normal secretory responsiveness, but following a high-fat diet (dashed), progress to a hyperexcitable, hypersecretory phenotype. Enhanced K_{ATP} channel activity also reduces excitability and hence reduces secretory responsiveness (as in neonatal diabetes). Conversely, heterozygous knockout of K_{ATP} or dominant-negative suppression, causes an approx. 70% decrease of K_{ATP} and hypersecretory responsiveness. A high-fat diet causes further enhancement of excitability, beyond the threshold that drives AAA islets 'over the top' (dashed) to undersecretion. K_{ATP} knockout islets (100% decrease of K_{ATP}) have maximally enhanced excitability, but spontaneously undersecrete even on a normal diet (solid) – a situation that is exacerbated after high-fat diet (dashed). Finally, wild-type islets can be reversibly driven through hypersecretion to undersecretion by chronic pharmacological suppression of K_{ATP} (short-dashed).

of the K_{ATP} channel have now been found to underlie human NDM [20]. All show enhanced activity at any given [ATP]/[ADP] ratio [19], typically due to a decrease in the apparent affinity of the ATP-binding pocket or increased open state stability of the Kir6.2 subunit, or enhanced Mg-nucleotide activation of the SUR1 subunit. Several Kir6.2 residues (i.e. I182, R201, R50), previously implicated as being in the ATP binding; and others (Y330 and F333) predicted to lie close to the phosphate tail of the ATP-binding pocket [21], have been found to be mutated in patients with NDM (fig. 1c). Other NDM mutations, located in both Kir6.2 and the TM0 domain of the SUR1 subunit, are involved in altered channel gating (detected in the absence of ATP) and allosterically result in reduction of ATP sensitivity without changes in ATP-binding affinity (e.g. I296L, V59G, Q52R, C42R; fig. 1c). Q52 and V59 residues are located within the 'slide helix' of Kir6.2 (fig. 1c), consistent with a role for this structure in linking ATP binding and gating.

The realization that NDM results from mutations in the K_{ATP} channel has rapidly shifted the therapy from insulin injections to oral sulfonylurea drugs: by directly inhibiting the overactive K_{ATP} channels, these drugs can provide successful control of blood glucose levels, and insulin requirements can be avoided (or reduced) in the majority of K_{ATP}-induced NDM [19]. The stimulation of endogenous insulin secretion by sulfonylureas may be augmented by the presence of potentiating hormones (glucagon and GLP-1) and by other K_{ATP}-independent mechanisms, such that insulin secretion becomes quasi-physiological in such treated patients and blood glucose control may be better than that afforded by insulin injections.

Finally, in addition to a direct causal role in NDM, it should be noted that a common amino acid polymorphism (E23K) in the Kir6.2 subunit of the channel, is one of the established risk factors for type 2 diabetes [22]. In this case, the polymorphism also causes a very weak loss of ATP-sensitivity [23], leading to reduced insulin secretion, even in nondiabetic carriers [24], that seems to underlie diabetes susceptibility.

Animal Models of Reduced ATP-Sensitive Potassium Channel Activity: Insights to Hyperinsulinemia

Naively, we expect reduced K_{ATP} channel activity to result in enhanced membrane depolarization, elevated $[Ca^{2+}]_I$, and hypersecretion of insulin. Consistent with this, loss-of-function mutations of K_{ATP} subunits underlie congenital hyperinsulinemia, while gain-of-function mutations cause undersecreting neonatal diabetes (see above and Stanley and Matschinsky [this vol., pp. 1–6]). Genetic manipulation of K_{ATP} channel subunits in mice has been carried out to probe the role of the channels in insulin secretion and the etiology of these diseases. Gain-of function transgenic mice reiterate the key features of neonatal diabetes and indeed predicted the human disease mechanism [19], but mice completely lacking SUR1 or Kir6.2 subunits do not reiterate the hyperinsulinemia disease in any simple way. In these animals, hypersecretion reportedly occurs immediately after birth, but rapidly progresses to a relative undersecretion with mild-to-severe glucose intolerance in adults and an overall loss of secretory capacity [25]. A full explanation for the complexity of the results has yet to be achieved, but in terms of modeling hyperinsulinemia, it is clear that post-neonatal mice with complete absence of beta-cell K_{ATP} channels are actually glucose-intolerant and neither persistently hyperinsulinemic nor hypoglycemic. Therefore, on the surface there is an apparent discrepancy between the outcome of genetic loss of K_{ATP} channels in mice and humans. One important potential caveat to consider is whether patients really have a complete loss of K_{ATP} channels, and therefore whether complete knockout mice provide the appropriate model for the disease. There is a very nonlinear dependence of electrical activity and secretion on K_{ATP} conductance, and significant reduction of K_{ATP} conductance can occur without big shifts in glucose-sensitivity of secretion. Mice expressing a dominant-negative Kir6.2[AAA] transgene in beta-cells, as well as mice heterozygous for either Kir6.2 or SUR1, show substantial (approx. 60–70%) reduction of K_{ATP} channel activity, but only a small shift in glucose-sensitivity (approx. 1–2 mM) [25].

We have therefore proposed [25] an 'inverse-U' model to explain the beta-cell response to hyperexcitability resulting from reduced K_{ATP} conductance (fig. 2b). Initially, any reduction of K_{ATP} will cause hyperexcitability that will lead to enhanced insulin secretion; however, above a threshold, enhanced excitability triggers a consequent failure of glucose-sensing and secretion (fig. 2b). K_{ATP} knockout animals may reach this threshold spontaneously, such that adult mice exhibit only basal secretion and are glucose-intolerant [26, 27]. Normally Kir6.$2^{+/-}$ or Kir6.2[AAA] mice do not reach this threshold, but when excitability is further enhanced, e.g. by dietary stress [28], a rapid progression to undersecretion ensues. The phenotype of many hyperinsulinemia mutations (see De León and Stanley [this vol., pp. 18–29]) would actually suggest that a reduced, but not complete, absence of K_{ATP} channels is likely to be the case in human patients, and persistent hyperinsulinism in humans might indeed typically reflect an incomplete loss of K_{ATP} conductance. Some hyperinsulinemia patients with K_{ATP} channel mutations must maintain some K_{ATP} channel activity since the patients are responsive to the K_{ATP} channel drugs tolbutamide and diazoxide [29], and carriers of loss-of-function K_{ATP} mutations may have enhanced glucose responsiveness and subclinical hyperinsulinism (comparable to Kir6.$2^{+/-}$ or $SUR1^{+/-}$ mice) [30]. A second implication is that in humans with more complete loss of K_{ATP} channels, a progression from hyperinsulinemia to glucose intolerance will be expected, and there are indeed reports that some nonsurgically treated hyperinsulinemia patients spontaneously progress to type 2 diabetes [31], i.e. onto the descending limb of the 'inverse-U' progression. Interestingly, the 'inverse-U' progression occurs in wild-type animals with chronic suppression of K_{ATP} activity: within a short period of treatment the animal progress from a hyperinsulinemic state to undersecretion, just like K_{ATP}

knockout animals [32]. However, complete reversibility of undersecretion following removal of glibenclamide suggests the possibility that suppression of excitability with diazoxide or dietary restriction may prove beneficial in controlling diabetes in such patients.

References

1 Nichols CG: K_{ATP} channels as molecular sensors of cellular metabolism. Nature 2006;440:470–476.

2 Tucker SJ, Ashcroft FM: Mapping of the physical interaction between the intracellular domains of an inwardly rectifying potassium channel, Kir6.2. J Biol Chem 1999;274:33393–33397.

3 Zerangue N, Schwappach B, Jan YN, Jan LY: A new ER trafficking signal regulates the subunit stoichiometry of plasma membrane K(ATP) channels. Neuron 1999;22:537–548.

4 Kuo A, Gulbis JM, Antcliff JF, Rahman T, Lowe ED, Zimmer J, Cuthbertson J, Ashcroft FM, Ezaki T, Doyle DA: Crystal structure of the potassium channel KirBac1.1 in the closed state. Science 2003;300:1922–1926.

5 Tao X, Avalos JL, Chen J, MacKinnon R: Crystal structure of the eukaryotic strong inward-rectifier K^+ channel Kir2.2 at 3.1 A resolution. Science 2009; 326:1668–1674.

6 Bryan J, Vila-Carriles WH, Zhao G, Babenko AP, Aguilar-Bryan L: Toward linking structure with function in ATP-sensitive K^+ channels. Diabetes 2004;53(Suppl 3):S104–S112.

7 Mikhailov MV, Campbell JD, de Wet H, Shimomura K, Zadek B, Collins RF, Sansom MS, Ford RC, Ashcroft FM: 3-D structural and functional characterization of the purified K_{ATP} channel complex Kir6.2-SUR1. EMBO J 2005;24:4166–4175.

8 Ashcroft SJ, Ashcroft FM: Properties and functions of ATP-sensitive K-channels. Cell Signal 1990;2: 197–214.

9 Inagaki N, Gonoi T, Clement JP 4th, Namba N, Inazawa J, Gonzalez G, Aguilar-Bryan L, Seino S, Bryan J: Reconstitution of IKATP: an inward rectifier subunit plus the sulfonylurea receptor (see comments). Science 1995;270:1166–1170.

10 Nichols CG, Shyng SL, Nestorowicz A, Glaser B, Clement JP, Gonzalez G, Aguilarbryan L, Permutt MA, Bryan J: Adenosine diphosphate as an intracellular regulator of insulin secretion. Science 1996;272: 1785–1787.

11 Enkvetchakul D, Nichols CG: Gating mechanism of K_{ATP} channels: function fits form. J Gen Physiol 2003;122:471–480.

12 Aguilar-Bryan L, Nichols CG, Wechsler SW, Clement JP 4th, Boyd AE 3rd, Gonzalez G, Herrera-Sosa H, Nguy K, Bryan J, Nelson DA: Cloning of the beta cell high-affinity sulfonylurea receptor: a regulator of insulin secretion. Science 1995;268:423–426.

13 Gribble FM, Tucker SJ, Ashcroft FM: The essential role of the Walker A motifs of SUR1 in K-ATP channel activation by Mg-ADP and diazoxide. EMBO J 1997;16:1145–1152.

14 Ueda K, Inagaki N, Seino S: MgADP antagonism to Mg^{2+}-independent ATP binding of the sulfonylurea receptor SUR1. J Biol Chem 1997;272:22983–22986.

15 Ueda K, Komine J, Matsuo M, Seino S, Amachi T: Cooperative binding of ATP and MgADP in the sulfonylurea receptor is modulated by glibenclamide. Proc Natl Acad Sci USA 1999;96:1268–1272.

16 Beguin P, Nagashima K, Nishimura M, Gonoi T, Seino S: PKA-mediated phosphorylation of the human K(ATP) channel: separate roles of Kir6.2 and SUR1 subunit phosphorylation. EMBO J 1999; 18:4722–4732.

17 Ashcroft FM, Gribble FM: ATP-sensitive K^+ channels and insulin secretion: their role in health and disease. Diabetologia 1999;42:903–919.

18 Sharma N, Crane A, Gonzalez G, Bryan J, Aguilar-Bryan L: Familial hyperinsulinism and pancreatic beta-cell ATP-sensitive potassium channels. Kidney Int 2000;57:803–808.

19 Remedi MS, Koster JC: K_{ATP} channelopathies in the pancreas. Pflugers Arch 2010;460:307–320.

20 Flanagan SE, Clauin S, Bellanne-Chantelot C, de Lonlay P, Harries LW, Gloyn AL, Ellard S: Update of mutations in the genes encoding the pancreatic beta-cell K(ATP) channel subunits Kir6.2 (KCNJ11) and sulfonylurea receptor 1 (ABCC8) in diabetes mellitus and hyperinsulinism. Hum Mutat 2009;30: 170–180.

21 Haider S, Antcliff JF, Proks P, Sansom MS, Ashcroft FM: Focus on Kir6.2: a key component of the ATP-sensitive potassium channel. J Mol Cell Cardiol 2005;38:927–936.

22 Florez JC: Newly identified loci highlight beta cell dysfunction as a key cause of type 2 diabetes: where are the insulin resistance genes? Diabetologia 2008; 51:1100–1110.

23 Schwanstecher C, Meyer U, Schwanstecher M: K(IR)6.2 polymorphism predisposes to type 2 diabetes by inducing overactivity of pancreatic beta-cell ATP-sensitive K(+) channels. Diabetes 2002;51:875–879.

24 Villareal DT, Koster JC, Robertson H, Akrouh A, Miyake K, Bell GI, Patterson BW, Nichols CG, Polonsky KS: Kir6.2 variant E23K increases ATP-sensitive K^+ channel activity and is associated with impaired insulin release and enhanced insulin sensitivity in adults with normal glucose tolerance. Diabetes 2009;58:1869–1878.

25 Nichols CG, Koster JC, Remedi MS: Beta-cell hyperexcitability: from hyperinsulinism to diabetes. Diabetes Obes Metab 2007;9(Suppl 2):81–88.

26 Miki T, Nagashima K, Tashiro F, Kotake K, Yoshitomi H, Tamamoto A, Gonoi T, Iwanaga T, Miyazaki J, Seino S: Defective insulin secretion and enhanced insulin action in K_{ATP} channel-deficient mice. Proc Natl Acad Sci USA 1998;95:10402–10406.

27 Seghers V, Nakazaki M, DeMayo F, Aguilar-Bryan L, Bryan J: Sur1 knockout mice. A model for K(ATP) channel-independent regulation of insulin secretion. J Biol Chem 2000;275:9270–9277.

28 Remedi M-S, Koster JC, Markova KP, Seino S, Miki T, Patton BL, McDaniel ML, Nichols CG: Diet-induced glucose intolerance in mice with decreased β-cell K_{ATP} channels. Diabetes 2004;53:3159–3167.

29 Henwood MJ, Kelly A, Macmullen C, Bhatia P, Ganguly A, Thornton PS, Stanley CA: Genotype-phenotype correlations in children with congenital hyperinsulinism due to recessive mutations of the adenosine triphosphate-sensitive potassium channel genes. J Clin Endocrinol Metab 2005;90:789–794.

30 Loechner KJ, Akrouh A, Kurata HT, Dionisi-Vici C, Maiorana A, Pizzoferro M, Rufini V, de Ville de Goyet J, Colombo C, Barbetti F, et al: Congenital hyperinsulinism and glucose hypersensitivity in homozygous and heterozygous carriers of Kir6.2 (KCNJ11) mutation V290M mutation: K(ATP) channel inactivation mechanism and clinical management. Diabetes 2011;60:209–217.

31 Huopio H, Shyng SL, Otonkoski T, Nichols CG: K(ATP) channels and insulin secretion disorders. Am J Physiol Endocrinol Metab 2002;283:E207–E216.

32 Remedi MS, Nichols CG: Chronic antidiabetic sulfonylureas in vivo: reversible effects on mouse pancreatic beta-cells. PLoS Med 2008;5:e206.

Colin G. Nichols, PhD
Department of Cell Biology and Physiology
Washington University School of Medicine
660 South Euclid Avenue
St. Louis, MO 63110 (USA)
Tel. +1 314 362 6630, E-Mail cnichols@wustl.edu

Stanley CA, De León DD (eds): Monogenic Hyperinsulinemic Hypoglycemia Disorders.
Front Diabetes. Basel, Karger, 2012, vol 21, pp 18–29

Pathophysiology of Diffuse ATP-Sensitive Potassium Channel Hyperinsulinism

Diva D. De León · Charles A. Stanley

Division of Endocrinology/Diabetes, The Children's Hospital of Philadelphia, Philadelphia, Pa., USA

Abstract

The most severe form of congenital hyperinsulinism (HI) is caused by inactivating mutations in the genes encoding the ATP-sensitive potassium (K_{ATP}) channels. In K_{ATP}HI, loss of functional channels results in inappropriate insulin responses to glucose. Thus, there is a failure to suppress insulin secretion when glucose levels fall, but there is also a blunting of glucose-stimulated insulin release. There are three distinct subtypes of diffuse K_{ATP}HI: (1) recessive (biallelic) diazoxide-unresponsive; (2) dominant (monoallelic) diazoxide-unresponsive; and (3) dominant (monoallelic) diazoxide-responsive. Mutations that prevent production of the channels or impair the trafficking of mature channels to the plasma membrane act recessively and result in severe hypoglycemia presenting shortly after birth. These children do not respond to medical therapy with diazoxide. The dominant defects allow the expression of channels on the plasma membrane as hetero-octamers comprised of both mutant and wild-type subunits; in those with sufficient partial function, the hypoglycemia may present later and respond to diazoxide. Our understanding of the natural history of K_{ATP}HI is incomplete, but progression to diabetes in children treated with surgical pancreatectomy is not uncommon. Whether the diabetes is a consequence of the treatment (pancreatectomy) or of dysregulated islet function itself is not fully known. Further exploration of genotype-phenotype correlations may facilitate appropriate management decisions and prediction of outcomes for affected children.

Introduction

Inactivating mutations of SUR1 or Kir6.2, the two subunits that form the beta-cell ATP-sensitive potassium (K_{ATP}) channel, are responsible for the most common and most severe form of congenital hyperinsulinism (HI), known as K_{ATP}HI. The chapters by Remedi and Nichols [pp. 7–17], Shyng et al. [pp. 30–42], and Suchi et al. [pp. 57–70] review the important role of the K_{ATP} channel in insulin secretion, the pathobiology of K_{ATP}HI mutations in in vitro expression, and the histopathology of K_{ATP}HI.

Table 1. Genotypes and phenotypes of diffuse K_{ATP}HI

Genotype	Birth weight percentile	Median age of presentation in days (range)	Diazoxide responsiveness	Parent of origin
Recessive (n = 48)	87% LGA	1 (1–9)	100% no	48/48 biallelic
Dominant diazoxide-unresponsive (n = 17)	65% LGA	1 (1–180)	100% no	5/17 maternal 1/17 paternal 9/17 de novo 2/17 not maternal
Dominant diazoxide-responsive (n = 13)	77% LGA	30 (1–1,215)	100% yes	5/13 maternal 4/13 paternal 4/13 de novo

LGA = Large for gestational age.

As discussed in the chapter by Arnoux et al. [pp. 43–56], K_{ATP} mutations are also associated with the focal form of congenital HI. This chapter will focus on the clinical manifestations and pathophysiology of K_{ATP}HI, focusing on the diffuse form (where all pancreatic beta-cells are affected).

Molecular Genetics

As shown in table 1, there are three distinctive subtypes of diffuse K_{ATP}HI: (1) recessive diazoxide-unresponsive, (2) dominant diazoxide-unresponsive, and (3) dominant diazoxide-responsive. Here, recessive mutations refer to biallelic defects in which heterozygous mutation carriers have no detectable abnormalities of insulin regulation. Dominant mutations refer to monoallelic defects in which mutation carriers have demonstrable abnormalities of insulin regulation. The clinical manifestations of the first two groups are identical. Affected infants are typically born large for gestational age due to the effects of in utero hyperinsulinemia. They usually present with severe hypoglycemia immediately after birth. These infants fail to respond to treatment with diazoxide, a K_{ATP} channel agonist that increases channel open probability to inhibit insulin secretion since no functional K_{ATP} channels exist (recessive defects) or are severely impaired (dominant defects). Therefore, they often require near-total pancreatectomy to control hypoglycemia. The third group (dominant diazoxide-responsive) manifests milder disease since K_{ATP} channel function is not completely absent. Their hypoglycemia may not be noted at birth and can be controlled medically with diazoxide.

Recessive K_{ATP}HI mutations (biallelic defects) act by interfering with the expression of K_{ATP} channels on the beta-cell plasma membrane. Recessive defects can be nonsense mutations or splicing defects of either the *ABCC8* or *KCNJ11* genes, and completely prevent the production of the sulfonylurea receptor 1 (SUR1) or the Kir6.2 subunit of the channel. Recessive defects can also be missense mutations which impair trafficking of the mutated subunit into mature channels on the plasma membrane. Since affected patients have essentially complete absence of plasma membrane K_{ATP} channels, they are incapable of responding to medical treatment with the channel agonist, diazoxide. Heterozygous carriers are not affected since the presence of the mutation does not interfere with expression of the normal allele and the production of channels composed entirely of wild-type subunits. Whether carriers have a reduced number of channels is not known.

Recessive K_{ATP}HI mutations are the most common defects identified in patients with congenital HI. They probably account for most of the estimated incidence of congenital HI (from 1 in 40,000 live births in Northern Europe [1] to 1 in 2,675 live births in Saudi Arabia where the frequency of consanguinity is high [2]).

As illustrated in figure 1, which shows mutations found in the large series of cases seen at The Children's Hospital of Philadelphia, a large number of recessive K_{ATP}HI mutations have been identified and many patients carry novel defects. The recessive K_{ATP} mutations are distributed throughout the coding regions of both *ABCC8* and *KCNJ11*, roughly consistent with the relative size of the coding regions of the two genes. A few common mutations have been identified in some ethnic groups. For example, in the Ashkenazi Jewish population, two *ABCC8* founder mutations are responsible for approximately 90% of cases: p.delPhe1388 and, especially, c.3992–9G>A [3]. The founder mutation, V187D, has been found in Finnish patients [4, 5] and R837X appears to be common in the Mexican population [6].

Dominant diazoxide-unresponsive K_{ATP} mutations (monoallelic defects) are missense amino acid substitutions that, unlike the recessive biallelic defects, allow normal trafficking of the mutated subunit to the plasma membrane to form hetero-octameric channels containing 0–4 mutant subunits. As shown in figure 1, to date, all of the dominant diazoxide-unresponsive mutations have involved only the SUR1 subunit. The defective subunit appears to act in a dominant-negative fashion to impair total channel activity in heterozygotes to the point that diazoxide is not effective in suppressing insulin release [7].

Dominant diazoxide-responsive K_{ATP} mutations (monoallelic defects) are also missense amino acid mutations, but they appear to cause a milder defect in channel activity so that clinical responsiveness to diazoxide is retained [8]. As shown in figure 1, dominant diazoxide-responsive mutations may affect the Kir6.2 and SUR1 channel subunits. As shown in figure 2 and discussed later, although affected patients may present with severe symptomatic hypoglycemia at birth, carriers may often escape recognition.

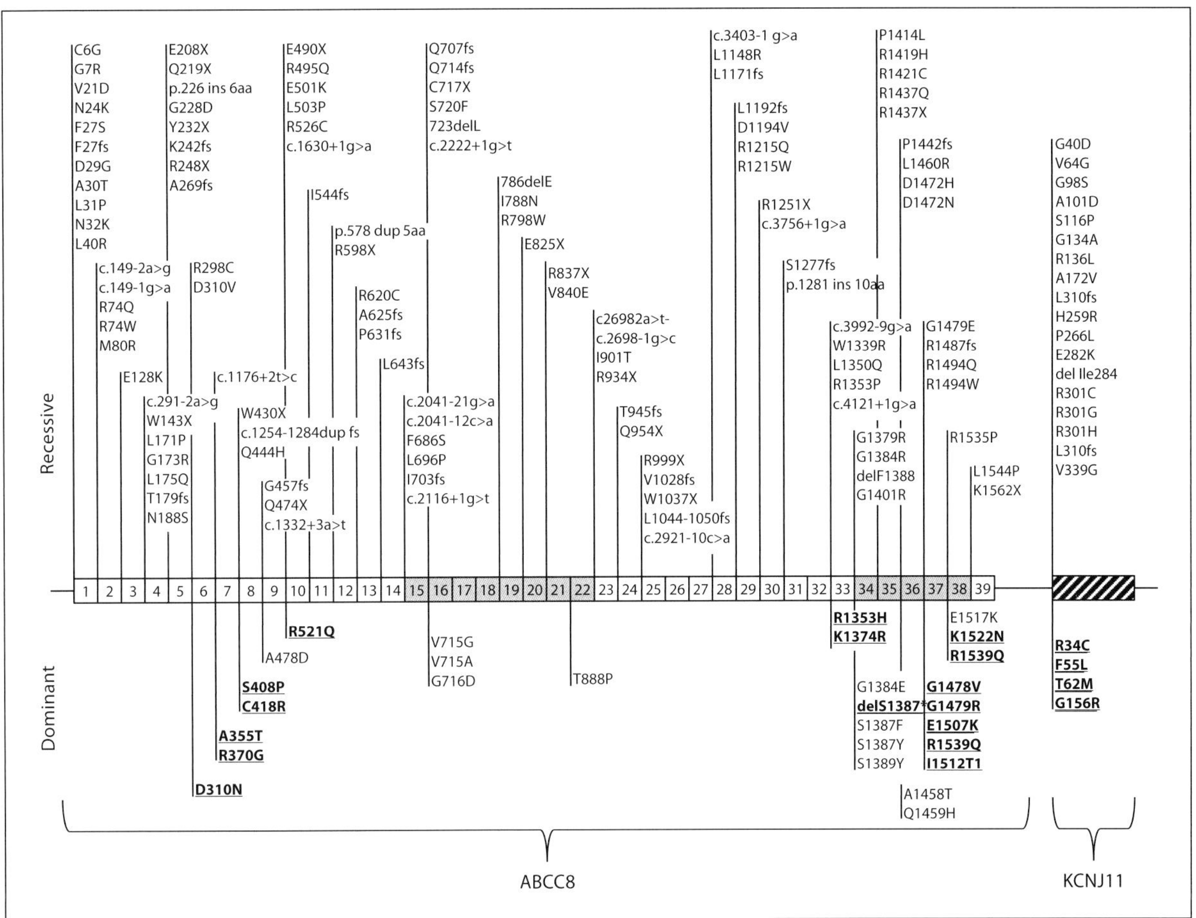

Fig. 1. Mutations of the *ABCC8* and *KCNJ11* genes. Recessive mutations are shown above the gene while dominant mutations are shown below. Dominant diazoxide-responsive mutations are indicated with bold-underlined letters. There are a total of 119 recessive mutations in *ABCC8* (56 missense, 40 nonsense/frameshift, 17 splicing, and 6 in-frame in/del) and 27 dominant mutations (26 missense mutations and 1 in-frame in/del). There are a total of 18 recessive mutations in *KNCJ11* (16 missense, 1 frameshift, and 1 in-frame in/del) and 4 dominant (4 missense) in *KCNJ11*. Nucleotide-binding folds 1 and 2 (NBF1 and NBF 2) in *ABCC8* are shown in gray. * In vitro expression studies indicate that the delS1387 mutation should be diazoxide responsive. However, we have seen both diazoxide-responsive and -unresponsive patients with this mutation.

Clinical Pathophysiology

The pathophysiology of the K_{ATP} channel HI defects has been illustrated by in vivo functional tests, as described below. Note that the physiologic defects seen in recessive K_{ATP}HI are also found in dominant K_{ATP}HI defects and in focal K_{ATP}HI, with one significant exception noted below.

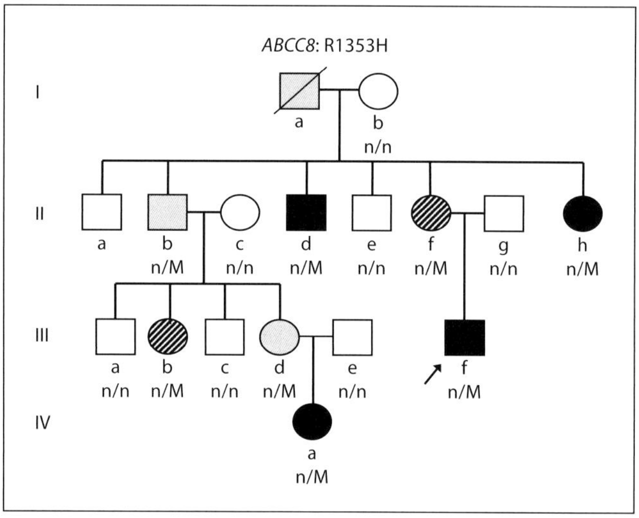

ABCC8: R1353H

I: a; b n/n

II: a; b n/M; c n/n; d n/M; e n/n; f n/M; g n/n; h n/M

III: a n/n; b n/M; c n/n; d n/M; e n/n; f n/M

IV: a n/M

Fig. 2. Pedigree of a family with dominant K_{ATP}HI due to a mutation in *ABCC8* (R1353H). Males are depicted as squares, females as circles. Arrow indicates proband. Deceased individuals are depicted with a slash. n/M = Mutation positive; n/n = mutation negative; filled black = hypoglycemia diagnosed; filled dashed = symptomatic but not diagnosed; gray = asymptomatic carrier.

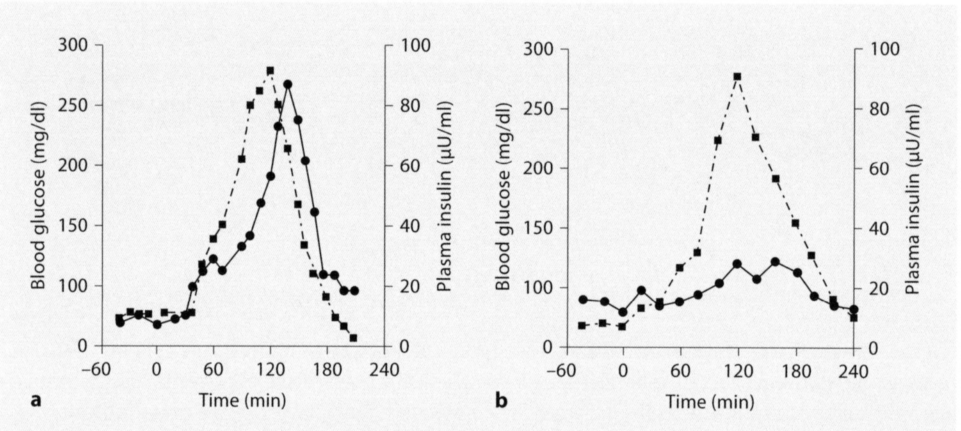

Fig. 3. Insulin response to graded glucose infusion in K_{ATP}HI. Blood glucose (black squares, dashed line) and plasma insulin (black circles, solid line) in response to an increasing and decreasing glucose ramp in a normal individual (**a**) and in an individual with recessive K_{ATP}HI (**b**). Reproduced with permission from [9].

Insulin Response to Graded Glucose Infusion

As shown in figure 3, patients with recessive K_{ATP}HI show a severely blunted insulin response to a glucose ramp, as well as a failure to completely suppress insulin at low glucose levels [9]. This reduced beta-cell sensitivity to glucose stimulation is consistent with in vitro observations in SUR1 knockout mouse islets [10] and in islets isolated from patients undergoing surgery, which show constitutive elevation of cytosolic calcium and insulin release [11]. Thus, children with K_{ATP}HI have a defect not only in suppressing insulin release at low blood glucose,

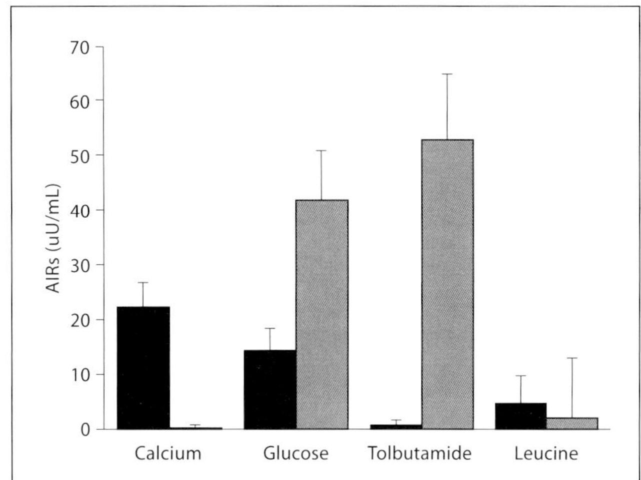

Fig. 4. AIRs in K_{ATP}HI. AIRs to calcium, glucose, tolbutamide, and leucine in children with recessive K_{ATP}HI (black bars) and normal controls (gray bars).

but also an impaired capacity to release insulin in response to a glucose challenge [9]. The former defect dominates clinical manifestations in early infancy, whereas the latter may play a role in later development of glucose intolerance and, possibly, diabetes. Insulin responses to glucose ramp stimulation have not been examined in dominant K_{ATP}HI, but presumably would be similar to recessive K_{ATP}HI.

Acute Insulin Responses to Intravenous Stimulation

Figure 4 shows the acute insulin responses (AIRs) to different secretagogues (calcium, glucose, tolbutamide, and leucine) in children with recessive K_{ATP}HI mutations. Inactivation of the K_{ATP} channels results in a markedly increased AIR to calcium [12]. AIR to tolbutamide is markedly impaired, consistent with the absence of channel activity and the lack of responsiveness to the channel agonist diazoxide. In focal HI, the AIR to tolbutamide may be positive [13] because of the responses by normal islets outside the focal lesion, but this is not sufficient to reliably differentiate between focal and diffuse HI [14]. Similar to the blunted response seen with graded glucose infusion (fig. 3), the AIR to glucose is much smaller compared to normal. This 'glucose blindness' in K_{ATP}HI is also manifested by the observation of impaired oral glucose tolerance tests in patients with either recessive or dominant K_{ATP}HI mutations who have not undergone pancreatectomy [5]. Heterozygous carriers of K_{ATP} recessive mutations exhibit normal AIRs to calcium, glucose, and tolbutamide [9].

The pattern of AIRs to calcium, glucose, and tolbutamide in individuals with dominant types of K_{ATP}HI is similar to that seen in recessive K_{ATP}HI. However, the latter had more severely impaired responses to glucose and tolbutamide stimulation than patients with dominant K_{ATP}HI [8].

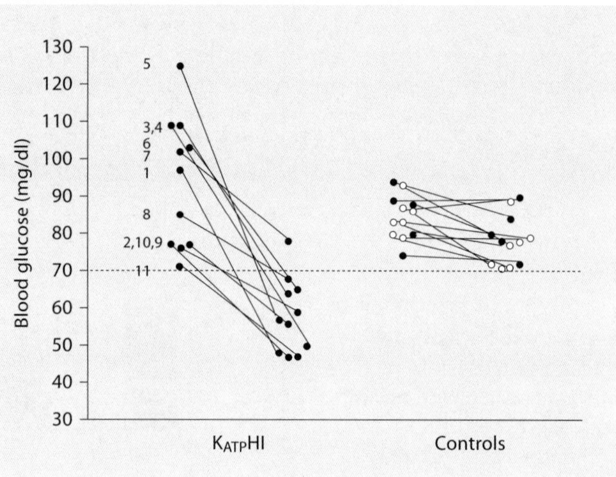

Fig. 5. Blood glucose response to oral protein tolerance test in $K_{ATP}HI$. Individual responses are shown for children with recessive $K_{ATP}HI$. Responses for healthy control subjects are indicated by black circles and for control children with ketotic hypoglycemia by white circles. Reproduced with permission from [16].

Responses to Protein and Leucine

In the past, leucine-sensitive hypoglycemia, protein-sensitive hypoglycemia, and congenital HI were commonly thought to be synonymous. However, it is now clear that leucine sensitivity is not a feature in all forms of congenital HI. Leucine, which triggers insulin release by allosteric activation of glutamate dehydrogenase, is a potent insulin secretagogue in patients with glutamate dehydrogenase HI, but, as shown in figure 4, has little effect in $K_{ATP}HI$ (see also the chapters by Smith [pp. 87–99] and Kelly et al. [pp. 100–111]) [15]. However, despite this lack of leucine sensitivity, protein-induced hypoglycemia is an important clinical feature of both recessive and dominant $K_{ATP}HI$ (fig. 5) [8, 16].

The mechanism of protein-sensitive hypoglycemia in $K_{ATP}HI$ appears to be due to an effect of amino acids, particularly glutamine, on the amplification pathway of insulin release when cytosolic calcium is elevated [17].

Clinical Manifestations Associated with ATP-Sensitive Potassium Channel Hyperinsulinism

As noted above, children with all three subtypes of $K_{ATP}HI$ are often large for gestational age at birth due to the growth promoting effects of insulin in utero. Many of the severe cases have hypertrophic cardiomyopathy, similar to infants of diabetic mothers, probably also as a consequence of fetal hyperinsulinemia [18]. Hypoglycemia in $K_{ATP}HI$ often requires extremely high glucose infusion rates, frequently 4–5 times higher than normal to control blood glucose. Feeding aversion and reflux are common, but it is unclear if this is a direct effect of the K_{ATP} channel defect (due to channel mutation effects in the central nervous system and/or gastrointestinal tract) or, more likely, an iatrogenic consequence of force-feeding in an effort to manage hypoglycemia.

The severity of the hypoglycemia and the age at presentation of dominantly inherited K_{ATP}HI (both diazoxide responsive and unresponsive forms) can vary among members of the same pedigree and some mutation carriers may be completely asymptomatic. Figure 2 depicts the pedigree of a family with dominant diazoxide-responsive K_{ATP}HI due to a mutation in *ABCC8* [8].

Recessive K_{ATP}HI is refractory to medical therapy with diazoxide, as are patients with dominant diazoxide-unresponsive mutations. These infants often require 95–98% near-total pancreatectomy within the first few weeks of birth to manage the hypoglycemia. On the other hand, diazoxide is very effective in controlling hypoglycemia in cases with dominant diazoxide-responsive K_{ATP}HI. Octreotide, a long-acting somatostatin analog, is a second-line medical therapy for infants unresponsive to diazoxide. The initial response to octreotide is usually good, but tachyphylaxis develops after 1–2 doses (due to downregulation of somatostatin receptors), often rendering therapy inadequate for long-term use in most cases. Furthermore, octreotide appears to increase the risk of necrotizing enterocolitis in neonates [19] and must be used with caution. Glucagon, as a continuous intravenous infusion, can help maintain euglycemia in infants awaiting surgery, but its long-term use as a subcutaneous infusion [20] is limited by crystallization of the glucagon and clogging in the tubing [21]. A nonsurgical approach in diazoxide-unresponsive HI consisting of octreotide in combination with continuous or frequent enteral feedings has been proposed [21]. This approach is challenging for home management of these children, as it requires feedings as frequently as every 2–3 h.

Prognosis and Outcome

Children with congenital HI are at risk for severe complications inherent to their disease and as a consequence of their therapy. Most long-term follow-up studies include data from heterogeneous cohorts, making it difficult to assess the outcome of specific forms of HI and of specific management approaches.

Neurodevelopmental Outcome

Brain injury due to hypoglycemia is particularly likely in K_{ATP}HI due to the severity of the hypoglycemia. In the experience of The Children's Hospital of Philadelphia, the prevalence of developmental delay in patients with HI is approximately 30%. Patients with K_{ATP}HI requiring surgical therapy have a higher incidence of neurodevelopmental problems than diazoxide-responsive patients [22]. A homogenous cohort of children with the known Ashkenazi mutations who were treated without surgery showed good neurological outcome by school age, based on parental reports, although earlier developmental deficits were present [23]. A higher rate (44%) of long-term neurodevelopmental retardation was reported in a large series of children (49 medically treated, 65 surgically treated) [24]. In another series of 90 patients, severe mental retardation was found in 8%, with milder disability in another 18%. Psychomotor delays were more common in patients with neonatal onset than in those with onset of hypoglycemia later in infancy presumably reflecting more severe hypoglycemia [25].

In general, the high risk of brain damage appears to be due to delays in diagnosis and treatment rather than a consequence of the K_{ATP} channel defect and, thus, potentially preventable.

Natural History of ATP-Sensitive Potassium Channel Hyperinsulinism and Possibility of Progression to Diabetes

The natural history of patients with K_{ATP}HI and their risk of developing diabetes, either with or without having had a surgical pancreatectomy, remain unclear and, to some extent, topics of controversy. In general, there appears to be a tendency for gradual improvement in the severity of the hypoglycemia in both the recessive and dominant forms K_{ATP}HI. For example, patients with recessive K_{ATP}HI treated solely with intensive medical treatment have been reported to be able to discontinue tube feedings at a mean age of about 10 years. In our own experience, where we operate on the majority of the diazoxide-unresponsive cases, we have seen a similar evolution in patients with K_{ATP}HI who were treated surgically but continued to require tube feedings and/or octreotide; these patients also appear to become easier to control in later childhood. In addition, patients with dominant diazoxide-responsive K_{ATP}HI usually require lower doses of diazoxide as they grow older and sometimes can discontinue therapy by their teenage years. However, it should be emphasized that, in our experience, both recessive and dominant K_{ATP}HI patients who have not undergone pancreatectomy usually continue to have problems with episodes of symptomatic hypoglycemia as adults. It is also important to note that some cases that have had pancreatectomy may not develop diabetes, but may continue to have hypoglycemia as adults.

There are conflicting data about the potential pathophysiologic basis for the natural history of K_{ATP}HI that we have described in a rather provisional fashion above. One suggestion is that the defect causes beta-cell apoptosis which ultimately leads to development of insulin-deficient diabetes mellitus, perhaps as a consequence of the chronic elevation of beta-cell cytosolic calcium. For example, transgenic mice overexpressing a dominant negative Kir6.2 mutation develop diabetes with histologic evidence of beta-cell apoptosis [26]. However, the beta-cell demise in this model is probably not simply due to elevated cytosolic calcium, but most likely involves nonspecific toxic effects of the transgene because *SUR1*$^{-/-}$ mice do not appear to develop diabetes or show increased beta-cell apoptosis. It has also been reported that sections of pancreas from infants operated on for K_{ATP}HI show increased beta-cell apoptosis by TUNEL staining – again, possibly due to elevated cytosolic calcium [27]. However, other investigators have not yet confirmed this finding. An additional problem in evaluating the natural history of K_{ATP}HI is that affected patients are inherently less sensitive to glucose-stimulated insulin secretion than normal (fig. 3, 4). Thus, evidence of impaired glucose tolerance on oral glucose testing cannot be interpreted as having the same implications regarding development of diabetes as normals. For example, Huopio et al. [5] suggested that the diazoxide-responsive dominant *ABCC8* E1506K mutation was a subtype of autosomal dominant diabetes in which many of the carrier adults developed diabetes, based on evidence of gestational diabetes or impaired oral glucose tolerance. However, in a larger series of dominant diazoxide-responsive K_{ATP}HI families, the prevalence of diabetes in mutation carriers was not different from the estimated prevalence in the United States population [8]. Thus, the abnormalities of glucose tolerance observed by Huopio et al. [5] are likely the result of 'glucose blindness' by K_{ATP}HI-defective beta-cells, rather than a state of insulin deficiency. Concordant with this, an Israeli group has reported that glucose intolerance, but not diabetes mellitus, is common in their group of nonsurgically managed children during follow-up for up to 23 years [23]. In our own experience, in several 20- to 30-year-old cases with recessive K_{ATP}HI that did not have surgery, persistent elevations of HbA_{1c} as high as 7.5% were noted when the patients became mildly insulin resistant due to overweight.

In contrast, diabetes is a common complication in K_{ATP}HI treated surgically. In one series, the incidence of diabetes mellitus was as high as 27% immediately after pancreatectomy and the highest rate was seen in patients who had undergone more than one surgical resection [24]. More commonly, diabetes develops later. The mean age of diabetes diagnosis after pancreatectomy in 25 children with K_{ATP}HI was reported to be 7.3 years (0.92–17.4) [28]. In our experience, diabetes in children with K_{ATP}HI is milder and the onset more gradual than is typical of type 1 diabetes. Frequently, patients develop notable glucose intolerance while continuing to have episodes of hypoglycemia. Some individuals eventually require complete insulin replacement therapy, but others may be well controlled for long periods of time with insulin sensitizers, such as metformin.

Conclusion

The in vivo and in vitro characterization of the effects of K_{ATP}HI-associated mutations has allowed for the identification of three distinct subtypes of diffuse K_{ATP}HI: recessive diazoxide-unresponsive, dominant diazoxide-unresponsive, and dominant diazoxide-responsive. The severity of the channel defect determines the severity of the phenotype, with defects affecting the production and trafficking of the K_{ATP} channels to the plasma membrane presenting earlier with severe hypoglycemia that does not respond to diazoxide. The pathophysiology in all subtypes is characterized by a failure of the beta-cells to regulate insulin secretion according to blood glucose levels; therefore, insulin secretion is not suppressed during hypoglycemia and there is also a failure to secrete insulin in response to a glucose challenge. This 'glucose blindness' has been misinterpreted as a progression from hypoglycemia to glucose intolerance and diabetes. Further studies of long-term outcomes in children with K_{ATP}HI are needed to better understand the natural progression of the disease and the results of the different intervention approaches.

Acknowledgements

This work was supported in part by grants from the NIH: R37-DK056268 (C.A.S.), R01-DK053012 (C.A.S.), DK-19525, UL1-RR024134, and by the Clifford and Katherine Goldsmith Philanthropic Fund.

References

1 Bruining GJ: Recent advances in hyperinsulinism and pathogenesis of diabetes mellitus. Curr Opin Pediatr 1990;2:758–765.

2 Mathew PM, Young JM, Abu-Osba YK, Mulhern BD, Hammoudi S, Hamdan JA, Sa'di AR: Persistent neonatal hyperinsulinism. Clin Pediatr (Phila) 1988; 27: Z148–151.

3 Nestorowicz A, Wilson BA, Schoor KP, Inoue H, Glaser B, Landau H, Stanley CA, Thornton PS, Clement JP 4th, Bryan J, Aguilar-Bryan L, Permutt MA: Mutations in the sulonylurea receptor gene are associated with familial hyperinsulinism in Ashkenazi Jews. Hum Mol Genet 1996;5: 1813–1822.

4 Otonkoski T, Ammala C, Huopio H, Cote GJ, Chapman J, Cosgrove K, Ashfield R, Huang E, Komulainen J, Ashcroft FM, Dunne MJ, Kere J, Thomas PM: A point mutation inactivating the sulfonylurea receptor causes the severe form of persistent hyperinsulinemic hypoglycemia of infancy in Finland. Diabetes 1999;48:408–415.

5 Huopio H, Reimann F, Ashfield R, Komulainen J, Lenko HL, Rahier J, Vauhkonen I, Kere J, Laakso M, Ashcroft F, Otonkoski T: Dominantly inherited hyperinsulinism caused by a mutation in the sulfonylurea receptor type 1. J Clin Invest 2000;106: 897–906.

6 Glaser B, Thornton P, Otonkoski T, Junien C: Genetics of neonatal hyperinsulinism. Arch Dis Child Fetal Neonatal Ed 2000;82:F79–F86.

7 Macmullen CM, Zhou Q, Snider KE, Tewson PH, Becker SA, Aziz AR, Ganguly A, Shyng SL, Stanley CA: Diazoxide-unresponsive congenital hyperinsulinism in children with dominant mutations of the β-cell sulfonylurea receptor SUR1. Diabetes 2011;60: 1797–1804.

8 Pinney SE, MacMullen C, Becker S, Lin YW, Hanna C, Thornton P, Ganguly A, Shyng SL, Stanley CA: Clinical characteristics and biochemical mechanisms of congenital hyperinsulinism associated with dominant K_{ATP} channel mutations. J Clin Invest 2008;118:2877–2886.

9 Grimberg A, Ferry RJ Jr, Kelly A, Koo-McCoy S, Polonsky K, Glaser B, Permutt MA, Aguilar-Bryan L, Stafford D, Thornton PS, Baker L, Stanley CA: Dysregulation of insulin secretion in children with congenital hyperinsulinism due to sulfonylurea receptor mutations. Diabetes 2001;50:322–328.

10 Shiota C, Larsson O, Shelton KD, Shiota M, Efanov AM, Hoy M, Lindner J, Kooptiwut S, Juntti-Berggren L, Gromada J, Berggren PO, Magnuson MA: Sulfonylurea receptor type 1 knock-out mice have intact feeding-stimulated insulin secretion despite marked impairment in their response to glucose. J Biol Chem 2002;277:37176–37183.

11 Henquin JC, Nenquin M, Sempoux C, Guiot Y, Bellanne-Chantelot C, Otonkoski T, de Lonlay P, Nihoul-Fekete C, Rahier J: In vitro insulin secretion deviates from model predictions in infants with diazoxide-resistant congenital hyperinsulinism. J Clin Invest 2011;121:3932–3942.

12 Ferry RJ Jr, Kelly A, Grimberg A, Koo-McCoy S, Shapiro MJ, Fellows KE, Glaser B, Aguilar-Bryan L, Stafford DE, Stanley CA: Calcium-stimulated insulin secretion in diffuse and focal forms of congenital hyperinsulinism. J Pediatr 2000;137:239–246.

13 Stanley CA, Thornton PS, Ganguly A, MacMullen C, Underwood P, Bhatia P, Steinkrauss L, Wanner L, Kaye R, Ruchelli E, Suchi M, Adzick NS: Preoperative evaluation of infants with focal or diffuse congenital hyperinsulinism by intravenous acute insulin response tests and selective pancreatic arterial calcium stimulation. J Clin Endocrinol Metab 2004;89:288–296.

14 Giurgea I, Laborde K, Touati G, Bellanne-Chantelot C, Nassogne MC, Sempoux C, Jaubert F, Khoa N, Chigot V, Rahier J, Brunelle F, Nihoul-Fekete C, Dunne MJ, Stanley C, Saudubray JM, Robert JJ, de Lonlay P: Acute insulin responses to calcium and tolbutamide do not differentiate focal from diffuse congenital hyperinsulinism. J Clin Endocrinol Metab 2004;89:925–929.

15 Kelly A, Ng D, Ferry RJ Jr, Grimberg A, Koo-McCoy S, Thornton PS, Stanley CA: Acute insulin responses to leucine in children with the hyperinsulinism/hyperammonemia syndrome. J Clin Endocrinol Metab 2001;86:3724–3728.

16 Fourtner SH, Stanley CA, Kelly A: Protein-sensitive hypoglycemia without leucine sensitivity in hyperinsulinism caused by K(ATP) channel mutations. J Pediatr 2006;149:47–52.

17 Li C, Buettger C, Kwagh J, Matter A, Daikhin Y, Nissim IB, Collins HW, Yudkoff M, Stanley CA, Matschinsky FM: A signaling role of glutamine in insulin secretion. J Biol Chem 2004;279: 13393–13401.

18 Bulbul A, Bolat F, Comert S, Demirin H, Tanik C, Bulbul L, Nuhoglu A, Dokucu AI: Persistent hyperinsulinemic hypoglycemia with left ventricular hypertrophy and dysrhythmia: a case report. Fetal Pediatr Pathol 2010;29:165–171.

19 Laje P, Halaby L, Adzick NS, Stanley CA: Necrotizing enterocolitis in neonates receiving octreotide for the management of congenital hyperinsulinism. Pediatr Diabetes 2010;11:142–147.

20 Mohnike K, Blankenstein O, Pfuetzner A, Potzsch S, Schober E, Steiner S, Hardy OT, Grimberg A, van Waarde WM: Long-term non-surgical therapy of severe persistent congenital hyperinsulinism with glucagon. Horm Res 2008;70:59–64.

21 Mazor-Aronovitch K, Landau H, Gillis D: Surgical versus non-surgical treatment of congenital hyperinsulinism. Pediatr Endocrinol Rev 2009;6: 424–430.

22 Steinkrauss L, Lipman TH, Hendell CD, Gerdes M, Thornton PS, Stanley CA: Effects of hypoglycemia on developmental outcome in children with congenital hyperinsulinism. J Pediatr Nurs 2005;20: 109–118.

23 Mazor-Aronovitch K, Gillis D, Lobel D, Hirsch HJ, Pinhas-Hamiel O, Modan-Moses D, Glaser B, Landau H: Long-term neurodevelopmental outcome in conservatively treated congenital hyperinsulinism. Eur J Endocrinol 2007;157:491–497.

24 Meissner T, Wendel U, Burgard P, Schaetzle S, Mayatepek E: Long-term follow-up of 114 patients with congenital hyperinsulinism. Eur J Endocrinol 2003;149:43–51.

25 Menni F, de Lonlay P, Sevin C, Touati G, Peigne C, Barbier V, Nihoul-Fekete C, Saudubray JM, Robert JJ: Neurologic outcomes of 90 neonates and infants with persistent hyperinsulinemic hypoglycemia. Pediatrics 2001;107:476–479.

26 Miki T, Tashiro F, Iwanaga T, Nagashima K, Yoshitomi H, Aihara H, Nitta Y, Gonoi T, Inagaki N, Miyazaki J, Seino S: Abnormalities of pancreatic islets by targeted expression of a dominant-negative K_{ATP} channel. Proc Natl Acad Sci USA 1997;94: 11969–11973.

27 Kassem SA, Ariel I, Thornton PS, Scheimberg I, Glaser B: Beta-cell proliferation and apoptosis in the developing normal human pancreas and in hyperinsulinism of infancy. Diabetes 2000;49: 1325–1333.

28 Ludwig A, Ziegenhorn K, Empting S, Meissner T, Marquard J, Holl R, Mohnike K: Glucose metabolism and neurological outcome in congenital hyperinsulinism. Semin Pediatr Surg 2011;20:45–49.

Charles A. Stanley, MD
Division of Endocrinology/Diabetes
The Children's Hospital of Philadelphia
34th Street and Civic Center Boulevard
Philadelphia, PA 19104 (USA)
Tel. +1 215 590 3420, E-Mail stanleyc@email.chop.edu

Stanley CA, De León DD (eds): Monogenic Hyperinsulinemic Hypoglycemia Disorders.
Front Diabetes. Basel, Karger, 2012, vol 21, pp 30–42

Molecular Defects of ATP-Sensitive Potassium Channels in Congenital Hyperinsulinism

Show-Ling Shyng · Jeremy D. Bushman · Emily B. Pratt · Qing Zhou

Department of Biochemistry and Molecular Biology, Oregon Health and Science University, Portland, Oreg., USA

Abstract

The beta-cell ATP-sensitive potassium (K_{ATP}) channel plays a key role in regulating insulin secretion by linking glucose metabolism to cell excitability. The channel is a protein complex composed of four Kir6.2 inwardly rectifying potassium channel subunits and four sulfonylurea receptor 1 subunits encoded by *KCNJ11* and *ABCC8,* respectively. K_{ATP} channel function in beta-cells is dependent on correct expression as well as proper gating of the channel by metabolic signals at the plasma membrane. Mutations in *ABCC8* or *KCNJ11* that perturb channel expression or gating can reduce channel function and lead to congenital hyperinsulinism. This chapter reviews recent advances in understanding the pathophysiology of mutant K_{ATP} channels from in vitro functional studies.

Loss of ATP-sensitive potassium (K_{ATP}) channel function owing to genetic mutations was linked to congenital hyperinsulinism (CHI) in 1995 following the cloning of *KCNJ11* and *ABCC8*, which encode the pore-forming Kir6.2 subunit and the regulatory sulfonylurea receptor 1 (SUR1) subunit, respectively [1]. More than 150 CHI-associated mutations have now been identified, with the majority in *ABCC8* [2]. To understand the mechanisms by which mutations disrupt channel function, detailed in vitro functional characterization of mutant channels are needed. To date, approximately two thirds of the known mutations have been analyzed by in vitro studies. These studies show that mutations can abolish or reduce channel activity by causing defects in channel gating, disrupting channel biogenesis or trafficking to the cell surface (collectively referred to as 'trafficking mutations' hereinafter), or disruption of both gating and surface expression [3–5]. The information gathered has greatly improved our understanding of genotype-phenotype relationships and has provided invaluable insights into the molecular mechanisms of channel regulation in health and disease.

Methods for in vitro Study of Mutant ATP-Sensitive Potassium Channels

To study the functional effects of K_{ATP} channel mutations, recombinant mutant channels are usually expressed in *Xenopus oocytes* or mammalian cell lines such as COS or HEK293. These heterologous expression systems offer a convenient experimental platform for genetic manipulations; moreover, they are devoid of endogenous channels which might confound data interpretation. Mutant channel proteins can be expressed either as a homogeneous population to mimic the homozygous state or coexpressed with the wild-type protein at a 1:1 ratio to simulate the heterozygous state.

Several approaches have been developed to study mutant channel function and expression, both in the context of the complex intracellular milieu as well as simpler controlled settings. A tracer ion efflux assay (using $^{86}Rb^+$ as a substitute for the physiological conduction ion K^+) is suitable for assessing if mutant channels respond to metabolic inhibition in intact mammalian cells. Metabolic inhibition lowers the intracellular ATP/ADP ratio and activates K_{ATP} channels. Reduced $^{86}Rb^+$ efflux therefore indicates loss of channel function and a causal role of a mutation in the disease. This assay is also used to test if mutant channels respond to pharmacological agents such as the potassium channel opener diazoxide. Electrophysiological recordings of mutant channels expressed in oocytes or mammalian cells offer a direct readout of channel activity. Using the inside-out patch-clamp recording configuration, solutions exposed to the cytosolic surface can be precisely controlled and channel gating by intracellular nucleotides and diazoxide can be easily monitored and quantified. To assess mutant channel protein biogenesis and trafficking, Western blotting and a surface labeling chemiluminescence assay are commonly employed. Western blots report the total steady-state channel protein levels and the glycosylation pattern of SUR1. The latter can be utilized to gauge K_{ATP} trafficking. SUR1 undergoes complex glycosylation in the Golgi, giving rise to an upper 'mature' band distinguishable from the lower 'immature' band that represents core-glycosylated SUR1 within the endoplasmic reticulum (ER; fig. 1c). Since channel proteins are allowed to exit the ER only when the RKR-ER retention motifs become hidden in assembled octameric complexes (see Remedi and Nichols [this vol., pp. 7–17]), the upper SUR1 band serves as a proxy measure for channels that have passed the ER quality control. The abundance of upper band, in general, correlates with surface channel expression; however, it is not a direct measure as mature SUR1 is present not only in the plasma membrane, but also in other post-Golgi intracellular secretory and endocytic membrane compartments. To measure surface channel expression directly, a chemiluminescence-based immunoassay has been developed [6]. Here, only mutant channel proteins (with an

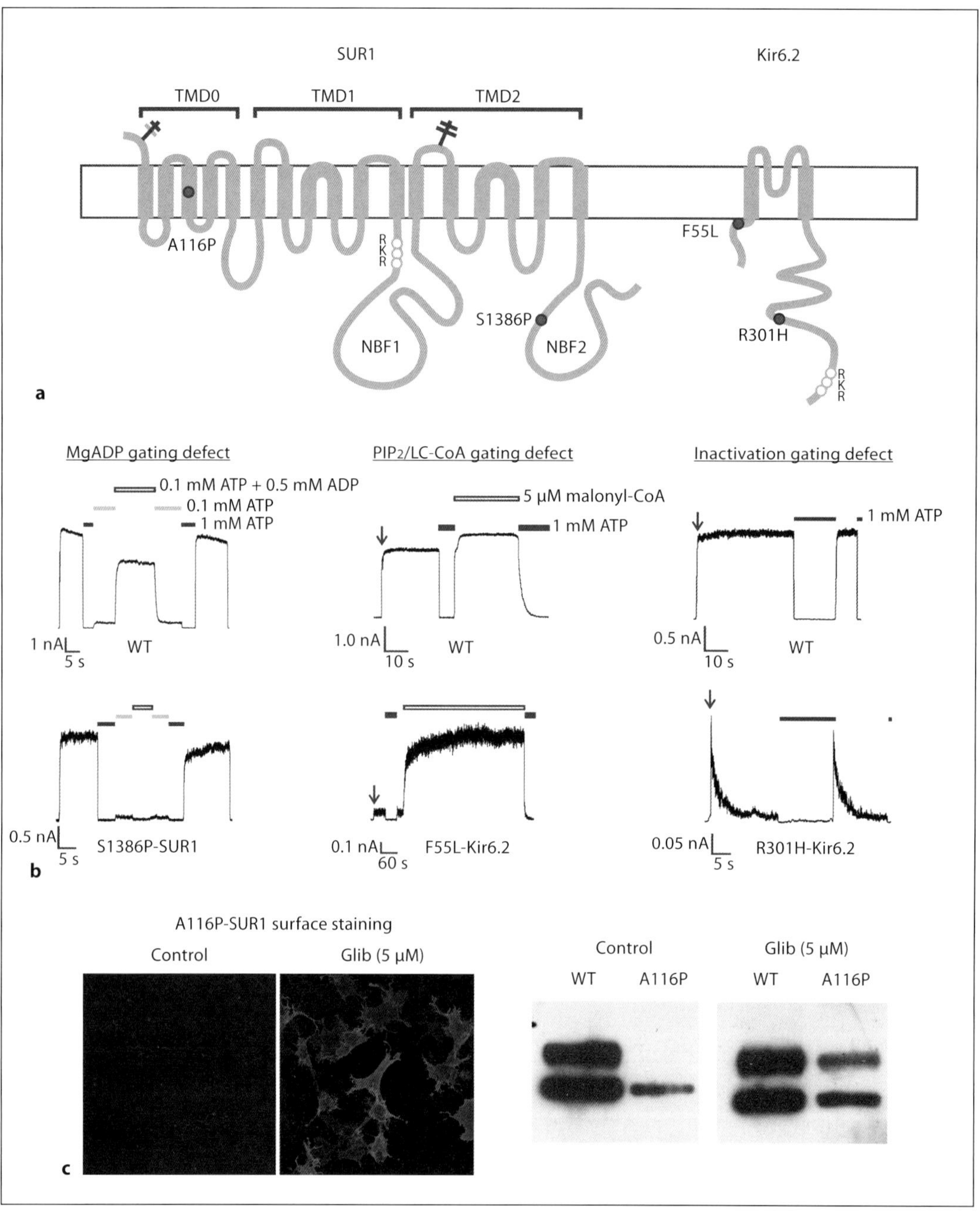

Fig. 1. K_{ATP} channel defects in CHI. **a** Membrane topology of SUR1 and Kir6.2. SUR1 has three transmembrane domains (TMD0, TMD1, and TMD2) and two nucleotide-binding folds (NBF1 and NBF2). Mutations that cause the gating or expression defects shown in **b** and **c** are marked. **b** Examples of gating defects caused by SUR1 or Kir6.2 mutations. Inside-out patch clamp recordings were made in COS cells transiently transfected with the mutant K_{ATP} channels. **c** A K_{ATP} trafficking mutant and its rescue by sulfonylureas. Left: Immunofluorescent staining of COS cells transiently transfected with A116P-SUR1 and Kir6.2 showing lack of surface expression (control) and recovery of surface expression upon glibenclamide treatment (Glib). Right: Corresponding Western blots of A116P-SUR1. (continued on p. 33)

engineered extracellular epitope tag) that are expressed at the cell surface become labeled with an antibody directed against the epitope tag; subsequently, an enzymatic reaction mediated by a HRP-conjugated secondary antibody produces a chemiluminescence signal that is detected by a luminometer – this signal is proportional to K_{ATP} channel surface expression.

Limitations exist when interpreting in vitro functional data in the literature. For example, studies using oocytes might not detect folding or trafficking defects as they are cultured at a lower temperature – a condition known to allow surface expression of some misfolded mutant channels [7]. Also, many studies have used rodent SUR1 and Kir6.2 (hamster, rat, or mouse) for expression, likely because they were cloned first and used in the initial functional reconstitution study [8]. Although human and rodent channel proteins are highly conserved and rodent channel subunits with human-equivalent mutations likely serve as adequate surrogates in most cases, potential functional differences due to small sequence variations cannot be ruled out. Despite these shortcomings, generally good correlations exist between disease phenotypes and channel defects revealed by in vitro studies.

Gating Defects

Early functional characterization of CHI mutations focused mostly on channel gating properties. The first K_{ATP} channel gating defect reported was loss of MgADP-mediated stimulation caused by a G1479R mutation in SUR1 [9]; this turns out to be by far the most common gating abnormality in CHI (fig. 1b, left). Not surprisingly, nearly all mutations with this gating defect are in SUR1, the subunit that confers the MgADP gating effect. Many of them are in or near the nucleotide-binding folds and may reduce MgADP stimulation by impairing nucleotide binding, hydrolysis, and/or subsequent conformational rearrangement between the two nucleotide-binding folds (see Remedi and Nichols [this vol., pp. 7–17]) [4, 9–13]. However, some of them lie outside the nucleotide-binding folds and likely diminish MgADP stimulation as a result of a transduction error caused by interference with functional coupling between SUR1 and the pore subunit Kir6.2 [4, 14, 15]. The only Kir6.2 mutation implicated in altering Mg-nucleotide sensitivity is T294M [16]. This mutation appears to reduce channel stimulation by MgADP only in the presence of ATP, leading to the proposal that T294M does not disrupt MgADP stimulation per se, but rather interferes with the ability of SUR1 to alleviate ATP inhibition in the presence of MgADP.

The prevalence of MgADP gating defects among CHI mutants demonstrates the indispensable role ADP plays in the activation of K_{ATP} channels during glucose

(fig. 1 continued from p. 32) WT-SUR1 is seen as both the core-glycosylated lower band present in the ER and the complex-glycosylated upper band that has passed the medial Golgi. A116P in contrast is only seen as the core-glycosylated form. Upon glibenclamide treatment, however, both lower and upper bands are present.

deprivation [9]. Interestingly, the extent of a MgADP gating defect for a given mutation generally parallels a defect in its response to the potassium channel opener diazoxide (table 1) [4, 9, 12, 17]. Consequently, patients expressing mutant channels with less severe MgADP gating defects also tend to respond to diazoxide treatment (table 1; diazoxide-responsive mutations) [9]. However, exceptions to this relationship exist. Some mutations have a slightly more severe MgADP gating defect than a diazoxide gating defect, or vice versa, and response to one agonist does not predict response to the other [18].

Recent identification and characterization of CHI-associated mutations in the Kir6.2 subunit have revealed less common gating defects related to the intrinsic gating properties conferred by Kir6.2. The F55L mutation, which is located in a structure called the slide helix and has been implicated in gating, markedly reduces the open probability of the channel by attenuating channel response to the membrane phospholipid PIP_2 (Remedi and Nichols [this vol., pp. 7–17]; fig. 1b, middle) [19]. Although F55L mutant channels exhibit greatly reduced activity, they are still inhibited by ATP and stimulated by MgADP and diazoxide like wild-type channels, suggesting the mutation does not disrupt functional coupling between Kir6.2 and SUR1 [19].

Another mutation, G156R, is heterozygous, dominant, and located in the second transmembrane helix of Kir6.2 lining the channel pore. It abolishes channel activity by preventing ion conduction [20]. Analyses of concatenated tandem Kir6.2 tetramers containing 0–4 mutant subunits indicate that just one G156R mutant is sufficient to reduce K_{ATP} conductance, and increasing the number of mutant subunits further reduces conduction [20]. This study demonstrates directly a dominant-negative effect of the mutation. Under the simulated heterozygous expression condition (wild-type to G156R mutant molar ratio of 1:1, unconcatenated subunits), K_{ATP} currents were reduced by more than 60%, yet the remaining currents responded to diazoxide stimulation, consistent with clinical response of the patient to the drug.

A different gating defect causing inactivation has been described in several CHI mutations, including those at residue R301 (to C, G, H, or P) and V290M. These mutations cause a rapid spontaneous current decay in the absence of inhibitory ATP, referred to as 'inactivation.' (fig. 1b, right) [21, 22]. The inactivation residues are predicted to lie at the Kir6.2 subunit-subunit interface where they interact with residues in an adjacent Kir6.2 subunit [23, 24]. This suggests that inactivation mutations destabilize K_{ATP} currents by disrupting subunit-subunit interactions, resulting in an inability of beta-cells to sustain a polarized membrane potential in the face of low-blood glucose.

Expression/Trafficking Defects

It is now clear that a large number of CHI mutations cause loss of channel function by preventing fully assembled channels from being expressed at the plasma membrane

Table 1. Dominant K_{ATP} channel gating mutations

Mutation[1]	Surface expression, % of wild-type	MgADP response, % of wild-type[2]	Diazoxide response, % of wild-type[3]	Reference
Diazoxide-responsive				
SUR1				
D310N	65	59	30	15
R370G	106	17	57	15
R1353H	90	62	77	37
K1374R	127	15	14	15
S1386P	91	2	3	15
G1478V	93	5	4	15
G1479R	74	19	13	9, 15
E1507K	98	1	4	12, 15
I1512T	96	12	12	15
Kir6.2				
F55L	94	99	99	15, 19
G156R[4]	110	–	–	15, 20
D204E[4]	80	–	–	15
Diazoxide-unresponsive				
SUR1				
Q474R	119	5	3	18
A478D	83	1	4	18
V715A	83	1	2	18
V715G	96	1	3	18
G716D	66	4	3	18
T888P	54	1	2	18
G1384E	101	0	2	18
S1387F	83	1	5	18, 27
S1387Y	83	4	3	18
S1389Y	70	2	2	18
A1458T	94	1	1	18
Q1459H	91	1	2	18
E1517K	72	3	3	18

[1] All are dominant heterozygous in diffuse disease. Functional data are from homomeric mutant channels. Only those mutations with complete surface expression, and MgADP and diazoxide response measurements are included.
[2] MgADP response was measured in 0.1 mM ATP and 0.5 mM ADP with free [Mg^{2+}] approx. 1 mM.
[3] MgADP response was measured in 0.1 mM ATP and 0.2 mM diazoxide with free [Mg^{2+}] approx. 1 mM.
[4] No currents were detectable when expressed as homomeric mutant channels, thus no MgADP or diazoxide response was available.

Table 2. K_{ATP} channel trafficking mutations

Mutation[1]	Disease	Surface expression % of wild-type	Clinical diazoxide response	Reference
SUR1				
G7R[1]	focal	35	no	5
N24K[1]	diffuse	45	no	5
F27S[1]	focal	18	no	5
R74W[1]	focal	2	no	5, 36
A116P[1]	unknown	6	unknown	1, 27, 29, 38
E128K[1]	diffuse	7	no	5, 36
V187D[1]	unknown	19	no	27, 29, 39
R495Q	diffuse	2	no	5
E501K	focal	4	no	5
L503P	focal	2	no	5
F686S	focal	1	no	5
G716V	diffuse	5	no	5
L1350Q	focal	4	no	5
F1388	diffuse	1	no	25, 40
D1472H	diffuse	8	no	5, 33
L1544P	diffuse	19	no	31
Kir6.2				
W91R[2]	unknown	–	no	1, 26
P254L	diffuse	0	no	34
E282K[2]	focal	–	unknown	32
R301G[3]	focal	26	no	21
R301H[3]	focal	20	no	21
R301P[3]	diffuse	4	no	21

[1] Trafficking defects that have been shown to be rescued by sulfonylureas.
[2] No direct surface expression measurement data is available.
[3] These mutations also cause inactivation gating defects. The R301P mutation is homozygous.

(table 2). In a few cases, mutations introduce premature stop codons, resulting in truncated nonfunctional proteins. In most cases, however, mutations lead to failure of the channel proteins to express at the cell surface by causing defective folding or assembly, and/or defective trafficking from the ER to the plasma membrane.

Proteins that are misfolded or that fail to assemble are usually retained in the ER. ER retention results in the lack or reduction of mature complex-glycosylated SUR1, the form representative of channels that have passed the ER quality control surveillance and trafficked to Golgi. The SUR1 A116P trafficking mutation is shown as an example of this in figure 1c. ER-retained proteins are often subject to ER-associated degradation via the ubiquitin-proteasome pathway. Susceptibility to degradation can be inferred by reduced steady-state protein levels in Western blots, as has been observed in many SUR1 and Kir6.2 trafficking mutants [5, 21, 25]. Alternatively, the degradation rate can be directly measured in metabolically (^{35}S[Met/Cys]) labeled mutant proteins. This approach has been used to demonstrate accelerated degradation of two SUR1 mutations, ΔF1388 and A116P, and one Kir6.2 mutation, W91R [26–28].

For most of the ER-retained SUR1 and Kir6.2 mutants, it is unclear whether the mutation interferes with folding, subunit assembly, or both. Two SUR1 mutants, A116P and V187D, have been reported to exhibit reduced association with Kir6.2 based on coimmunoprecipitation data, implying impaired subunit assembly [29]; however, another study showed that they are able to form functional channels with Kir6.2 once rescued to the cell surface by chemical chaperones (see below) [27]. Also, ΔF1388 of SUR1 and W91R of Kir6.2 have been shown to form complexes with their respective assembly partners, but the complexes are short-lived and the mutant subunits dissociate from the complexes to be degraded [26]. Recently, a CHI mutation of an extracellular cysteine residue in SUR1, C26S, was shown to disrupt intramolecular disulfide bond formation, leading to SUR1 misfolding and ER retention [30].

In addition to the above mechanisms, mutations may disrupt signals that regulate forward trafficking of the assembled channel complex. For example, the L1544P SUR1 mutation has been proposed to cause incomplete shielding of the RKR ER-retention motifs in the channel complex to prevent trafficking out of the ER [31]. Another Kir6.2 mutation, E282K, is thought to diminish surface expression of K_{ATP} channels by disrupting a diacidic ER exit signal (Kir6.2 ^{280}DLE^{282}) [32]. Clearly, there are many mechanisms that can prevent channels from reaching the plasma membrane. More work is needed to gain better understanding of how channel folding, assembly, and trafficking are regulated and how mutations affect these regulatory processes.

Correlating in vitro Functional Data with Clinical Phenotype

Mutant channel defects uncovered by in vitro functional studies provide the basis for understanding clinical phenotypes. Because each functional K_{ATP} channel contains four SUR1 and four Kir6.2 subunits that can originate from either allele, it is necessary to consider the genetic context of a mutation when making genotype-phenotype correlations. In focal CHI, there is a loss of heterozygosity (see Arnoux et al. [this vol., pp. 43–56]). Thus, channel defects in expression, gating, or both caused by the paternally inherited SUR1 or Kir6.2 mutation are well correlated with clinical phenotype.

In diffuse disease, mutations follow recessive or dominant modes of inheritance. Large-scale studies have revealed general characteristics of recessive and dominant mutations. Recessive mutations such as ΔF1388 of SUR1 result in inability of the channel to traffic to the cell surface (table 2) [15, 25]. Individuals heterozygous for such mutations are asymptomatic; only when the mutation is present in both alleles is the loss of channel expression and function manifested clinically. This suggests that in heterozygous patients, the wild-type allele is able to give rise to sufficient number of functional channels to spare them of the disease. Interestingly, by studying the ΔF1388-SUR1 and W91R-Kir6.2 recessive trafficking mutations, Crane and Aguilar-Bryan [26] observed that although mutant subunits form complexes with their respective wild-type assembly partners, they quickly dissociate and become degraded, leading to the idea that mutant proteins are weeded out in the ER allowing wild-type channels to reach the cell surface.

In contrast, dominant mutations tend to traffic to the plasma membrane, but cause loss-of-function gating defects (table 2) [15]. In heterozygous conditions, mutant subunits incorporate into octameric channel complexes to disrupt normal gating. As discussed above, clinical diazoxide responsiveness and disease severity often, but not always, vary with the extent of channel gating defect [18]. In addition to SUR1 dominant mutations, several Kir6.2 dominant mutations including F55L, G156R, and D204E have been identified (table 1) [15]. Like SUR1 dominant mutations, these Kir6.2 mutations do not affect channel trafficking. Unlike SUR1 mutations that disrupt MgADP response, they impair intrinsic gating properties endowed by the Kir6.2 subunit in the absence of nucleotides. Further, simulated heterozygous conditions result in decreased activities but retention of diazoxide stimulation – an effect mediated by the SUR1 subunit [19, 20]. This correlates well with the clinical diazoxide response seen in patients heterozygous for dominant Kir6.2 mutations [15, 20].

In addition to the genotypes discussed above, compound heterozygous mutations on the same or different alleles have been reported [30, 33, 34]. In these rare cases, one or both mutations may contribute to the clinical phenotype. Continued functional characterization of disease-associated mutations should uncover the full spectrum of genotype-phenotype relationships.

In vitro Rescue of Mutant ATP-Sensitive Potassium Channel Defects and Therapeutic Implications

Improved understanding of the molecular mechanisms by which K_{ATP} mutations disrupt channel function has led to attempts to correct channel defects and expand the limited pharmacological treatment options for CHI. Several studies have reported in vitro rescue of dysfunctional channels using pharmacological or genetic approaches. For example, inactivation of the RKR ER retention signal by mutating it to AAA in SUR1 or Kir6.2 can partially correct trafficking defects caused by ΔF1388 and L1544P mutations in SUR1 [25, 31]. More clinically germane, pharmacological chaperones have been explored to rescue mutant channels that are retained in the ER. Sulfonylureas such as glibenclamide and tolbutamide are highly effective in correcting trafficking defects of some mutations [27]. For example, in COS cells transfected with Kir6.2 and the trafficking mutant SUR1 A116P, overnight treatment with glibenclamide significantly improved maturation efficiency of the mutant SUR1 as seen by the increase in the complex-glycosylated band and surface expression of the channel (fig. 1c). It is interesting that studies of over 20 trafficking mutants distributed throughout the SUR1 protein have shown only mutations located in TMD0 are effectively rescued by sulfonylureas (table 2) [5, 27]. It remains to be determined whether sulfonylureas can also correct trafficking defects caused by Kir6.2 CHI mutations.

The ability to correct the expression defect caused by certain mutations raises the possibility that channel function may be restored. Indeed, some SUR1 mutations that are rescued by pharmacological chaperones have normal nucleotide sensitivity, such as A116P and V187D rescued by the reversible sulfonylurea tolbutamide [27, 35]. The potential use of currently available sulfonylureas as pharmacological chaperones in the treatment of CHI is challenging as they also inhibit channel activity. Although diazoxide would be an ideal pharmacological chaperone since it also stimulates channel activity, it is ineffective in rescuing ER-retained mutant channels tested so far [5, 27]. Not all CHI trafficking mutants rescued to the cell surface with pharmacological chaperones display normal gating properties. For example, ΔF1388 and L1544P mutant channels rescued to the cell surface showed diminished MgADP stimulation, indicating that they will not be physiologically functional [25, 31]. Two SUR1 TMD0 trafficking mutations, R74W and E128K, after being rescued to the cell surface by reversible sulfonylureas actually exhibit significantly reduced ATP-sensitivity – a gating defect characteristic of neonatal diabetes-causing mutations [36]. These latter two mutations represent extreme examples of how surface expression can dictate disease phenotype and highlight the importance of in vitro functional studies in identifying mutations suitable for chaperone therapy.

In addition to efforts directed towards restoring channel expression, a number of studies have employed strategies attempting to correct channel gating defects. In isolated membrane patches, the reduced open probability gating defect caused by the F55L mutation in Kir6.2 is reversed by PIP_2 or malonyl-CoA applied to the cytoplasmic face [19]. The same manipulation also reversed the inactivation gating defect observed in channels bearing mutations at the R301 residue in Kir6.2 [21]. These studies suggest that upregulation of PIP_2 or long-chain CoA concentrations in cells may overcome select gating defects. For the G156R Kir6.2 mutation which abolishes potassium ion conduction, normal conduction was restored by introducing a second mutation, N160D, roughly one helical turn down the transmembrane alpha-helix lining the conduction pathway – an effect likely brought about via electrostatic interactions between the two mutated amino acids [20]. The G156R/N160D doubly mutant channel exhibited normal conductance and sensitivity to ATP inhibition and MgADP stimulation. Although not immediately clinically applicable, this study provides proof of principle that gating defects caused by Kir6.2 pore mutations can be overcome by manipulating the chemical environment surrounding the mutated pore residue.

Conclusions and Perspectives

The past 15 years have seen significant progress towards understanding the pathophysiology of K_{ATP} channels in CHI. While generally in vitro functional data obtained in heterologous expression systems provide adequate explanation for the disease phenotype, allowing better diagnosis and treatment, there are exceptions that remain enigmatic. It is possible that a lack of genotype-phenotype correlation in some cases is due to the expression system or species of channel protein used. For example, some channel regulatory mechanisms involving protein phosphorylation and interaction with other proteins may occur only in beta-cells. An important future effort is to better understand channel regulation in beta-cells and to study mutant channels in their native environment. Some mutations seem to only cause disease in a subset of carriers or cause disease of variable severity. Insufficient clinical information for definitive diagnosis in some carriers could explain the apparent variability in mutation penetrance, highlighting the importance of complete clinical data. A possible role of epigenetic regulation or genetic modifiers in disease manifestation is also a challenging question that needs to be tackled in the future. Finally, continued efforts on identifying strategies to rescue channel expression and/or gating defects in vitro will undoubtedly provide insight for future drug design and lead to expansion of disease treatment options.

Acknowledgements

This work is supported by NIH grants DK57699 and DK66485 (S.L.S), F31NS065688 (J.D.B.), and F30DK081305 (E.B.P.).

References

1 Aguilar-Bryan L, Bryan J: Molecular biology of adenosine triphosphate-sensitive potassium channels. Endocr Rev 1999;20:101–135.

2 Flanagan SE, et al: Update of mutations in the genes encoding the pancreatic beta-cell K(ATP) channel subunits Kir6.2 (KCNJ11) and sulfonylurea receptor 1 (ABCC8) in diabetes mellitus and hyperinsulinism. Hum Mutat 2009;30:170–180.

3 Marthinet E, et al: Severe congenital hyperinsulinism caused by a mutation in the Kir6.2 subunit of the adenosine triphosphate-sensitive potassium channel impairing trafficking and function. J Clin Endocrinol Metab 2005;90:5401–5406.

4 Shyng SL, et al: Functional analyses of novel mutations in the sulfonylurea receptor 1 associated with persistent hyperinsulinemic hypoglycemia of infancy. Diabetes 1998;47:1145–1151.

5 Yan FF, et al: Congenital hyperinsulinism associated ABCC8 mutations that cause defective trafficking of ATP-sensitive K+ channels: identification and rescue. Diabetes 2007;56:2339–2348.

6 Zerangue N, et al: A new ER trafficking signal regulates the subunit stoichiometry of plasma membrane K(ATP) channels. Neuron 1999;22:537–548.

7 Yang K, et al: Low temperature completely rescues the function of two misfolded K ATP channel disease-mutants. FEBS Lett 2005;579:4113–4118.

8 Inagaki N, et al: Reconstitution of IKATP: an inward rectifier subunit plus the sulfonylurea receptor. Science 1995;270:1166–1170.

9 Nichols CG, et al: Adenosine diphosphate as an intracellular regulator of insulin secretion. Science 1996;272:1785–1787.

10 Matsuo M, et al: Functional analysis of a mutant sulfonylurea receptor, SUR1-R1420C, that is responsible for persistent hyperinsulinemic hypoglycemia of infancy. J Biol Chem 2000;275:41184–41191.

11 Cartier EA, Shen S, Shyng SL: Modulation of the trafficking efficiency and functional properties of ATP-sensitive potassium channels through a single amino acid in the sulfonylurea receptor. J Biol Chem 2003;278: 7081–7090.

12 Huopio H, et al: Dominantly inherited hyperinsulinism caused by a mutation in the sulfonylurea receptor type 1. J Clin Invest 2000;106: 897–906.

13 Reimann F, et al: Characterisation of new K(ATP)-channel mutations associated with congenital hyperinsulinism in the Finnish population. Diabetologia 2003;46:241–249.

14 Abdulhadi-Atwan M, et al: Novel de novo mutation in sulfonylurea receptor 1 presenting as hyperinsulinism in infancy followed by overt diabetes in early adolescence. Diabetes 2008;57:1935–1940.

15 Pinney SE, et al: Clinical characteristics and biochemical mechanisms of congenital hyperinsulinism associated with dominant KATP channel mutations. J Clin Invest 2008;118:2877–2886.

16 Shimomura K, et al: Adjacent mutations in the gating loop of Kir6.2 produce neonatal diabetes and hyperinsulinism. EMBO Mol Med 2009;1:166–177.

17 Shyng S, Ferrigni T, Nichols CG: Regulation of KATP channel activity by diazoxide and MgADP. Distinct functions of the two nucleotide binding folds of the sulfonylurea receptor. J Gen Physiol 1997;110:643–654.

18 Macmullen CM, et al: Diazoxide-unresponsive congenital hyperinsulinism in children with dominant mutations of the β-cell sulfonylurea receptor SUR1. Diabetes 2011;60:1797–1804.

19 Lin YW, et al: A novel KCNJ11 mutation associated with congenital hyperinsulinism reduces the intrinsic open probability of beta-cell ATP-sensitive potassium channels. J Biol Chem 2006;281:3006–3012.

20 Bushman JD, et al: Characterization and functional restoration of a potassium channel Kir6.2 pore mutation identified in congenital hyperinsulinism. J Biol Chem 2011;285:6012–6023.

21 Lin YW, et al: Destabilization of ATP-sensitive potassium channel activity by novel KCNJ11 mutations identified in congenital hyperinsulinism. J Biol Chem 2008;283:146–156.

22 Loechner KJ, et al: Congenital hyperinsulinism and glucose hypersensitivity in homozygous and heterozygous carriers of Kir6.2 (KCNJ11) mutation V290M mutation: K(ATP) channel inactivation mechanism and clinical management. Diabetes 2011;60:209–217.

23 Kuo A, et al: Crystal structure of the potassium channel KirBac1.1 in the closed state. Science 2003;300:1922–1926.

24 Nishida M, MacKinnon R: Structural Basis of Inward Rectification. Cytoplasmic Pore of the G Protein-Gated Inward Rectifier GIRK1 at 1.8 A Resolution. Cell 2002;111:957–965.

25 Cartier EA, et al: Defective trafficking and function of KATP channels caused by a sulfonylurea receptor 1 mutation associated with persistent hyperinsulinemic hypoglycemia of infancy. Proc Natl Acad Sci U S A 2001;98:2882–2887.

26 Crane A, Aguilar-Bryan L: Assembly, maturation, and turnover of K(ATP) channel subunits. J Biol Chem 2004;279:9080–9090.

27 Yan F, et al: Sulfonylureas correct trafficking defects of ATP-sensitive potassium channels caused by mutations in the sulfonylurea receptor. J Biol Chem 2004;279:11096–11105.

28 Yan FF, et al: Role of ubiquitin-proteasome degradation pathway in biogenesis efficiency of {beta}-cell ATP-sensitive potassium channels. Am J Physiol Cell Physiol 2005;289:C1351–C1359.

29 Chan KW, Zhang H, Logothetis DE: N-terminal transmembrane domain of the SUR controls trafficking and gating of Kir6 channel subunits. Embo J 2003;22:3833–3843.

30 Fukuda Y, et al: Conserved intramolecular disulfide bond is critical to trafficking and fate of ATP-binding cassette (ABC) transporters ABCB6 and sulfonylurea receptor 1 (SUR1)/ABCC8. J Biol Chem 2010;286:8481–8492.

31 Taschenberger G, et al: Identification of a familial hyperinsulinism-causing mutation in the sulfonylurea receptor 1 that prevents normal trafficking and function of KATP channels. J Biol Chem 2002;277: 17139–17146.

32 Taneja TK, et al: Sar1-GTPase-dependent ER exit of KATP channels revealed by a mutation causing congenital hyperinsulinism. Hum Mol Genet 2009;18: 2400–2413.

33 Muzyamba M, et al: Complex ABCC8 DNA variations in congenital hyperinsulinism: lessons from functional studies. Clin Endocrinol (Oxf) 2007;67: 115–124.

34 Tornovsky S, et al: Hyperinsulinism of infancy: novel ABCC8 and KCNJ11 mutations and evidence for additional locus heterogeneity. J Clin Endocrinol Metab 2004;89:6224–6234.

35 Partridge CJ, Beech DJ, Sivaprasadarao A: Identification and pharmacological correction of a membrane trafficking defect associated with a mutation in the sulfonylurea receptor causing familial hyperinsulinism. J Biol Chem 2001;276:35947–35952.
36 Pratt EB, et al: Sulfonylurea receptor 1 mutations that cause opposite insulin secretion defects with chemical chaperone exposure. J Biol Chem 2009; 284:7951–7959.
37 Magge SN, et al: Familial leucine-sensitive hypoglycemia of infancy due to a dominant mutation of the beta-cell sulfonylurea receptor. J Clin Endocrinol Metab 2004;89:4450–4456.
38 Babenko AP, Bryan J: SUR domains that associate with and gate KATP pores define a novel gatekeeper. J Biol Chem 2003;26:26.
39 Otonkoski T, et al: A point mutation inactivating the sulfonylurea receptor causes the severe form of persistent hyperinsulinemic hypoglycemia of infancy in Finland. Diabetes 1999;48:408–415.
40 Yan FF, et al: Role of Hsp90 in biogenesis of the beta-cell ATP-sensitive potassium channel complex. Mol Biol Cell 2010;21:1945–1954.

Prof. Show-Ling Shyng, PhD
Department of Biochemistry and Molecular Biology
Oregon Health and Science University
3181 S.W. Sam Jackson Park Road
Portland, OR 97239 (USA)
Tel. +1 503 494 2694, E-Mail shyngs@ohsu.edu

Stanley CA, De León DD (eds): Monogenic Hyperinsulinemic Hypoglycemia Disorders.
Front Diabetes. Basel, Karger, 2012, vol 21, pp 43–56

Molecular Mechanisms and Clinical Pathophysiologies of Focal ATP-Sensitive Potassium Channel Hyperinsulinism and Beckwith-Wiedemann Syndrome

Jean-Baptiste Arnoux[a] · Virginie Verkarre[b] · Sylvie Rossignol[d] · Yves Aigrain[c] · Pascale de Lonlay[a]

[a]Centre de Référence des Maladies Héréditaires du Métabolisme de l'Enfant et l'Adulte, [b]Département d'Anatomopathologie, [c]Service de Chirurgie Viscérale Pédiatrique, Hôpital Necker-Enfants Malades, AP-HP, Université Paris Descartes, and [d]Laboratoire d'Explorations Fonctionnelles, Hôpital Trousseau, AP-HP, Université Pierre et Marie Curie, Paris, France

Abstract

One of the major advances in the care of patients with congenital hyperinsulinism was the discovery of focal adenomatous hyperplasia since patients can be definitively cured after a limited pancreatectomy. The histological features include hyperplasia and an increased beta-cell mass within the focal lesion. These findings were already reported in the pancreas of patients with Beckwith-Wiedemann syndrome (BWS), a condition which is known to be associated with hyperinsulinism. However, the pathophysiology of focal hyperinsulinism (FoHI) is more complex and includes a 'two hits' mechanism: (1) a paternally inherited mutation of an ATP-sensitive potassium (K_{ATP}) channel gene located on the 11p15 chromosome; and (2) in a pancreatic endocrine progenitor, a deletion of the maternally inherited 11p15 chromosomal region, compensated by a paternal uniparental disomy as observed in some cases of BWS. The loss of heterozygosity in the imprinted 11p15.5 region bearing genes involved in tumor suppression and cell proliferation explains the histopathological findings of FoHI, while the paternally inherited K_{ATP} channel mutation reduced to homozygosity within the beta-cells of the focal lesion causes hyperinsulinemic hypoglycemia unresponsive to diazoxide.

The discovery of the molecular mechanism of focal hyperinsulinism (FoHI) was initially triggered by the striking similarity between the histological findings observed in FoHI and in a particular condition known to cause hyperinsulinemic hypoglycemia: the Beckwith-Wiedemann syndrome (BWS). Indeed, both conditions bear a common chromosomal rearrangement: a paternal uniparental disomy (pUPD) involving the 11p15.5 chromosomal region with a variable extent from the telomere toward the centromere. However, specific to FoHI, a second mechanism explains the usual diazoxide-unresponsiveness of FoHI patients: a paternally inherited mutation of an ATP-sensitive potassium (K_{ATP}) channel gene (located in 11p15.1) is reduced to homozygosity within the focal form because of the pUPD. This chapter will describe the molecular mechanisms underlying BWS and, more specifically, the 11p15 pUPD, to give light on the pathophysiology of FoHI.

Beckwith-Wiedemann Syndrome

BWS (OMIM 130650) is a model disorder for the study of imprinting, growth dysregulation, and tumorigenesis. BWS results from various genetic and epigenetic anomalies in the imprinted 11p15.5 region that causes overexpression of paternally expressed genes or a lack of expression of maternally expressed genes. BWS has an incidence of 1 in 13,700. The clinical features as described by Beckwith [1] and Wiedemann in 1969 include the characteristic growth disorder with macrosomia, macroglossia, visceromegaly, abdominal wall defects including omphalocele and umbilical hernia, neonatal hypoglycemia, ear creases/pits, body asymmetry, and an increased risk for embryonal tumor development. Close to 50% of neonates with BWS present with hypoglycemia.

Pathophysiology of Beckwith-Wiedemann Syndrome

Molecular mechanisms that lead to BWS are various, but have in common an imbalance in gene expression on chromosome 11p15.5. Most autosomal genes are equally expressed from both alleles, the paternally inherited as well as the maternally inherited one. However, some genes are subjected to imprinting and are thus expressed only with regard to their parent of origin (mother or father).

The 11p15.5 region includes a cluster of several imprinted genes controlled by two imprinting centers (IC1 and IC2), which are differentially methylated on the two parental alleles. These imprinting centers define two domains (fig. 1). One is the telomeric domain controlled by IC1 (paternally methylated), which includes the paternally expressed fetal growth factor IGF2 gene and the maternally expressed H19 gene, considered as a transregulator of genes involved in fetal growth. The other is the centromeric domain controlled by IC2 (maternally methylated), which includes the maternally expressed CDKN1C (cyclin-dependent kinase inhibitor acting as a negative regulator of cell proliferation) and KCNQ1 (potassium channel voltage gated) genes, as well as the paternally expressed KCNQ1OT1 (gene silencer) gene.

Cytogenetic, Genetic, and Epigenetic Causes of Beckwith-Wiedemann Syndrome

Familial BWS accounts for about 15% of all cases and are explained by rare cytogenetic abnormalities, with the common finding of involvement of the 11p15 chromosomal region. This consists of (1) maternally inherited translocations or inversions or

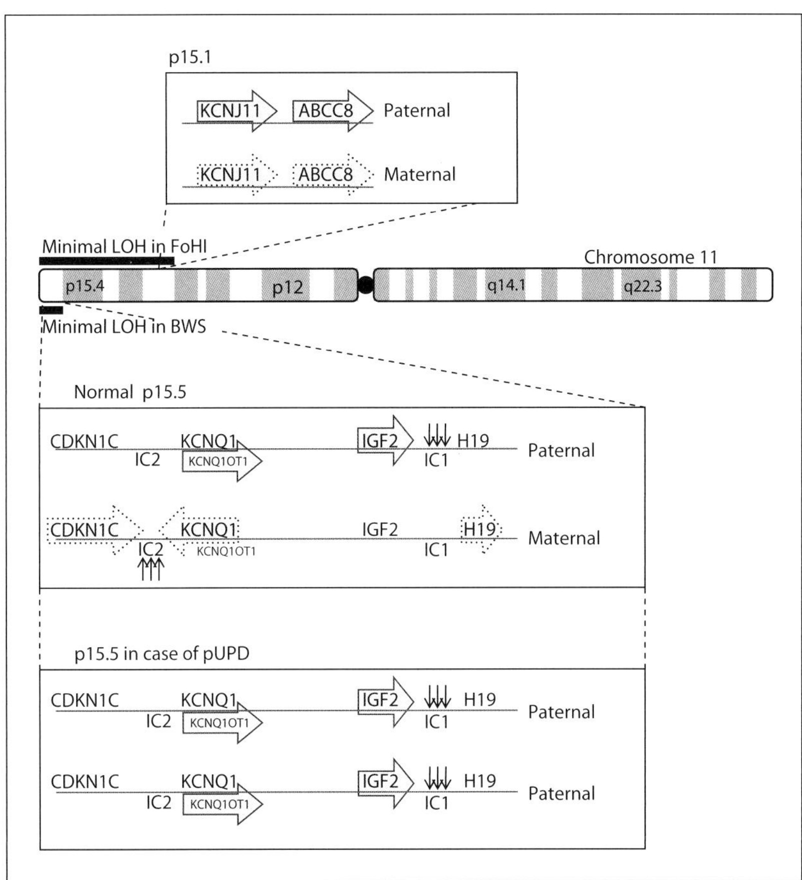

Fig. 1. Diagrammatic representation of the chromosome 11. Relevant genes leading to the clinicopathological features of BWS are gathered in the 11p15.5 region. Only alleles represented in large arrows are expressed. Other alleles are silent. In the 11p15.5 region, genes are subdued to imprinting. The triplet arrows over an imprinting center (IC) indicate its methylation. However, genes in the 11p15.1 *(ABCC8* and *KCNJ11)* are expressed from both alleles. The minimal extent of the maternal LOH (thick black lines) is indicated for BWS and for FoHI.

(2) paternal duplications (trisomy with a double dose of the paternal 11p15 region) resulting from duplications or unbalanced reciprocal translocation involving the 11p15 region. Familial BWS can also be explained by point mutations of the maternal allele of *CDKN1C* leading to a loss or a reduced expression of the active allele. In 85% of cases, BWS is sporadic and results from the following: an epigenetic error of one or more of the 11p15.5 imprinted gene clusters, loss of methylation at the imprinting center 2 (IC2 or KvDMR; 50–60% of cases) on the maternal allele leading to the biallelic expression of KCNQ1OT1 and loss of CDKN1C expression, gain of methylation at the imprinting center 1 (IC1 or H19DMR; 5–10%) on the paternal allele leading to the biallelic expression of IGF2 and loss of H19 expression, or from a mosaic paternal 11p15 isodisomy (pUPD, 20% of cases) [2] leading to the overexpression of

paternally expressed genes (IGF2 and KCNQ1OT1) and loss of maternally expressed genes (H19 and CDKN1C).

Beckwith-Wiedemann Syndrome and Paternal Uniparental Disomy
pUPD appears to be a postzygotic somatic recombination event since BWS patients with 11p15 pUPD always show mosaicism. The extent of the pUPD always spans from the telomere to a variable breakpoint. It always includes the whole 11p15.5 chromosomal region which contains the genes involved in the pathophysiology of BWS (IGF2, H19, CDKN1C). Recently, a SNP-array study performed on 9 patients did not provide any evidence of a recombination hotspot because all patients had different extent of pUPD (in 4 patients the pUPD spanned from 11p15.5 to different breakpoints in 11p11.2; in 1 patient to 11p12; in 2 patients to 11p13; and in 2 other patients pUPD was restricted to the 11p15.5 region alone) [3]. During meiosis, specific hotspots for chromosomal recombination are observed; however, the highly variable location of the breakpoints on the short arm of chromosome 11 in BWS patients does not support the hypothesis of a molecular event occurring during meiosis. Finally, the pUPD may be subsequent to an abnormal recombination between nonsister chromatids during mitosis or by a deletion of a region and the further duplication of its homologous region on the other chromosome. The cause of the loss of the maternal allele is not known. Actually, neither gene mutations nor specific DNA sequences are known to provoke or facilitate the loss of the maternal allele.

Some cases with mosaic pUPD for all of chromosome 11 were also described and the clinical finding did not differ from patients with pUPD restricted to a small part of 11p. Cells with pUPD may have a growth advantage. Some exceptional cases of maternal UPD of the 11p15 region have been reported in patients with Silver-Russel syndrome, consistent with the clinical findings of this syndrome (poor fetal growth, etc.). Thus, pUPD of the 11p15.5 region is expected to destabilize the physiological balance between imprinted genes controlling cell growth, thereby permitting overgrowth and tumor growth. The main genes suspected to explain the pathophysiology of BWS are:

- *IGF2,* a paternally expressed gene which has proliferative and antiapoptotic effects. It is mostly expressed during embryogenesis, then its expression drops [4].
- *H19*, a maternally expressed transregulator of genes involved in fetal growth. This gene is expressed only during fetal development and early postnatal growth in mice. The loss of the H19 active allele in mice leads to a fetal overgrowth and probably deregulates *IGF2* expression. A recent report by Gabory et al. [5], in the mouse model of BWS, showed that, apart from a cis-effect, the H19 noncoding RNA also regulates the expression of IGF2 by a trans-acting mechanism.
- *CDKN1C*, also a maternally expressed tumor suppressor gene. The encoded protein is an inhibitor of G1 cyclin/Cdk complexes and acts as a negative regulator of cell proliferation. Mutations in this gene were reported in BWS and sporadic cancers.

- *KCNQ1OT1*, a paternally expressed gene that is thought to be noncoding. It may act as a chromatin regulatory RNA (gene silencer) and/or a methylation regulator. It may prevent the expression of *CDKN1C* from the paternally inherited allele.

pUPD of 11p is expected to increase *IGF2* and decrease *H19* and *CDKN1C* expression, thus bestowing a growth advantage to islet cell progenitors which proliferate and ultimately give rise to the histological findings observed in FoHI and the pancreas from BWS patients.

Some genotype-phenotype correlations exist with pUPD. A clear association exists between mosaic pUPD and hemihypertrophy, and between organ enlargement and the proportion of cells with pUPD within each organ [2]. In addition, it has been clearly shown that neoplasias and Wilms tumors are more frequent in BWS with pUPD and gain of methylation (i.e. patients with an overexpression of IGF2) than in patients with other molecular defects.

Pancreatic Histology in Beckwith-Wiedemann Syndrome

In the original description by Beckwith [1] in 1969, the pancreas was about 3 times heavier than normal in 2 of the 6 patients. Since then, very little information has been published about pancreatic histology in BWS. The pancreas in BWS is characterized by a florid hyperplasia of ducts, acini, and islets. The pancreatic islets are well organized but abnormally large and have a marked proliferation of beta- and alpha-cells, and a moderate increase of pancreatic polypeptide cells and somatostatin cells [6]. No genotype histology correlation has been published yet. Therefore, it is not known whether the pancreatic histology in BWS is different according to the molecular defect (mosaic pUPD, point mutation in CDKN1C, etc.). Pancreatoblastoma is reported as a rare complication of BWS, and occurs mostly in patients with hemihypertrophy.

Hypoglycemia in Beckwith-Wiedemann Syndrome

In 2000, DeBaun et al. [7] reported a series of 263 patients with a clinical diagnosis of BWS. Among them, 52% presented with hypoglycemia at birth. In another series of patients, hypoglycemia required extra feeds or intravenous glucose, with a glucose infusion rate greater than 10 mg/kg/min to maintain euglycemia [8]. Insulin levels were inappropriate in hypoglycemia, ketone bodies were low, and a glycemic response to glucagon injection was found. Thus, hyperinsulinism explains the hypoglycemia observed in BWS. The hypoglycemia usually resolves within the first few days of life. However, in 20% of the patients, hypoglycemia persisted more than 1 week, even beyond the first month of life in 4% of patients and sometimes for several years [7]. Intellectual disabilities were correlated with the severity of hypoglycemia.

Usually hyperinsulinemic hypoglycemia in BWS is easily treated with diazoxide. However, several cases of diazoxide-unresponsive hyperinsulinism have been described in BWS, with some even resistant to octreotide and requiring surgery. In the report by Hussain et al. [9], the patient was diazoxide- and octreotide-unresponsive, required a glucose infusion rate of 20 mg/kg/day, and finally underwent a pancreatectomy. After surgery, hypoglycemia resolved without any treatment at 14 months of age. However, the relation between BWS and hyperinsulinism was not clear in this case because 11p15 pUPD was found in blood cells, but not in the pancreatic beta-cells.

The mechanism of hyperinsulinism related to BWS is still unclear. Hyperplasia of the beta-cells has been suggested to explain hypoglycemia. This hyperplasia may be due to the overexpression of a growth factor gene *(IGF2)* observed in 20% of patients [10] and/or an imbalance between *IGF2* and tumor suppressor genes *(H19, CDKN1C)* [11]. IGF2 is known to weakly bind the insulin receptor. However, mice models of BWS overexpressing IGF2 display clinical features of BWS except hypoglycemia. Another hypothesis is that the duplication of the region containing the insulin locus (11p15.5) leads to an overexpression of the *INS* gene. However, no evidence of duplication of *INS, HRAS1,* and *IGF2* [12], or overexpression of the *INS* and *IGF2* genes [13], has been found to cause hyperinsulinism in BWS. Thus, it is not known whether the cause of hyperinsulinism in BWS is either the increased mass of the beta-cells, dysregulation of the insulin secretion by the beta-cells, or a combination of these two hypotheses.

The role, level, and influence of paracrine secretions from the other cells types of the hyperplastic pancreatic islets (glucagon, somatostatin) on the beta-cells are not known.

Abnormalities of the Ploidy

We reported 2 cases of unusual BWS associated with mosaic abnormalities of the ploidy [14]. Both cases were suspected to unbalance the 11p15 region and were diazoxide-unresponsive, leading to surgery despite the absence of K_{ATP} channel gene mutations. The histological features of the focal lesions were unusual, and one was suspected of malignancy. A genome-wide loss of the maternal alleles and a paternal isodisomy was found in the lesional pancreas of the first patient, whereas we observed a triploidy with one maternal allele and two distinct or identical paternal alleles within the lesions of the second patient.

Focal Hyperinsulinism

When hyperinsulinism is resistant to all available treatments (diazoxide, octreotide, and diet), surgery is required to avoid recurrent severe hypoglycemia and a risk of subsequent neurological disabilities. In the mid-1980s, pathologists studied very severe patients who were surprisingly cured after a hemipancreatectomy. Surprisingly, the histological analysis of the pancreas was normal. A careful second look, using anti-insulin antibodies, revealed a small focal endocrine 'tumor-like' lesion which showed evidence of beta-cell proliferation. By contrast, other hyperinsulinism patients, now classified as diffuse hyperinsulinism (DiHI), had in their pancreatic islets a normal number of beta-cells, which exposed signs of hyperactivity. Thus, the two distinct types of pancreatic beta-cell involvement, focal and diffuse, were described for the first time [1, 15].

In 1997, we found a striking similarity between beta-cell proliferation in FoHI and what was observed in the pancreas of BWS patients [16]. This observation led us to investigate whether the genes in the 11p15.5 region (especially the proliferation and tumor suppressor genes) were involved in FoHI.

The focal adenomatous hyperplasia of the pancreatic islets in FoHI does not suggest a tumor since it does not invade or push at the margins and has no pseudocapsule. It is more likely that it suggests an abnormal developmental process because an organoid pattern remains and other endocrine cells are present within the foci (positive immunohistochemistry with antisomatostatin antibodies). Finally, this hyperplastic lesion is restricted to a small portion of the pancreas and is surrounded by normal tissue, suggesting a clonal process. The common histological features between BWS and FoHI led to the search for a common mechanism.

Loss of the Maternal Allele from the 11p15 Chromosomal Region

A variable loss of maternal chromosomal material was detected at the expense of the short arm of chromosome 11 [16]. Microsatellite studies of other chromosomes were normal, confirming the exclusive involvement of chromosome 11 in FoHI. This loss of heterozygosity (LOH) was not found in the surrounding normal pancreas, but was restricted to the pancreatic focal lesion, consistent with a proliferative monoclonal lesion. Moreover, the maternal 11p LOH was not found in islets cells from DiHI [16].

The studies by our team (10 patients) [16] and by Suchi et al. (11 patients) [17] using microsatellite markers showed a constant loss of the maternal alleles in the 11p15.1 region, which contains the *ABCC8* and *KCNJ11* genes. Some evidence from hyperinsulinism as well as from BWS led to the hypothesis of a unique (but variable in its location) breakpoint on the short arm of chromosome 11 leading to the loss of the telomeric extremity. The extent of this LOH is variable, but involves: *constantly* (1) subtelomeric microsatellites (e.g. D11S922 in 11pter), (2) the 11p15.5 region (e.g. D11S1758, D11S569) where the genes involved in BWS are located and that contains imprinted domains, and (3) the 11p15.1 region which contains the nonimprinted *ABCC8* and *KCNJ11* genes (e.g. D11S902, D11S921); and *variably* a seemingly random extent toward the centromere. The loss of the maternal allele was observed almost constantly in the 11p14 region and, in 3 out of 10 patients on the long arm of the 11 chromosome (e.g. D11S1365 in 11q14.1). In these 3 patients, the LOH involved almost two thirds of the whole maternal chromosome.

As a consequence, the expression of maternal genes appears decreased or absent as shown by the loss of $p57^{kip2}$ expression demonstrated by immunohistochemistry [17]. This protein is encoded by the imprinted and maternally expressed *CDKN1C* gene from the 11p15.5 region. Using $p57^{kip2}$ antibody, Suchi et al. [17] showed a moderate labeling of normal tissues, whereas 48 out of 56 FoHI exposed a clear loss of the

$p57^{kip2}$ expression in the endocrine cells of the foci. Moreover, the expression of the imprinted and maternally expressed *H19* gene was also assessed by RT-PCR in five FoHI and was found decreased within the lesion compared to the result obtained from the adjacent normal pancreas [11].

Paternal Unidisomy
At this stage, it was not clear whether FoHI resulted from an isolated deletion of a variable fragment of chromosome 11, or whether there was also a compensatory duplication of the paternal chromosome resulting in UPD as observed in BWS.

Damaj et al. [18] showed pUPD in four FoHI in immunohistochemistry and microsatellite analysis. Beta-cells were detected by using anti-insulin fluorescent antibodies: (1) beta-cells from the focus and in the normal pancreas were diploid as a FISH analysis of the 11q telomeres found two copies of this region in each nucleus; (2) within the focus, FISH analysis with a probe spanning the *ABCC8* gene and a second probe spanning the *CDKN1C* gene showed two copies of the *ABCC8* and of the *CDKN1C* genes in each nucleus; and (3) the study of microsatellites markers located in 11p15.5, in 11p15.1, and within the *ABCC8* gene showed the absence of the maternal allele in the beta-cells from the focus, whereas it is present in the normal pancreas. No other allele but the paternally inherited one was noticed within the focus. A further study by quantitative PCR of microsatellite markers from the 11p15.5 region [11] confirmed that the maternal allele was absent and that the quantity of the paternal allele was double. Thus, it was clear that the two copies of the *ABCC8* and *CDKN1C* genes detected by FISH analysis were from the paternally inherited allele, whereas the maternal allele was lacking, which correspond to the definition of pUPD.

Unbalanced Expression of 11p15-Imprinted Genes
In 2001, in a series of five cases of FoHI [11], the expression of imprinted genes from the 11p15.5 region was assessed by determining the mRNA concentrations in normal pancreas and in the hyperplastic FoHI. The paternally expressed *IGF2* gene was not found overexpressed, but there was a clear decrease in the expression of the maternally expressed *H19* gene within the hyperplastic focus compared to the level of expression in the normal pancreas. Moreover, as seen earlier, the drop in the expression of the maternally expressed *CDKN1C* gene was also shown by using $p57^{kip2}$ antibodies, as this staining was negative in FoHI [17].

Mutations in the ATP-Sensitive Potassium Channel Genes
As seen earlier, the minimal region of LOH in FoHI encompasses the 11p15.1 region which bears the *ABCC8* and *KCNJ11* genes, both known to be responsible for diazoxide-unresponsive hyperinsulinism [19]. Moreover, in 1996, the K^{+}_{ATP} channel activity was shown to be not only deficient in DiHI, but also in FoHI, suggesting a mechanism involving the K_{ATP} channel genes [20].

In the white blood cells and the normal pancreas of the patients, one mutation in either of these two genes was found. This mutation was inherited from the father. In 1998, with PCR single-strand conformation polymorphism, the signal of the paternally inherited mutated allele was found clearly enhanced when performed on beta-cells from FoHI compared to results on normal adjacent pancreas. Moreover, the normal and maternally inherited allele was absent in the FoHI, consistent with the LOH [21]. These results were confirmed by a large series of 56 patients with FoHI [17]. Eight of these patients had no identifiable mutation in either the K_{ATP} genes (but data on MLPA analysis to screen for deletion were lacking), while in the recent series of Bellanné-Chantelot et al. [22] in 2010, all patients with FoHI had one mutation in either of the K_{ATP} genes. Thus, pUDP unmasked a heterozygous paternal mutation leading to a somatic recessive disorder within the focus.

Knudson's 'Two Hit' Mechanism

The LOH may be regarded as the 'second hit' according to Knudson's model based on the paradigm of retinoblastoma [19], whereas the germ-line inherited mutation may be regarded as the 'first hit'. Unlike mutations of genes involved in cell growth or DNA repair, the germ-line K_{ATP} gene mutation is not expected to trigger the 'second hit' [21]. Though FoHI is more likely to be sporadic, a recurrence of FoHI among siblings had already been reported (fig. 2) [23].

Focal Hyperinsulinism: An Abnormal Developmental Process

pUPD in FoHI is similar to that observed in BWS, which explains the common hyperplastic aspect of the pancreatic islets cells in both conditions; however, (1) pUPD is restricted to the beta-cells of the focal lesion (the potential involvement of the other cell types of the focal form is not known) and (2) the minimal extent of pUPD in FoHI is larger, as it always encompass the 11p15.1 region, while the larger extent is probably the same (the whole chromosome 11).

FoHI may be considered as a very restricted BWS because the mosaic 11p chromosome pUPD involves only some pancreatic endocrine cells. Thus, the cause of the hyperinsulinemic hypoglycemia appears double in FoHI since: (1) BWS is known to cause hyperinsulinism and (2) pUPD reduces a paternally inherited mutation of a K_{ATP} gene to homozygoty, besides explaining the diazoxide-unresponsiveness of FoHI [24].

The unbalanced expression of the 11p15.5 genes secondary to pUPD explains the histological aspect. Indeed, *IGF2* is differentially regulated in normal tissues: the paternal allele is transiently expressed during embryogenesis and its expression decreases after birth [4]. Therefore, the somatic event (pUPD) probably occurred during the early stage of organogenesis. This may explain (1) the normal *IGF2* expression in the hyperplastic beta-cells from the focus of operated children, and (2) the histological pattern of the FoHI which exposes a clear increased number of beta-cells without

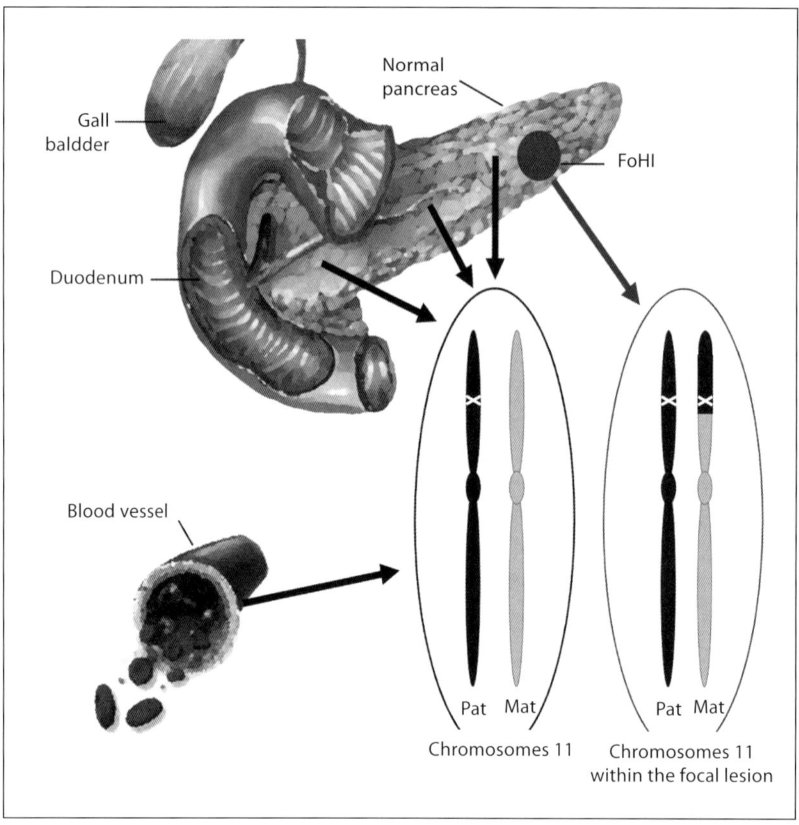

Fig. 2. Two hits' mechanism in focal form of hyperinsulinism: the paternally inherited chromosome 11 is colored in black and the maternally inherited chromosome in gray. In patients with a FoHI, the paternally inherited mutation (white cross) in the *ABCC8* or *KCNJ11* gene is present in all the cells. Thus, molecular analysis performed on a blood sample will find one mutation inherited from the patient's father. However, within the focal pancreatic lesion, this heterozygous mutation is reduced to homozygoty because the loss of the maternal 11p15 region is compensated by an isodisomy of the paternal allele.

any sign of malignancy, consistent with an abnormal developmental process during embryogenesis.

Cases of Multifocal Hyperinsulinism

Patients with FoHI usually have one single and small-sized (2–5 mm in diameter) pancreatic lesion. The area of abnormal pancreatic development can also be multilobular and can have satellites in the nearby pancreas that necessitates intraoperative margin analysis to ensure complete excision and avoid recurrence. However, some patients may have unusual focal lesions, i.e. multifocal lesions (two focal lesions or more within the same pancreas) and/or a large or very large focal lesion which may involve a large portion of the pancreas.

All patients with bifocal hyperinsulinism had symptomatic and severe hypoglycemia since birth. In a series of 2 patients with bifocal hyperinsulinism and 1 patient with a very large focal form, one single and paternally inherited mutation of the ABCC8 gene was found [24]. The deletion breakpoints were determined by using microsatellite markers as described above. It appeared that the breakpoint was different in each focal lesion. On the other hand, the study of the giant focal form found the same breakpoint in distinct tissue samples. In both patients with bifocal hyperinsulinism, the foci were close to each other. In the first patient, one focus was in the lower part of the head of the pancreas and the second focus was in the anterior wall of the duodenum, 15 mm from the head of the pancreas. In the second patient, the first focus was in the anterior portion of the isthmus of the pancreas and the second focus was behind the portal vein, outside of the pancreas. In both cases, pancreatic venous sampling localized only one focus at a time.

Multifocal and ectopic FoHI [25, 26] were also reported, with a focus in the pancreas and another focus in ectopic pancreatic tissues of various localizations (jejunum and abdominal cavity) which were diagnosed on PET-scan imaging. However, no further investigation was performed to determine whether all the foci of this patient shared the same chromosomal breakpoint.

There are still two hypotheses: the second lesion may be a satellite from the first one, or it may be a second and independent FoHI in the same patient. No risk or triggering factor has been discovered yet for the LOH, but one may exist as there are preferential chromosomal sites for UPD (BWS and Silver-Russel syndrome: 11p15.5 chromosome; Prader-Willi syndrome: 15q chromosome; etc.).

Familial Recurrent Focal Hyperinsulinism and Genetic Counseling

The LOH is a rare sporadic event, as suggested by discordant identical twins, the absence of hyperinsulinism in the patients' fathers, and the negligible risk of recurrence of focal form among siblings. The latter was reported only once and the location of the focal lesions was different in both siblings (isthmus and head of pancreas) [23]. The physiological cause of the 11p15 instability, giving a risk for LOH, is not known. There is no genetic or environmental factor known to increase the risk of LOH.

The frequency of hyperinsulinism in out-bred communities is about 1/40,000 to 1/50,000 births. This equates to about 1/90,000 FoHI and 1/90,000 DiHI. Since the carrier frequency of K_{ATP} channel gene mutation is close to 1/150, the risk (R_{UPD}) for pUPD to occur in a pancreatic endocrine cell during embryogenesis is also around 1/300 ($1/2 \times 1/150 \times R_{UPD} = 1/90,000$). In case of a newborn with a diagnosed FoHI: (1) its siblings bear a risk of $1/2 \times 1/300 = 1/600$ of also having a FoHi (risk of receiving the mutated allele from its father: 1/2; risk of developing a pUPD in the beta-cells: 1/300), (2) the risk for itself to bear a second and independent focus is 1/300 (it already bears the paternally inherited K_{ATP} gene mutation, so risk = 1/1, and risk to develop pUPD = 1/300).

Only one family has been reported with the coexistence of both focal and diffuse neonatal hyperinsulinism in siblings [27]. The first child carried a paternally inherited *ABCC8* mutation associated with a LOH for the maternal wild-type chromosome in the lesion. The focal form was proven by the concomitant positive proinsulin staining in the beta-cells from the focus and the absence of expression of the $p57^{KIP2}$ protein in the same cells. Despite a reassuring genetic counseling, the parents' next pregnancy resulted in the birth of a child with severe hypoglycemia. The same *ABCC8* gene mutation as its sibling was found in the peripheral blood, but homozygous. He underwent subtotal pancreatectomy, with histology showing the typical findings of DiHI. The genetic testing of the parents found they were heterozygous for the same *ABCC8* gene mutation and it appeared they were inbred.

Focal Hyperinsulinism and Risk of Pancreatic Tumor
Patients with BWS caused by a pUPD are at risk for Wilms tumor, hepatoblastoma, pancreatoblastoma, and are generally more at risk of developing tumors than in the other genetic or epigenetic abnormalities causing BWS. An 11p15.5 pUPD has already been reported in isolated tumors, including Wilms tumors. Thus, as FoHI are caused by pUPD of this critical region, one can hypothesize that it likely leads to a higher risk for insulinoma.

Conclusion

The concept of FoHI is extremely important, as it accounts for about half of the patients with severe diazoxide-unresponsive hyperinsulinism who are candidates for a definitive cure after a limited pancreatic resection, with no risk to develop diabetes mellitus. The 11p15 chromosomal region is an unstable area both cytogenetically and epigenetically. The discovery of its involvement in hyperinsulinism has led to a better understanding of the pathological pattern of the focal lesions.

References

1 Beckwith JB: Macroglossia, omphalocele, adrenal cytomegay, gigantism, and hyperplastic visceromegaly. Birth Defects Original Articles 1969;5: 188–196.

2 Itoh N, Becroft DM, Reeve AE, Morison IM: Proportion of cells with paternal 11p15 uniparental disomy correlates with organ enlargement in Wiedemann-Beckwith syndrome. Am J Med Genet 2000;92:111–116.

3 Romanelli V, Meneses HN, Fernández L, Martínez-Glez V, Gracia-Bouthelier R, F Fraga M, Guillén E, Nevado J, Gean E, Martorell L, Marfil VE, García-Miñaur S, Lapunzina P: Beckwith-Wiedemann syndrome and uniparental disomy 11p: fine mapping of the recombination breakpoints and evaluation of several techniques. Eur J Hum Genet 2011; 19:416–421.

4 Randhawa R, Cohen P: The role of the insulin-like growth factor system in prenatal growth. Mol Genet Metab 2005;86:84–90.

5 Gabory A, Ripoche MA, Le Digarcher A, Watrin F, Ziyyat A, Forné T, Jammes H, Ainscough JF, Surani MA, Journot L, Dandolo L: H19 acts as a trans regulator of the imprinted gene network controlling growth in mice. Development 2009;136:3413–3421.
6 Stefan Y, Bordi C, Grasso S, Orci L: Beckwith-Wiedemann syndrome: a quantitative, immunohistochemical study of pancreatic islet cell populations. Diabetologia 1985;28:914–919.
7 DeBaun MR, King AA, White N: Hypoglycemia in Beckwith-Wiedemann syndrome. Semin Perinatol 2000;24:164–171.
8 Chitayat D, Friedman JM, Dimmick JE: Neuroblastoma in a child with Wiedemann-Beckwith syndrome. Am J Med Genet 1990;35:433–436.
9 Hussain K, Cosgrove KE, Shepherd RM, Luharia A, Smith VV, Kassem S, Gregory JW, Sivaprasadarao A, Christesen HT, Jacobsen BB, Brusgaard K, Glaser B, Maher EA, Lindley KJ, Hindmarsh P, Dattani M, Dunne MJ: Hyperinsulinemic hypoglycemia in Beckwith-Wiedemann syndrome due to defects in the function of pancreatic beta-cell adenosine triphosphate-sensitive potassium channels. J Clin Endocrinol Metab 2005;90:4376–4382.
10 Slavotinek A, Gaunt L, Donnai D: Paternally inherited duplications of 11p15.5 and Beckwith-Wiedemann syndrome. J Med Genet 1997;34: 819–826.
11 Fournet JC, Mayaud C, de Lonlay P, Gross-Morand MS, Verkarre V, Castanet M, Devillers M, Rahier J, Brunelle F, Robert JJ, Nihoul-Fékété C, Saudubray JM, Junien C: Unbalanced expression of 11p15 imprinted genes in focal forms of congenital hyperinsulinism: association with a reduction to homozygosity of a mutation in ABCC8 or KCNJ11. Am J Pathol 2001;158:2177–2184
12 Henry I, Jeanpierre M, Barichard F, Serre JL, Mallet J, Turleau C, de Grouchy J, Junien C: Duplication of HRAS1, INS, and IGF2 is not a common event in Beckwith-Wiedemann syndrome. Ann Genet 1988; 31:216–220.
13 Spritz RA, Mager D, Pauli RM, Laxova R: Normal dosage of the insulin and insulin-like growth factor II genes in patients with the Beckwith-Wiedemann syndrome. Am J Hum Genet 1986;39: 265–273.
14 Giurgea I, Sanlaville D, Fournet JC, Sempoux C, Bellanné-Chantelot C, Touati G, Hubert L, Groos MS, Brunelle F, Rahier J, Henquin JC, Dunne MJ, Jaubert F, Robert JJ, Nihoul-Fékété C, Vekemans M, Junien C, de Lonlay P: Congenital hyperinsulinism and mosaic abnormalities of the ploidy. J Med Genet 2006;43:248–254.
15 Rahier J, Guiot Y, Sempoux C: Morphologic analysis of focal and diffuse forms of congenital hyperinsulinism. Semin Pediatr Surg 2011;20:3–12.
16 de Lonlay P, Fournet JC, Rahier J, Gross-Morand MS, Poggi-Travert F, Foussier V, Bonnefont JP, Brusset MC, Brunelle F, Robert JJ, Nihoul-Fékété C, Saudubray JM, Junien C: Somatic deletion of the imprinted 11p15 region in sporadic persistent hyperinsulinemic hypoglycemia of infancy is specific of focal adenomatous hyperplasia and endorses partial pancreatectomy. J Clin Invest 1997;100: 802–807.
17 Suchi M, MacMullen CM, Thornton PS, Adzick NS, Ganguly A, Ruchelli ED, Stanley CA: Molecular and immunohistochemical analyses of the focal form of congenital hyperinsulinism. Mod Pathol 2006;19: 122–129
18 Damaj L, le Lorch M, Verkarre V, Werl C, Hubert L, Nihoul-Fékété C, Aigrain Y, de Keyzer Y, Romana SP, Ballanné-Chantelot C, de Lonlay P, Jaubert F: Chromosome 11p15 paternal isodisomy in focal forms of neonatal hyperinsulinism. Clin Endocrinol Metab 2008;93: 4941–4947.
19 Knudson AG Jr: Genetic predisposition to cancer. Cancer Detect Prev 1984;7:1–8.
20 Kane C, Shepherd RM, Squires PE, Johnson PR, James RF, Milla PJ, Aynsley-Green A, Lindley KJ, Dunne MJ: Loss of functional KATP channels in pancreatic beta-cells causes persistent hyperinsulinemic hypoglycemia of infancy. Nat Med 1996;2: 1344–1347.
21 Verkarre V, Fournet JC, de Lonlay P, Gross-Morand MS, Devillers M, Rahier J, Brunelle F, Robert JJ, Nihoul-Fékété C, Saudubray JM, Junien C: Paternal mutation of the sulfonylurea receptor (ABCC8) gene and maternal loss of 11p15 imprinted genes lead to persistent hyperinsulinism in focal adenomatous hyperplasia. J Clin Invest 1998;102: 1286–1291.
22 Bellanné-Chantelot C, Saint-Martin C, Ribeiro MJ, Vaury C, Verkarre V, Arnoux JB, Valayannopoulos V, Gobrecht S, Sempoux C, Rahier J, Fournet JC, Jaubert F, Aigrain Y, Nihoul-Fékété C, de Lonlay P: ABCC8 and KCNJ11 molecular spectrum of 109 patients with diazoxide-unresponsive congenital hyperinsulinism. J Med Genet 2010;47:752–759.
23 Ismail D, Smith VV, de Lonlay P, Ribeiro MJ, Rahier J, Blankenstein O, Flanagan SE, Bellanné-Chantelot C, Verkarre V, Aigrain Y, Pierro A, Ellard S, Hussain K: Familial focal congenital hyperinsulinism. J Clin Endocrinol Metab 2011;96:24–28.
24 Giurgea I, Sempoux C, Bellanné-Chantelot C, Ribeiro M, Hubert L, Boddaert N, Saudubray JM, Robert JJ, Brunelle F, Rahier J, Jaubert F, Nihoul-Fékété C, de Lonlay P: The Knudson's two-hit model and timing of somatic mutation may account for the phenotypic diversity of focal congenital hyperinsulinism. J Clin Endocrinol Metab 2006;91: 4118–4123.

25 Hussain K, Seppänen M, Näntö-Salonen K, Adzick NS, Stanley CA, Thornton P, Minn H: The diagnosis of ectopic focal hyperinsulinism of infancy with [18F]-dopa positron emission tomography. J Clin Endocrinol Metab 2006;91:2839–2842.
26 Peranteau WH, Bathaii SM, Pawel B, Hardy O, Alavi A, Stanley CA, Adzick NS: Multiple ectopic lesions of focal islet adenomatosis identified by positron emission tomography scan in an infant with congenital hyperinsulinism. J Pediatr Surg 2007;42:188–192.
27 Valayannopoulos V, Vaxillaire M, Aigrain Y, Jaubert F, Bellanné-Chantelot C, Ribeiro MJ, Brunelle F, Froguel P, Robert JJ, Polak M, Nihoul-Fékété C, de Lonlay P: Coexistence in the same family of both focal and diffuse forms of hyperinsulinism. Diabetes Care 2007;30:1590–1592.

Pascale de Lonlay, MD, PhD
Centre de Référence des Maladies Héréditaires du Métabolisme de l'Enfant et l'Adulte
Hôpital Necker-Enfants Malades, AP-HP
Université Paris Descartes
149 rue de Sèvres
FR–75015 Paris (France)
Tel. +33 1 44 49 48 52, E-Mail pascale.delonlay@nck.aphp.fr

Stanley CA, De León DD (eds): Monogenic Hyperinsulinemic Hypoglycemia Disorders.
Front Diabetes. Basel, Karger, 2012, vol 21, pp 57–70

Pancreatic Histopathology of Hyperinsulinism

Mariko Suchi[a,b] · Tricia R. Bhatti[c] · Eduardo D. Ruchelli[c,d]

[a]Department of Pathology, Medical College of Wisconsin, [b]Department of Pathology and Laboratory Medicine, Children's Hospital of Wisconsin, Milwaukee, Wisc., [c]Department of Pathology and Laboratory Medicine, The Children's Hospital of Philadelphia, and [d]Department of Pathology and Laboratory Medicine, University of Pennsylvania School of Medicine, Philadelphia, Pa., USA

Abstract

Several genetic abnormalities are known to cause hyperinsulinism. The formerly held concept that congenital hyperinsulinism results from abnormal pancreatic development, termed 'nesidioblastosis', is no longer accepted. The pathology of pancreases resected from individuals with inactivating mutations in the ATP-sensitive potassium channel is best studied and classified into diffuse and focal forms with their respective genetic alterations. A few variations within this group have been observed. The knowledge of the different histologic features aids surgical management by intraoperative frozen section evaluation along with preoperative imaging studies. Surgical intervention is less frequently applied to patients with other genetic abnormalities, including glucokinase and glutamate dehydrogenase abnormalities; therefore, systematic analyses are sparse. The pancreases of various genetic forms of hyperinsulinism may show different histologies from one another. Published reports along with our experience on this topic are summarized. Histology of the developing pancreas in young infants differs from that of normal adult pancreas. These features are the source of confusion in the earlier observations. Careful examination of the resected pancreases considering the age of the patients is necessary to describe and categorize the morphologic features, as well as and identify unrecognized patterns.

The genetic etiology of hyperinsulinism is manifold as discussed in the previous and following chapters. Clinical manifestation and symptom severity are also heterogeneous, ranging from severe hyperinsulinism presenting in the neonatal period to milder and medically manageable hyperinsulinism presenting later in life. Pancreatic pathology in cases with hyperinsulinism has been studied by examining the resection specimens from medically unmanageable individuals who undergo a partial or total pancreatectomy (table 1). Inactivating mutations in the ATP-sensitive potassium (K_{ATP}) channel comprise the vast majority of patients who require a pancreatectomy

Table 1. Findings in pancreas resected from children with hyperinsulinism at The Children's Hospital of Philadelphia (1983–2010, n = 321)

Histology of pancreas	Percentage of children affected
Diffuse endocrine abnormality (large nuclei in islets)	45.5
Adenomatosis/adenomatous hyperplasia (focal, multifocal, or generalized)	46.5
Adenoma (insulinoma)	1.6
Normal	2.8
Equivocal/difficult to classify	3.7

All known and unknown underlying genetic abnormalities inclusive.

for control of blood glucose levels, and it is in this group that the pathology is best described and categorized. Pancreases are only occasionally resected from individuals with other genetic diseases, such as abnormalities in glucokinase, glutamate dehydrogenase, and short-chain 3-hydroxylacyl-CoA dehydrogenase. Of note, approximately 5% of individuals with Beckwith-Wiedemann syndrome have hyperinsulinism that extends beyond the neonatal period, and rarely requires a partial pancreatectomy. This chapter describes the pancreatic histomorphology of each of the diseases mentioned above.

Hyperinsulinism with Beta-Cell ATP-Sensitive Potassium Channel Abnormalities

Three genetic mechanisms result in the loss of function of the K_{ATP} channel and cause hyperinsulinism. They are biallelic recessive mutations, paternally inherited mutations with somatic loss of maternal 11p15, and dominant mutations in the genes encoding the high-affinity sulfonylurea receptor 1 *(ABCC8*, formerly *SUR1)* and its regulated iron pore, potassium inward rectifier 6.2 *(KCNJ11*, formerly *Kir6.2)*.

Hyperinsulinism Caused by Biallelic Recessive ATP-Sensitive Potassium Channel Mutations Associated with Diffuse Histologic Abnormality (Diffuse Hyperinsulinism)

Diffuse hyperinsulinism is one of the most common forms of hyperinsulinism (table 1). The pathophysiology is discussed in the chapter by De León and Stanley [pp. 79–86]. The pancreatic histology is characterized by the presence of abnormally large islet cell nuclei that are distributed throughout the pancreas (fig. 1). The mean total endocrine area and volume density of beta-cells are not increased [1, 2]. The frequency of large islet cell nuclei varies from case to case. A large nucleus is empirically defined as a nucleus four times that of the nearby acinar cells [3] or a nucleus occupying an area more than three times larger than the

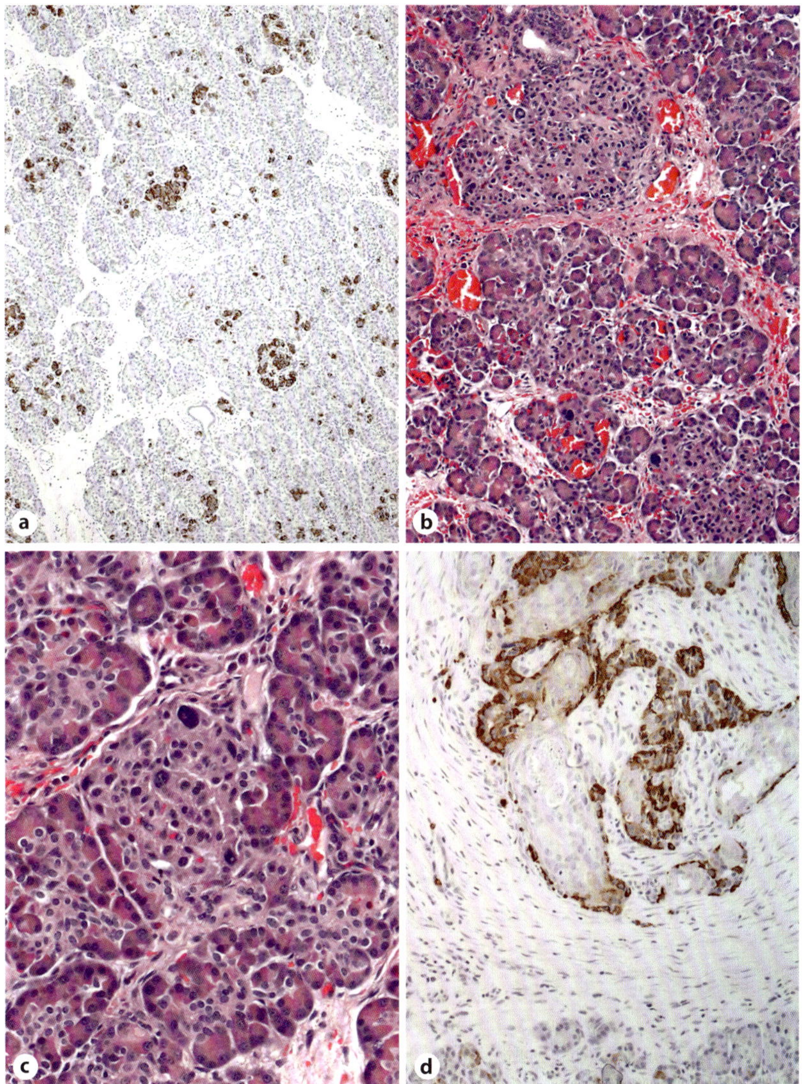

Fig. 1. K_{ATP} channel hyperinsulinism, diffuse form. **a** Quantity of endocrine component is not significantly different from pancreas of normoglycemic individuals of similar age (2 months; immunohistochemistry for insulin; original magnification ×50). **b** On a low-to-medium power field, a few large and hyperchromatic endocrine cell nuclei can be spotted (hematoxylin and eosin stain, original magnification ×200). **c** Enlarged islet cell nuclei are defined as those occupying an area at least three times larger than the neighboring endocrine nuclei, for diagnostic purposes (hematoxylin and eosin stain, original magnification ×400). **d** Ductuloinsular aggregates may be present in some cases, but they are seen too seldom to use as a diagnostic criterion (immunohistochemistry for chromogranin A, original magnification ×200). Reprinted with permission from Wolters Kluwer/Lippincott Williams and Wilkins [27, p 768].

surrounding islet cell nuclei [4]. Cytologic changes include crescent-shaped or ovoid nuclei with occasional nuclear pseudoinclusions (intranuclear cytoplasmic invagination). Morphometric analysis revealed that the mean nuclear radius of the 50 largest endocrine cell nuclei of diffuse hyperinsulinism is significantly larger than that of islet cell nuclei that are outside the adenomatous (focal) lesions in focal hyperinsulinism (described below) [2]. Ductuloinsular complexes composed of endocrine cells in the epithelium of the ducts and in connection with the endocrine cell clusters may be present (fig. 1). This feature, however, is also present in the normal developing pancreas of the neonates and is not specific for the hyperinsulinism pancreas.

Beta-cell proliferation rates as measured by the percentage of Ki-67-positive cells were not statistically higher as compared to a control group composed of age-matched autopsy materials or donated organs in one study [5], but was increased in another study [6]. In normal control pancreas, the frequency of apoptotic beta-cells identified by the terminal deoxynucleotidyl transferase-mediated dUTP-X 3′ nick-end labeling technique increases in the perinatal period (between 2 months before birth to 2 months of age). Kassem et al. [6] reported that the apoptotic rate of beta-cells in diffuse hyperinsulinism individuals older than 3 months is higher than in the control group. A similar increase in beta-cell apoptosis was observed in the adenomatous foci of the focal lesions. Although not proven on available tissue materials, the authors propose that the net rate of apoptosis may be greater than that of proliferation, thus explaining a slow decrease in the severity of hyperinsulinism over the years in patients with K_{ATP} channel hyperinsulinism who are managed medically.

To reiterate the variable frequency of large nuclei among cases, it is important to note that not all islets contain abnormal nuclei and the number of islets with characteristic nuclei may be small. We have recently observed 7 cases that may be a subset of diffuse hyperinsulinism, but are clinically and potentially genetically distinct. In these cases, although there are large islet cell nuclei in the pancreas, the islets with nuclear enlargement are confined to a region of the pancreas and not distributed throughout the pancreas. The postoperative course was significantly different from that of diffuse hyperinsulinism in that all were endocrinologically controlled or cured. In addition, no mutations have been identified in the *ABCC8* or *KCNJ11* genes. A proposal has been made to designate this pattern as 'localized islet cell nuclear enlargement' (LINE) [7]. Further studies, including laser capture microdissection of the abnormal islet cell nuclei, may be helpful to define the genetic basis of this condition.

Hyperinsulinism Caused by Paternally Inherited ATP-Sensitive Potassium Channel Mutations together with Somatic Loss of Maternal 11p15 Associated with Focal Histologic Abnormality (Focal Hyperinsulinism)

This histologically distinct form of hyperinsulinism results from a paternally inherited mutation in the channel genes *(ABCC8* and *KCNJ11)* together with a sporadic somatic loss of the maternal 11p15 which contains imprinted genes involved in cell

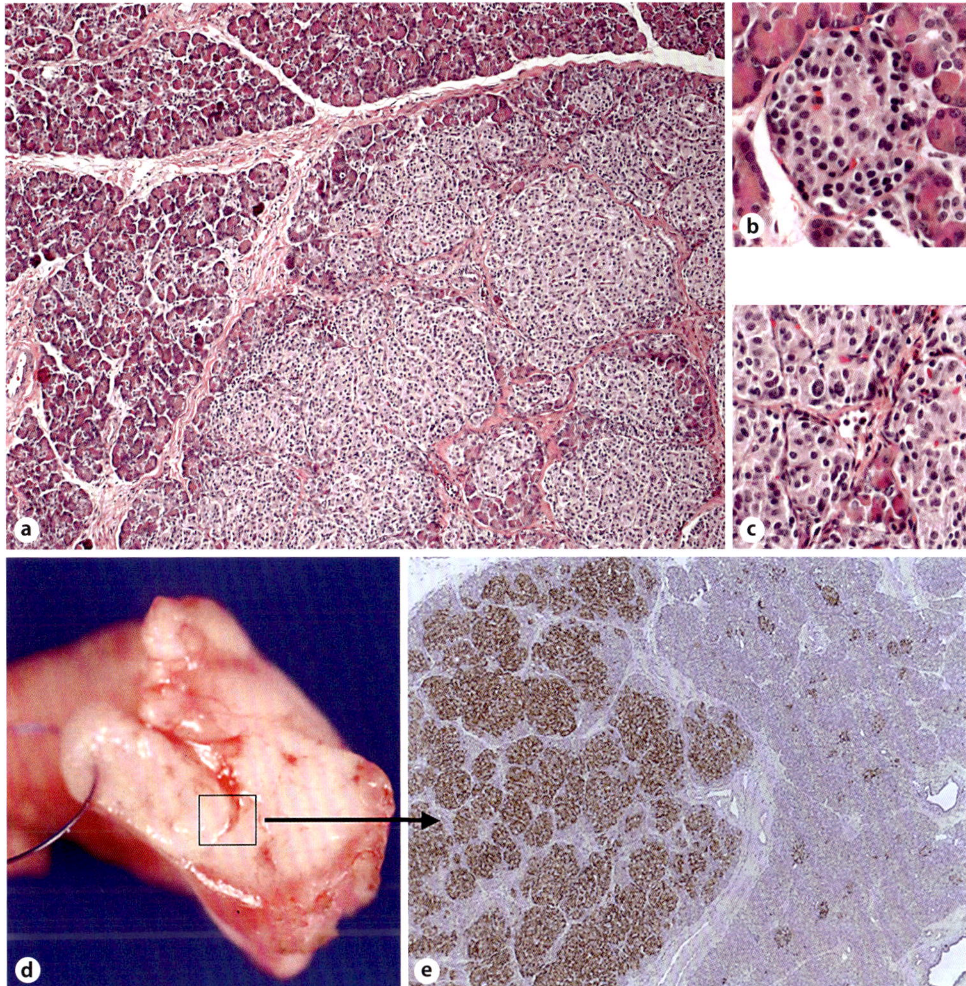

Fig. 2. K_{ATP} channel hyperinsulinism with loss of maternal 11p15 (focal form). **a** Much of the lobule in the right lower half is occupied by endocrine tissue (adenomatosis; hematoxylin and eosin stain, original magnification ×200). **b** Islets outside the adenomatous lesion contain nuclei of normal size. **c** There may be large endocrine cell nuclei within the adenomatosis (**b**, **c** hematoxylin and eosin stain, original magnification ×400). **d** The adenomatous lesion is difficult to distinguish from the neighboring pancreas grossly. **e** Immunohistochemistry confirms the abundance (>40%) of endocrine elements within the lobules (immunohistochemistry for chromogranin A, original magnification ×200). **a–c** Reprinted with permission from Wolters Kluwer/Lippincott Williams and Wilkins [27, p 769]. **d, e** Reprinted with permission from Elsevier [28].

proliferation (see Arnoux et al. [this vol., pp. 43–56]). This form was once thought to comprise a minority of hyperinsulinism. However, it is in fact equally as common as diffuse hyperinsulinism (table 1). Pancreatic histology is characterized by a lesion formed by the confluence of hyperplastic islets occupying more than 40% of the cross-sectional area of pancreatic lobules (fig. 2). All endocrine cell types

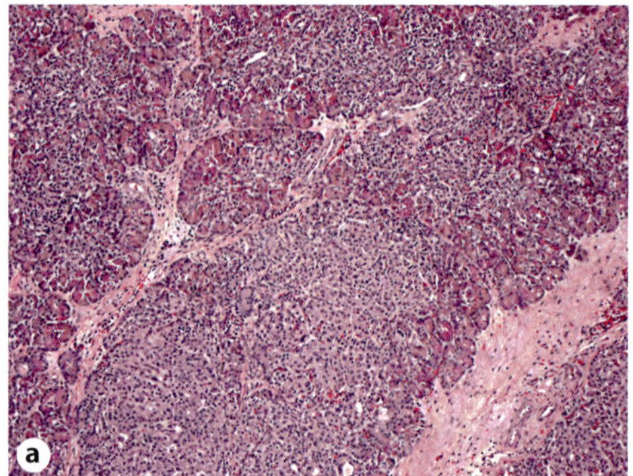

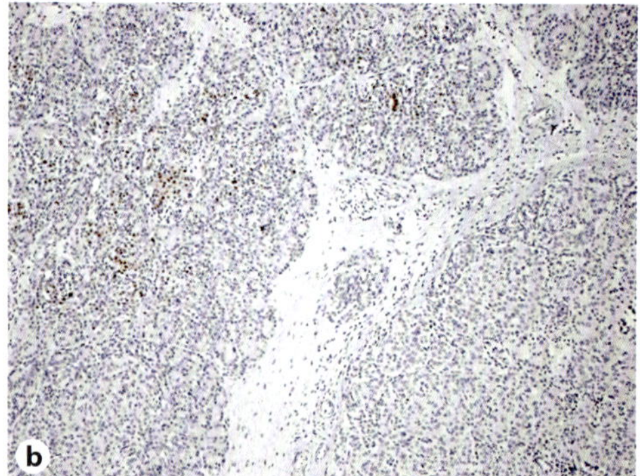

Fig. 3. K_{ATP} channel hyperinsulinism with loss of maternal 11p15 and focal histologic abnormality (focal hyperinsulinism). **a** Endocrine cells occupy more than 40% of lobules in a focus of adenomatous hyperplasia (adenomatosis) in the right lower half of the field (hematoxylin and eosin stain, original magnification ×200). **b** Endocrine cell nuclei within the focus of adenomatosis are negative for $p57^{kip2}$, while islet cell nuclei in the normal area (upper left corner) are positively labeled. A small number of duct epithelial cells and acinar cells also show nuclear labeling (immunohistochemistry for $p57^{kip2}$, original magnification ×200). Reprinted with permission from Wolters Kluwer/Lippincott Williams and Wilkins [27, www.stocker-pediatricpathology3.com].

(alpha-cell, beta-cell, and delta-cell) are represented within the overgrowth in relatively normal proportions. Distribution of hormone-producing cells within the endocrine proliferation recapitulates normal islet organization, best seen by the peripheral arrangement of alpha-cells [1]. The lesion appears to push the exocrine elements aside, but at the same time haphazardly incorporates them. These lesions are also called adenomatosis and adenomatous hyperplasia. The histologic differential diagnosis includes insulinoma (adenoma) which is generally well demarcated (thus can be appreciated grossly), does not have intermixed acinar elements, and is composed of tumor cells arranged in trabeculae and cords, similar to other endocrine neoplasms.

The loss of maternal 11p15 in the lesions can be visualized by the absence of immunohistochemical reaction to $p57^{kip2}$. $p57^{kip2}$ is the product of one of the imprinted genes (*CDKN1C*) on 11p15 that are normally expressed from the maternal allele [8]. Figure 3 demonstrates that endocrine cell nuclei within the proliferated focus are negative for $p57^{kip2}$, while islet cell nuclei in the normal area are positively labeled.

Identification of this form of disease has major clinical implications because the lesion can be surgically excised and the hyperinsulinism is cured without performing a near-total pancreatectomy. However, the lesions are difficult to identify grossly because they do not distort the normal lobular architecture (fig. 2). On microscopic examination, the boundary between the uninvolved portion of the pancreas and the lesion may be sharp (fig. 2), but it may also be vague and ill-defined. The lesions are generally small, thus their designation as 'focal hyperinsulinism'. In one series, 24 of 35 lesions were less than 1 cm in the greatest dimension [9]. However, the lesion may be multifocal and/or occupy a large portion of the pancreas and may even involve the entire pancreas [1, 10]. The genetic pathogenesis of the latter is the same as smaller typical lesions, as demonstrated by the loss of expression of $p57^{kip2}$ [8]. In these rare cases, the pathology may be described as 'generalized adenomatosis' in order to avoid the usage of either 'diffuse' or 'focal' [1].

Although there are large nuclei in the confluent islet tissue of the adenomatous focal lesions, the islets in uninvolved portions of pancreas have a 'resting' appearance with beta-cells containing a small amount of cytoplasm and small nuclei [3]. Beta-cell nuclear crowding expressed as the number of beta-cell nuclei/1,000 μm^2 of beta-cell cytoplasm is higher in islets outside of focal lesions as compared to islets of the diffuse hyperinsulinism [2]. This difference may be subtle and is not appreciated by other retrospective studies without morphometric measurements [4, 11].

In a limited number of institutions, intraoperative frozen sections are performed to identify patients with the focal form and further guide the extent of pancreatic resection [3, 10]. The presence of islet cell nuclear abnormalities in more than two areas of the pancreas (e.g. enlarged more than three times, 'bizarre' shaped) suggests diffuse hyperinsulinism, and a near-total pancreatectomy is advised. The absence of nuclear enlargement and the recognition of 'resting' morphology in islets are suggestive of the focal form and a search for a focal lesion continues until the lesion is identified. Most recently, preoperative diagnosis of patients with the focal form is aided by fluorine-18 L-3,4-dihydroxyphenylalanine ([^{18}F]-DOPA) positron emission tomography (PET) [12, 13]. This technique localizes the lesion within the pancreas and has also been used to detect extrapancreatic ectopic lesions [14]. The details of PET are discussed in the chapter by States and Adzick [this vol., pp. 71–78].

Hyperinsulinism Caused by Dominant ATP-Sensitive Potassium Channel Mutations

A dominantly expressed *ABCC8* missense mutation was originally described in a large pedigree presenting with a mild form of hyperinsulinism managed by long-term diazoxide treatment [15]. Although many of the dominant *ABCC8* and *KCNJ11* mutations similarly cause diazoxide-responsive hyperinsulinism with a later median age of onset [16], subsequent identification and characterization of additional mutations revealed that some dominant *ABCC8* mutations can cause diazoxide-unresponsive hyperinsulinism requiring a pancreatectomy [17] (see De León and Stanley [this vol., pp. 18–29]). All of the pancreases resected from the latter group demonstrate microscopic features indistinguishable from diffuse hyperinsulinism, i.e. large islet cell nuclei throughout the pancreas [17].

Most patients with diazoxide-responsive disease do not undergo surgery, but rare pancreatectomy specimens from this category also show histologic features similar to those in diffuse hyperinsulinism. In the report of the original pedigree, there is an

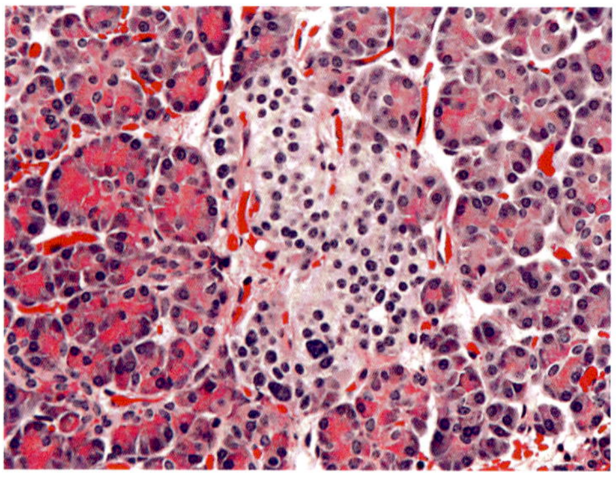

Fig. 4. Glucokinase hyperinsulinism. Islet with a few cells containing large hyperchromatic nuclei. Nucleomegaly in individual islets is indistinguishable from the same changes seen in the diffuse form of K_{ATP} channel hyperinsulinism (hematoxylin and eosin stain, original magnification ×400).

increase in the mean radius of 50 selected beta-cell nuclei and a low index of beta-cell nuclear crowding [15].

Hyperinsulinism Caused by Defects of Other Genes

Hypersinsulinism Caused by Glucokinase Mutations

The clinical manifestation of this disease is variable. Although surgical management is usually not required, hyperinsulinism is, in some cases, severe enough to warrant a pancreatectomy in order to control hypoglycemia. Since surgical specimens are rare, there are few reports in the literature describing the pancreatic pathology of patients with a gain of function mutation in the glucokinase gene *(GCK)*. While the pancreases of 4 patients were described as normal in three reports, in two additional cases in which quantitative histologic analysis was performed, there were moderately enlarged islet cell nuclei and an increase in the mean islet size compared to the pancreases of age-matched controls and patients with K_{ATP} channel hyperinsulinism [18]. Our own experience is limited to 3 patients. Although we have not performed quantitative histologic analysis, the pancreas of these patients had only rare septal islets that were twice as large in diameter as the largest islets of age-matched controls. We did observe islet cell nucleomegaly (fig. 4), but the number of cells with this change was lower than in most cases of diffuse hyperinsulinism.

Hyperinsulinism Caused by Glutamate Dehydrogenase Mutations

As hypoglycemia in patients with mutations of the glutamate dehydrogenase gene resulting in the hyperinsulinism/hyperammonemia syndrome can be medically controlled in the vast majority of cases, knowledge of the pancreatic pathology is rather limited. In one report, the pancreas was described as showing unusual islet cells arranged in a ribbon pattern [19]. Our own experience consists of one case with

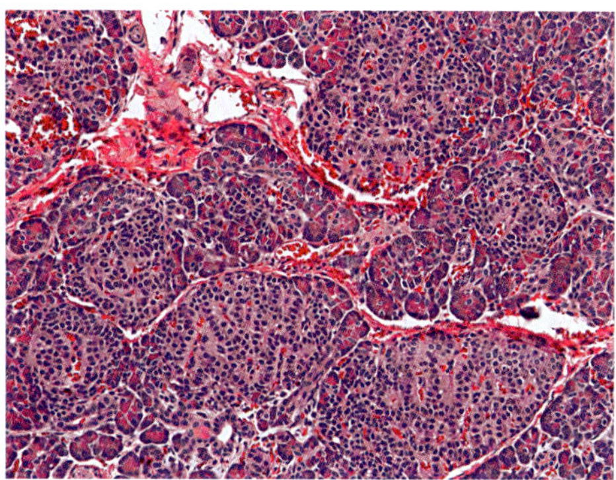

Fig. 5. Pancreas in Beckwith-Wiedemann syndrome. Islets are enlarged and occupy the majority of the lobule throughout the pancreas. Beta-cells are arranged in a trabecular architectural pattern. Significant nucleomegaly is not identified (hematoxylin and eosin stain, original magnification ×200).

diffuse islet cell nucleomegaly similar to that seen in the diffuse form of K_{ATP} channel hyperinsulinism.

Hyperinsulinism Caused by Short-Chain 3-Hydroxyacyl-CoA Dehydrogenase Mutations

One autopsy case of a patient with short-chain 3-hydroxyacyl-CoA dehydrogenase deficiency at our institution showed no abnormalities in quantity or distribution of endocrine tissue or nuclear size. In this case, the patient's hyperinsulinism had been medically managed and she succumbed to respiratory failure secondary to hypertrophic cardiomyopathy.

Beckwith-Wiedemann Syndrome

As hypoglycemia resolves during the first few weeks of life in the majority of cases of Beckwith-Wiedemann syndrome [20], knowledge of the pancreatic histology is usually limited to the rare severe cases in which the patient died or had a partial pancreatectomy. Pancreases show a variable degree of increased endocrine tissue distributed throughout the entire gland [21]. The majority of islets have an insular or trabecular architectural pattern composed of cells with medium-to-large nuclei and abundant eosinophilic cytoplasm. In many cases, the islets are confluent and constitute a large proportion of the involved lobule (fig. 5). The abundance of endocrine tissue forming irregular nodules and aggregates is different from the adenomatous hyperplasia of focal hyperinsulinism in that the abnormality in Beckwith-Wiedemann syndrome is present throughout the pancreas. Scattered, smaller islet cell clusters can also be seen. By immunohistochemistry, the islet-like aggregates recapitulate the normal islet topography with insulin-positive beta-cells centrally, glucagon-positive alpha-cells at the periphery, and cells reactive for somatostatin and pancreatic polypeptide interspersed throughout the islets [22]. In one of our cases, the islet cell proliferation harbored an incidental pancreatoblastoma, a tumor known to have increased incidence in Beckwith-Wiedemann syndrome. One report by Sotelo-Avila and Gooch

[23] describes islet cell hyperplasia in 5 children who died of their disease-associated tumors, even though the earlier hypoglycemia had been transient.

Normal Developing Pancreas, Nesidioblastosis, and Hyperinsulinism

Histologic evaluation of the pancreas of children with hyperinsulinism requires an understanding that the histology of the normal developing pancreas has many features that are different from those of the normal adult pancreas. The amount of endocrine tissue present at birth is roughly estimated to be 10% of the pancreas. This value decreases during the phase of acinar development to 5% by 6 months of age, and then gradually becomes the adult volume of 1–2% [1, 21]. There is also regional variation with a portion of the head of pancreas, which is derived from the ventral primordium, being particularly rich in islets (fig. 6). The endocrine tissue in the developing pancreas is closely associated with the ductal system from which it buds (fig. 6). In addition, the extrainsular component comprises a significant portion of endocrine tissues at term. The better-formed islets reside near the stalk of the lobule while smaller aggregates and single cells tend to be located in association with more peripheral centroacinar tissues [1] (fig. 7). Occasional large islets, mainly septal, can be noted (fig. 6). All these histologic features may be seen in the pancreas resected from individuals with hyperinsulinism, as the pancreases are usually from young infants; however, these features are likely not related to hyperinsulinism, but are those of a developing normal pancreas.

The cells that bud off the duct epithelium to build islets were called 'nesidioblasts' (islet builders) by Laidlaw [24]. He used this term to explain the origin of islet cell tumors of the pancreas because he observed the close association of duct epithelium and a group of islet cell tumor cells similar to the continuity of duct epithelium and islet cells in normal pancreas. He further proposed a name 'nesidioblastoma' for adenoma of islet cells, and another term 'nesidioblastosis' to describe a condition wherein a diffuse or disseminated proliferation of islet cells becomes a cause of hypoglycemia. Yakovac et al. [25] investigated the histopathology of 'idiopathic hypoglycemia of infancy', and reported that a defining feature was beta-cell nesidioblastosis. Nesidioblastosis was thereafter used to support the hypothesis that neonatal hypoglycemia-hyperinsulinism is a developmental problem.

'Nesidioblastosis' subsequently acquired a clinical meaning, essentially making it synonymous with the disorder presenting with persistent neonatal hypoglycemia [26]. The term has also been used frequently to describe the diverse histopathology found among pancreases obtained from patients with hyperinsulinism. The histologic features observed were what we understand currently as diffuse hyperinsulinism (large islet cell nuclei) and focal hyperinsulinism (a lesion formed by the confluence of hyperplastic but apparently normally structured islets), but also included features

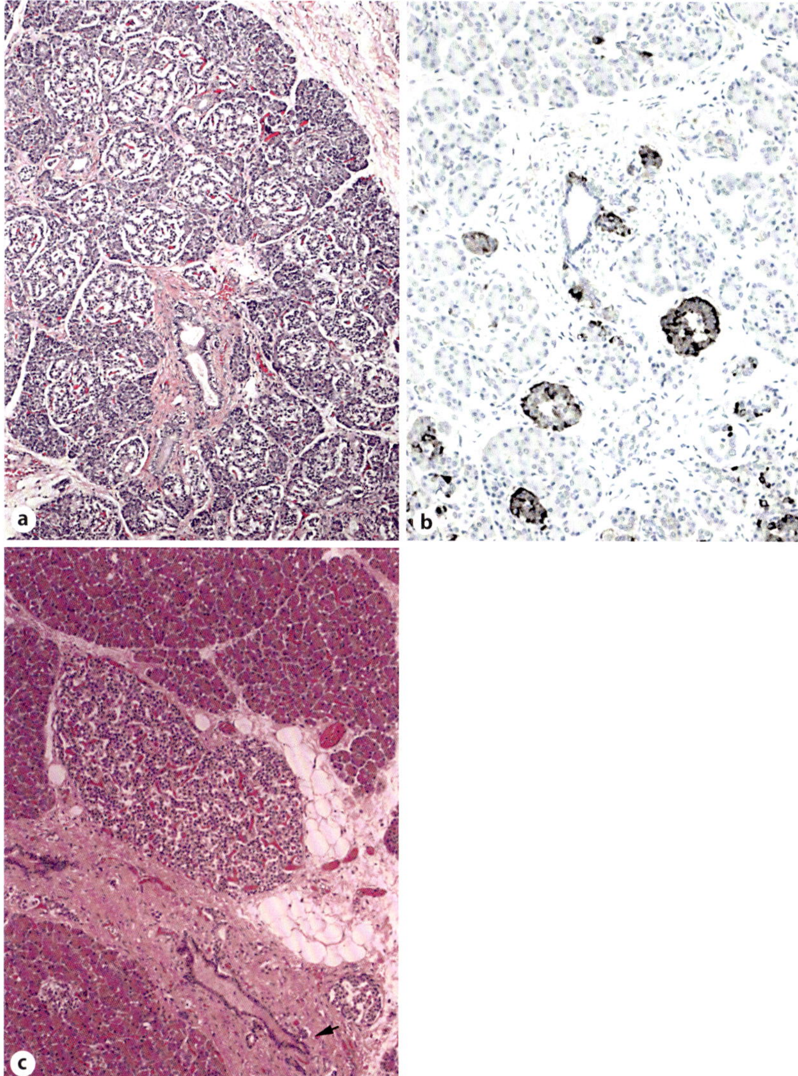

Fig. 6. Histologic features of pancreas from individuals less than 2 years of age. **a** Abundant islets/endocrine tissue is seen in the pancreas of a 5-month-old normoglycemic infant, especially in the head (hematoxylin and eosin stain, original magnification ×100). **b** Endocrine cells budding off a duct (nesidioblastosis) in an 8-day-old infant born at 40 weeks of gestation (immunohistochemistry for chromogranin A, original magnification ×200). **c** Very large septal islets, such as this one in a 22-month-old child, are not uncommon. A small cluster of endocrine cells is budding off a duct (nesidioblastosis) in the lower right corner (arrow; hematoxylin and eosin stain, original magnification ×100). Reprinted with permission from Wolters Kluwer/Lippincott Williams and Wilkins [27, p. 761].

observed in the normal neonatal pancreas different from those of adult pancreas as described above, i.e. abundant endocrine tissue as compared to the acinar component, the presence of endocrine cells continuous with the duct epithelium, single cells and small clusters of endocrine cells, and large septal islets. As a result, it has become

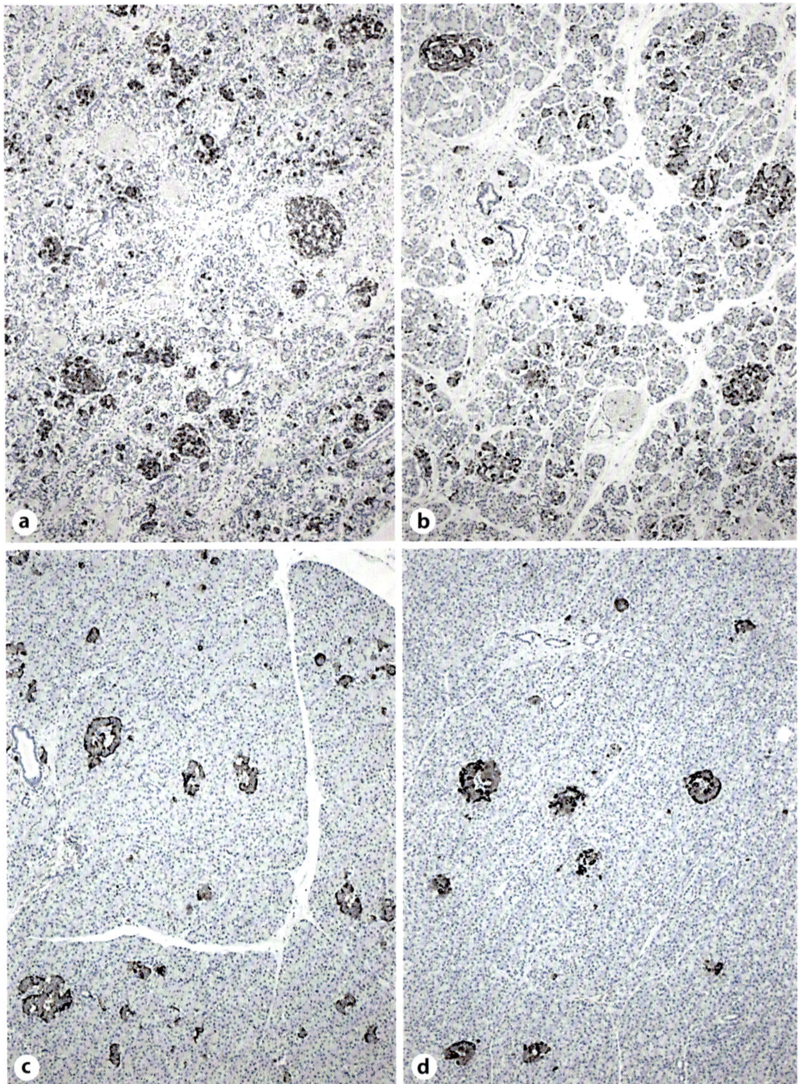

Fig. 7. Distribution of endocrine cells, which are revealed by immunohistochemistry for chromogranin A. Respective survival dates are as follows: stillbirth at 25 weeks (**a**); 40 weeks of gestation, 8 days of postnatal survival (**b**); 22 months (**c**), and 8 years (**d**) (original magnifications ×100). Reprinted with permission from Wolters Kluwer/Lippincott Williams and Wilkins [27, p 760].

increasingly difficult to grasp the exact morphology when a pathologic description is given such as 'the pancreas showed nesidioblastosis'.

Other terms, e.g. 'islet cell dysplasia' and 'nesidiodysplasia', were proposed in order to discourage the use of nesidioblastosis in the context of hyperinsulinism, but they did not seem to prevail. Meanwhile, pathologists who recognized the frequent association of endocrine cells and ducts in fetal and pediatric materials from nonhyperinsulinism individuals started to challenge the conventional wisdom regarding the pathologic basis of congenital hyperinsulinism [1, 2]. They were followed by endocrinologists, biochemists, and geneticists who further delineated an understanding that hyperinsulinism is a functional defect in insulin regulation, one not simply due to abnormal islet development.

Although K_{ATP} channel hyperinsulinism accounts for most cases of hyperinsulinism managed by surgical intervention, several forms of non-K_{ATP} channel hyperinsulinism have been described in the past decade, and the knowledge regarding this group is expanding rapidly. When pancreases are removed, careful and non-prejudiced examination should be performed as the pancreatic histology may vary according to the underlying causes. In addition to an unusual clinical presentation, pancreatic histology showing deviation from typical diffuse hyperinsulinism or focal hyperinsulinism may prompt investigation into an unrecognized mechanism of disease. For example, analysis of cases of localized islet cell nuclear enlargement (LINE) [7] may lead to the discovery of a new genetic pathway for hyperinsulinism. Lumping various histologic changes into a single term such as 'nesidioblastosis' is not only unscientific, but also limits an evolving clinical and pathologic understanding of this complex disease.

References

1 Jaffe R, Hashida Y, Yunis EJ: Pancreatic pathology in hyperinsulinemic hypoglycemia of infancy. Lab Invest 1980;42:356–365.

2 Rahier J, Guiot Y, Sempoux C: Persistent hyperinsulinaemic hypoglycaemia of infancy: a heterogeneous syndrome unrelated to nesidioblastosis. Arch Dis Child Fetal Neonatal Ed 2000;82: F108–F112.

3 Rahier J, Sempoux C, Fournet JC, Poggi F, Brunelle F, Nihoul-Fekete C, Saudubray JM, Jaubert F: Partial or near-total pancreatectomy for persistent neonatal hyperinsulinaemic hypoglycaemia: the pathologist's role. Histopathology 1998;32:15–19.

4 Suchi M, MacMullen C, Thornton PS, Ganguly A, Stanley CA, Ruchelli ED: Histopathology of congenital hyperinsulinism: retrospective study with genotype correlations. Pediatr Dev Pathol 2003;6: 322–333.

5 Sempoux C, Guiot Y, Dubois D, Nollevaux MC, Saudubray JM, Nihoul-Fekete C, Rahier J: Pancreatic B-cell proliferation in persistent hyperinsulinemic hypoglycemia of infancy: an immunohistochemical study of 18 cases. Mod Pathol 1998;11:444–449.

6 Kassem SA, Ariel I, Thornton PS, Scheimberg I, Glaser B: Beta-cell proliferation and apoptosis in the developing normal human pancreas and in hyperinsulinism of infancy. Diabetes 2000;49: 1325–1333.

7 Ernst LE, Suchi M, Stanley CA, Adzick NS, MacMullen C, Ruchelli ED: Localized islet cell nuclear enlargement in congenital hyperinsulinism: a distinct clinicopathologic entity. Mod Pathol 2007; 20:287.

8 Suchi M, MacMullen CM, Thornton PS, Adzick NS, Ganguly A, Ruchelli ED, Stanley CA: Molecular and immunohistochemical analyses of the focal form of congenital hyperinsulinism. Mod Pathol 2006;19: 122–129.

9 Stanley CA, Thornton PS, Ganguly A, MacMullen C, Underwood P, Bhatia P, Steinkrauss L, Wanner L, Kaye R, Ruchelli ED, Suchi M, Adzick NS: Preoperative evaluation of infants with focal or diffuse congenital hyperinsulinism by intraoperative acute insulin response tests and selective pancreatic arterial calcium stimulation. J Clin Endocrinol Metab 2004;89:288–296.

10 Suchi M, Thornton PS, Adzick NS, MacMullen C, Ganguly A, Stanley CA, Ruchelli ED: Congenital hyperinsulinism: intraoperative biopsy interpretation can direct the extent of pancreatectomy. Am J Surg Pathol 2004;28:1326–1335.

11 Jack MM, Walker RM, Thomsett MJ, Cotterill AM, Bell JR: Histologic findings in persistent hyperinsulinemic hypoglycemia of infancy: Australian experience. Pediatr Dev Pathol 2000;3:532–547.

12 Otonkoski T, Nanto-Salonen K, Seppanen M, Veijola R, Huopio H, Hussain K, Tapanainen P, Eskola O, Parkkola R, Ekstrom K, Guiot Y, Rahier J, Laakso M, Rintala R, Nuutila P, Minn H: Noninvasive diagnosis of focal hyperinsulinism of infancy with [^{18}F]-DOPA positron emission tomography. Diabetes 2006;55:13–18.
13 Hardy OT, Hernandez-Pampaloni M, Saffer JR, Suchi M, Ruchelli E, Zhuang H, Ganguly A, Freifelder R, Adzick NS, Alavi A, Stanley CA: Diagnosis and localization of focal congenital hyperinsulinism by ^{18}F-fluorodopa PET scan. J Pediatr 2007;150:140–145.
14 Hussain K, Seppanen M, Nanto-Salonen K, Adzick NS, Stanley CA, Thornton P, Minn H: The diagnosis of ectopic focal hyperinsulinism of infancy with [^{18}F]-dopa positron emission tomography. J Clin Endocrinol Metab 2006;91:2839–2842.
15 Huopio H, Reimann F, Ashfield R, Komulainen J, Lenko HL, Rahier J, Vauhkonen I, Kere J, Laakso M, Ashcroft F, Otonkoski T: Dominantly inherited hyperinsulinism caused by a mutation in the sulfonylurea receptor type 1. J Clin Invest 2000;106: 897–906.
16 Pinney SE, MacMullen C, Becker S, Lin YW, Hanna C, Thornton P, Ganguly A, Shyng SL, Stanley CA: Clinical characteristics and biochemical mechanisms of congenital hyperinsulinism associated with dominant K_{ATP} channel mutations. J Clin Invest 2008;118:2877–2886.
17 Macmullen CM, Zhou Q, Snider KE, Tewson PH, Becker SA, Aziz AR, Ganguly A, Shyng SL, Stanley CA: Diazoxide-unresponsive congenital hyperinsulinism in children with dominant mutations of the β-cell sulfonylurea receptor SUR1. Diabetes 2011;60: 1797–1804.
18 Kassem S, Bhandari S, Rodriguez-Bada P, Motaghedi R, Heyman M, Garcia-Gimeno MA, Cobo-Vuilleumier N, Sanz P, Maclaren NK, Rahier J, Glaser B, Cuesta-Munoz AL: Large islets, beta-cell proliferation, and a glucokinase mutation. N Engl J Med 2010;362:1348–1350.
19 Weinzimer SA, Stanley CA, Berry GT, Yudkoff M, Tuchman M, Thornton PS: A syndrome of congenital hyperinsulinism and hyperammonemia. J Pediatr 1997;130:661–664.
20 Elliott M, Bayly R, Cole T, Temple IK, Maher ER: Clinical features and natural history of Beckwith-Wiedemann syndrome: presentation of 74 new cases. Clin Genet 1994;46:168–174.
21 Jaffe R, Hashida Y, Yunis EJ: The endocrine pancreas of the neonate and infant. Perspect Pediatr Pathol 1982;7:137–165.
22 Stefan Y, Bordi C, Grasso S, Orci L: Beckwith-Wiedemann syndrome: a quantitative, immunohistochemical study of pancreatic islet cell populations. Diabetologia 1985;28:914–919.
23 Sotelo-Avila C, Gooch WM 3rd: Neoplasms associated with the Beckwith-Wiedemann syndrome. Perspect Pediatr Pathol 1976;3:255–272.
24 Laidlaw GF: Nesidioblastoma, the islet tumor of the pancreas. Am J Pathol 1938;14:125–134.
25 Yakovac WC, Baker L, Hummeler K: Beta cell nesidioblastosis in idiopathic hypoglycemia of infancy. J Pediatr 1971;79:226–231.
26 Milner RD: Nesidioblastosis unravelled. Arch Dis Child 1996;74:369–372.
27 Suchi M: The pancreas; in Stocker JT, Dehner LP, Hussain AN (eds): Stocker and Dehner's Pediatric Pathology, ed 3. Philadelphia, Wolters Kluwer/Lippincott Williams and Wilkins, 2011, pp 743–778.
28 Adzick NS, Thornton PS, Stanley CA, Kaye RD, Ruchelli E: A multidisciplinary approach to the focal form of congenital hyperinsulinism by partial pancreatectomy. J Pediatr Surg 2004;39:270–275.

Mariko Suchi, MD, PhD
Department of Pathology
Medical College of Wisconsin
Children's Hospital of Wisconsin
9000 W. Wisconsin Avenue
Milwaukee, WI 53226 (USA)
Tel. +1 414 266 2526, E-Mail msuchi@mcw.edu

Stanley CA, De León DD (eds): Monogenic Hyperinsulinemic Hypoglycemia Disorders.
Front Diabetes. Basel, Karger, 2012, vol 21, pp 71–78

Localization of a Focal Lesion of Congenital Hyperinsulinism: Imaging and Surgery

Lisa J. States · N. Scott Adzick

Department of Radiology, The Children's Hospital of Philadelphia, Philadelphia, Pa., USA

Abstract

Approximately half of the infants with congenital hyperinsulinism who require surgical pancreatectomy for glucose control have a potentially curable focal lesion. Molecular imaging with [^{18}F]-L-3,4-dihydroxyphenylalanine ([^{18}F]-DOPA) PET has revolutionized the diagnostic evaluation of infants and neonates with focal congenital hyperinsulinism. Since 2003, [^{18}F]-DOPA PET has been investigated for its ability to detect and accurately localize a focal lesion and thus distinguish focal from diffuse disease. This technique utilizes the uptake and decarboxylation of the amine precursors (APUD) pathway, a unique neuroendocrine property of the pancreatic islet beta-cell. Compared with prior diagnostic studies using interventional radiology techniques, this procedure is less invasive, safer, and easier to perform and interpret. To date, the two largest published series [Ribeiro et al: Eur J Nucl Med Mol Imaging 2007;34:2120–2128; Hardy et al: J Clin Endocrinol Metab 2007;92:4706–4711] of surgically proven focal disease have revealed an [^{18}F]-DOPA PET sensitivity of 75–100% for detection of a focal lesion with 100% accuracy in anatomic localization of detected lesions. Identification and accurate localization of a focal lesion can be used to create a more focused preoperative plan, resulting in a limited pancreatic resection and decreased surgical morbidity. In combination with surgical expertise, [^{18}F]-DOPA PET can offer an outcome with preservation of pancreatic function and cure of this devastating disease.

As detailed in other chapters, approximately half of the infants with hyperinsulinism (HI) that cannot be controlled medically will have a focal lesion of islet adenomatosis that is potentially curable by surgical excision. This chapter reviews the preoperative imaging evaluation and surgery in the treatment of infants with potential focal congenital HI.

Imaging Techniques

Conventional imaging techniques, such as CT or MRI, are unable to detect focal lesions of beta-cell adenomatosis [1, 2]. Invasive interventional radiology techniques

Table 1. Published results of interventional radiology studies with surgery and histology diagnosis

Author, procedure, year	Patients with surgery and histology	Sensitivity (detection of a focal lesion)	Specificity (detection of diffuse disease)	Accuracy of anatomic localization
De Lonlay-Debeney et al. [3], PVS, 1999	45	17/19 (89%)	17/26 (65%)	17/19 (89%)
Chigot et al. [4], ASVS, 2001	12	5/6 (83%)	2/6 (33%)	(100%)
Stanley et al. [5], ASVS, 2004	46	24/33 (73%)	4/13 (31%)	24/33 (73%)

Values represent the number of patients. PVS = Transhepatic portal venous sampling; ASVS = arterial calcium stimulation with venous sampling.

using transhepatic portal venous sampling or arterial calcium stimulation with venous sampling, developed to identify acquired insulinomas in adults, were previously the only diagnostic imaging techniques available to document the presence of a focal lesion. As shown in table 1, with either of these techniques, the accuracy of focal lesion localization and the ability to distinguish diffuse disease is poor and the procedures are highly invasive, requiring prolonged general anesthesia, multiple blood samples (sometimes requiring transfusion), and meticulous glucose control for safety and accuracy [3–5]. The most important disadvantage of these procedures is their inability to provide the surgeon with specific anatomic details regarding location. As detailed below, [^{18}F]-DOPA PET scans have proven to be a much more satisfactory method for detection of a focal lesion as well as high accuracy of localization [1, 2, 6].

[^{18}F]-DOPA PET Imaging

The mechanism for [^{18}F]-DOPA uptake by the beta-cells is via the APUD pathway (fig. 1). The dopaminergic pathway is expressed in pancreatic endocrine cells, including DOPA decarboxylase (DDC) [7] and DOPA, dopamine, the plasma membrane dopamine transporter, and the vesicular dopamine transporter [8]. In humans, immunohistochemistry of focal HI lesions reveals dense staining for DDC, colocalized with insulin and proinsulin, in association with weak staining in the surrounding normal beta-cells. Pancreatic specimens from humans with a normal pancreas or diffuse HI reveal no difference in the diffuse weak DDC staining of the beta-cells. The mechanism of increased F-DOPA uptake in a focal lesion of beta-cell adenomatosis, compared with surrounding normal tissue, is thought to be due the increased number of densely packed beta-cells, not increased insulin secretory activity [9]. Further

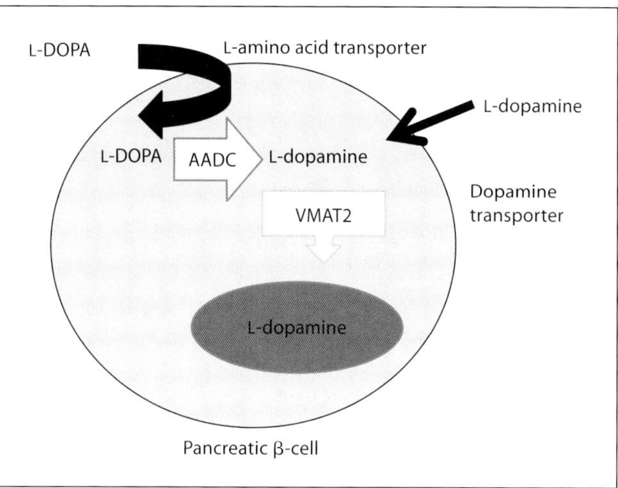

Fig. 1. L-DOPA enters the islet cells through an L-amino acid transporter for large neutral amino acids. In the cell, L-DOPA, is converted to L-dopamine, using the enzyme L-aromatic amino acid decarboxylase (AADC). L-dopamine is then taken up into cytoplasmic vesicles using a vesicular dopamine transporter 2 (VMAT2). L-dopamine formed in other endocrine or exocrine cells can be transported into the cell using dopamine transporter.

evidence that islet cell [^{18}F]-DOPA uptake involves the APUD pathway is shown with the use of the DDC inhibitor carbidopa in humans, which results in absent pancreatic uptake on [^{18}F]-DOPA PET scans [1]. Because it is uncertain whether medications such as diazoxide and octreotide might interfere with [^{18}F]-DOPA uptake, it is suggested that diazoxide be discontinued for 5 days and octreotide for 2 days prior to [^{18}F]-DOPA [1, 2, 10]. However, in 2 subjects who underwent two [^{18}F]-DOPA PET scans performed with and without octreotide and diazoxide, there was no change in qualitative or quantitative analysis of the two scans [1].

[^{18}F]-DOPA PET Scan Interpretation

The sensitivity, specificity, and localization data from the three largest series evaluating [^{18}F]-DOPA PET scans for preoperative localization of focal congenital HI are shown in table 2. Only cases with surgical resection and histological confirmation are included. The sensitivity of the test to detect a focal lesion ranged from 75 to 100%, and the specificity to correctly diagnose diffuse disease was 100% in all series [1, 2, 6]. Most importantly, the [^{18}F]-DOPA PET scan provided accurate information on the location of the focal lesion in 92–100% of detected lesions [1, 2, 6]. The following paragraphs summarize some of the techniques for interpreting the [^{18}F]-DOPA PET scans gained from our experience of over 170 cases.

Qualitative analysis of PET images begins with an initial review using a 3D rotating maximum intensity projection (MIP) image which gives an overview of the pancreatic morphology. Coregistered images with a contrast-enhanced CT or MRI are used to assess the location of a focal lesion and its position with respect to the splenic and superior mesenteric arteries, portal venous system, common

Table 2. Published results of [^{18}F]-DOPA PET scans with surgery and histology diagnosis

Author, year	Patients with surgery and histology	Sensitivity (detection of a focal lesion)	Specificity (detection of diffuse disease)	Accuracy of anatomic localization
Otonkoski et al. [6], 2006	9	5/5 (100%)	4/4 (100%)	100%
Ribeiro et al. [1], 2007	25	16/16 (100%)	7/7 (100%)*	92%
Hardy et al. [2], 2007	50	18/24 (75%)	24/24 (100%)*	100%

Values represent the number of patients.
* Two were atypical and not included.

bile duct, and duodenum. These images can be used to measure the distance of the focal lesion from a stable vascular structure such as the portal venous confluence, giving the surgeon the exact location of a lesion. Image fusion with a CT angiogram or dynamic 3D contrast-enhanced MR angiogram improves image localization and creates a visual road map for the surgeon. A focal lesion appears as a 'bright spot' of increased activity in a background of diffuse low-level pancreatic activity (fig. 2a). Sometimes when a lesion is present in the body or tail, there is mild increased activity in the pancreatic head giving the appearance of two areas of increased uptake. Semiquantitative analysis using standardized uptake values, a measure of activity, may help confirm the presence of a focal lesion. A standardized uptake values ratio of activity in the 'suspected' lesion versus background pancreatic activity of >1.2 [1] or ≥1.5 [6] is considered diagnostic for a focal lesion, and <1.2 is considered diagnostic for diffuse disease [1]. In most cases, however, simple visual analysis should be adequate for interpretation and localization of a focal lesion.

The [^{18}F]-DOPA pattern for diffuse disease is usually uniformly homogeneous, but may show increased activity in the head with respect to the rest of the pancreas due to greater tissue volume. Similarly, variability in the shape of the pancreas may cause patchy or nonuniform uptake (fig. 3), simulating multiple lesions. This is a common pitfall for the inexperienced reader. In our experience, focal lesions that were not identifiable included very small lesions, a peculiar flat leaf-like shape on the surface of the pancreas, and a large lesion involving almost the entire pancreas. The adjacent kidney can obscure focal lesions (fig. 2b). In one case, ectopic satellite focal lesions were detected in the small bowel [11].

Other forms of hyperinsulinemic hypoglycemia that may be indistinguishable from focal congenital HI include Beckwith-Wiedemann syndrome and acquired insulinomas such as in von Hippel-Lindau disease or tuberous sclerosis. In our experience, [^{18}F]-DOPA PET scans in patients with Beckwith-Wiedemann syndrome may show a large region of increased uptake due to large areas of beta-cell adenomatosis.

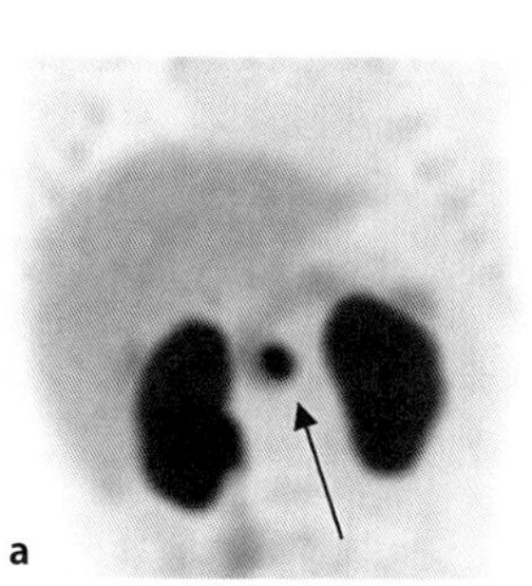
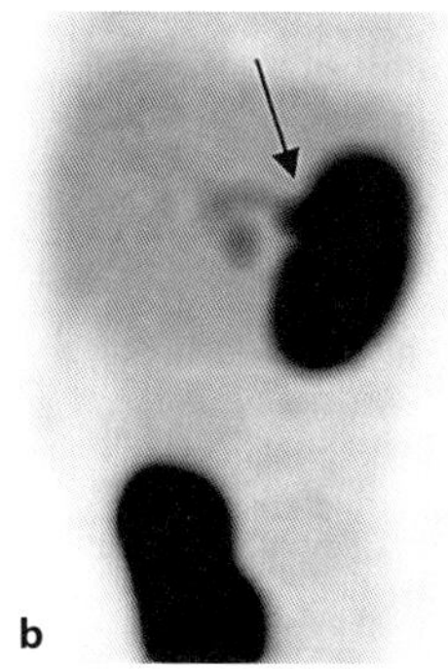
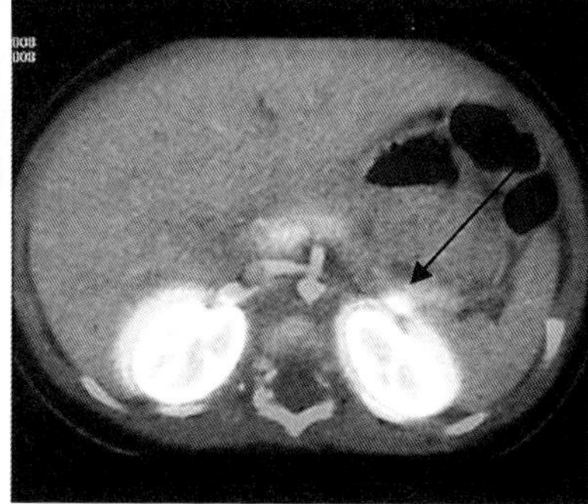

Fig. 2. **a** Frontal view of a 3D MIP showing a focal lesion in the uncinate process (arrow). Note the normal liver and renal uptake and mild growth plate uptake in the anterior ribs. **b** Oblique 3D MIP image demonstrates a 'bump' on the anterior surface of the left upper pole. An axial image of the PET image fused with a contrast-enhanced CT shows a small focal lesion (arrow) on the posterior surface of the pancreas abutting the left kidney.

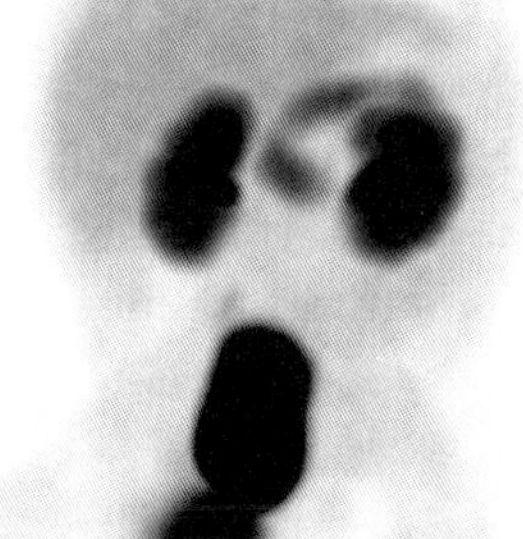

Fig. 3. Frontal view of a 3D MIP shows a non-uniform pattern of uptake in diffuse disease with areas of increased activity in the pancreatic head and body, and a bulbous pancreatic tail.

Insulinomas can sometimes be detected by [^{18}F]-DOPA PET scans, but are usually identifiable on contrast-enhanced CT or MRI. Atypical histology patterns have been reported (see discussion of localized islet cell nuclear enlargement in the chapter by Suchi et al. [pp. 57–70]), but are most often diffuse on [^{18}F]-DOPA PET scans [1, 2].

Current limitations of [^{18}F]-DOPA PET scans are related to the resolution of the scanner. Even with the newest hybrid PET/CT scanners, small lesions in the pancreatic head may be impossible to detect. High densities of glucagon-like peptide-1 receptors on pancreatic beta-cells provide a promising target for imaging using radiolabeled glucagon-like peptide-1 agonists such as exendin 4 (reviewed in the chapter by De León [pp. 79–86]).

Surgery

Surgical exploration of infants with HI requires technical expertise and experience. Using the standard intra-abdominal approach, the search for a focal lesion begins with a visual and tactile search followed by systematic biopsy of the tail, body, and head. Accurate preoperative localization can greatly facilitate this process since focal lesions are usually small, <10 mm in size, and frequently irregularly shaped. Although focal lesions may maintain a lobular structure similar to that of the normal pancreas, subtle visual clues ranging from a slightly reddish color to a marble-like appearance may permit visual detection of the lesion intraoperatively. In some cases, the lesion will feel firmer than the surrounding normal pancreas. However, a tiny focal lesion can be buried within the pancreas and impossible to see or feel. Certainly, greater operative experience has led to more frequent intraoperative visualization or palpation of a focal lesion. Expert pediatric pathologic interpretation of frozen section biopsies is vitally important since the distinction between focal and diffuse disease must be made during surgery [12]. When the biopsies demonstrate normal pancreatic histology, additional biopsies of suspicious areas are obtained until the focal lesion is diagnosed by frozen section. If no lesion is found, a further search for the focal lesion using the preoperative localization data is conducted. Once a focal lesion is identified, a partial pancreatectomy is performed using frozen sections of margins to ensure a complete resection.

The surgical approach varies depending on the location of the lesion. For periductal lesions in the body and tail, a distal pancreatectomy is performed. With pancreatic head lesions close to the common bile duct or pancreatic duct, it can be tricky to excise the entire lesion, particularly if there are tentacles of diseased tissue that emanate from the lesion. To ensure complete lesion resection in these challenging cases, most or all of the pancreatic head is removed followed by Roux-en-Y pancreaticojejunostomy to drain the remaining pancreatic body and tail [13]. In this way, the endocrine and exocrine function of the remaining normal pancreas is saved. Early initial experience, due to reluctance to use this approach in neonates and infants, led to inadequate resection in a few cases, which necessitated either another resection or continued medical therapy. Although rare, a focal lesion in the head can extend into the duodenal wall, in which case a Whipple procedure may be needed. After the surgery, all frozen samples are processed for routine histology and confirmation of findings based on paraffin-embedded sections and insulin immunohistochemistry.

Because [^{18}F]-DOPA PET scan localization of focal lesions has proven to be so accurate, focal lesions on the anterior surface of the body and tail can be resected using laparoscopic techniques. To facilitate pancreatic body and tail exposure during laparoscopy, it is useful to sew the stomach up to the anterior abdominal wall using 2–3 transabdominal sutures to the anterior gastric wall close to the greater curvature. The carbon dioxide pneumoperitoneum then suspends the stomach anteriorly. This technique makes it easy to expose and dissect the pancreatic body and tail. The laparoscopic procedure is performed via four 3- to 5-mm ports, which permits biopsies, complete resection of a visible peripherally located focal lesion, or distal pancreatectomy if needed. Attempts to resect focal lesions in the pancreatic head are hindered by the inability to accurately visualize the course of the common bile duct within the pancreatic head without consequent risk of ductal injury. The drawback to the laparoscopic approach is that there is no tactile feedback to help locate a nonvisible focal lesion.

Intraoperative high-resolution sonography is used to evaluate detection of a suspected focal lesion identified with [^{18}F]-DOPA PET, or if the PET scan shows diffuse disease and random intraoperative pancreatic biopsies demonstrate normal pancreatic tissue. A focal lesion can have a variable sonographic echotexture and blurred margins. Intraoperative sonography may also be helpful for the identification of vital structures such as the common bile duct.

Postoperative Care and Follow-Up

Postoperative management has been standardized by a clinical care pathway utilizing the glucose infusion rate (GIR) to quantitate the patient's glucose needs. For the initial postoperative period, blood glucose values are determined hourly. The GIR begins at 2 mg/kg/min immediately after the operation, is increased to a GIR of 5 on the morning of postoperative day 1, and then usually advances to a GIR of 8 by the evening of the first postoperative day. It is not unusual for an intravenous insulin infusion to be needed for the first few postoperative days. After hospital discharge, a complete response at follow-up is defined as no requirement for glycemic medications, no continuous tube feedings, no diabetes mellitus, and the ability to tolerate an 18-hour fast without hypoglycemia.

In our entire experience, 95% of babies with the focal form of HI are cured after limited pancreatectomy. The vast majority had a <50% pancreatectomy. For babies with diffuse HI treated with near-total pancreatectomy (95–98%), our current data reveal the following outcomes: 16% require no glycemic medications, 37% require insulin to treat diabetes, and 47% require a glycemic medication. Long-term follow-up is needed for all of these children, particularly with regard to neurodevelopmental issues.

Conclusion

Over the past 10 years, more than 300 patients with HI have been treated with pancreatectomy at The Children's Hospital of Philadelphia. The [^{18}F]-DOPA PET scan has become the 'GPS' (global positioning system) for directing the surgeon to the proper location of a focal lesion that cannot be seen or palpated. The current published data support the hypothesis that [^{18}F]-DOPA PET imaging provides a clinically useful guide to surgical resection of focal adenomatosis and should be considered in all patients requiring surgical management. Preoperative plans can change drastically based on the finding of a focal lesion that is amenable to laparoscopic resection. It must be remembered, however, that some focal lesions are not detected on [^{18}F]-DOPA PET scans. Of upmost importance is that surgery offers a chance of cure in patients with a focal lesion.

References

1 Ribeiro MJ, Boddaert N, Bellanne-Chantelot C, Bourgeois S, Valayannopoulos V, Delzescaux T, Jaubert F, Nihoul-Fékété C, Brunelle F, De Lonlay P: The added value of [^{18}F]fluoro-L-DOPA PET in the diagnosis of hyperinsulinism of infancy: a retrospective study involving 49 children. Eur J Nucl Med Mol Imaging 2007;34:2120–2128.

2 Hardy OT, Hernandez-Pampaloni M, Saffer JR, Scheuermann JS, Ernst LM, Divgi C, Alavi A, Stanley CA: Accuracy of [^{18}F]fluorodopa positron emission tomography for diagnosing and localizing focal congenital hyperinsulinism. J Clin Endocrinol Metab 2007;92:4706–4711.

3 de Lonlay-Debeney P, Poggi-Travert F, Fournet J, Sempoux C, Vici C, Brunelle F, Touati G, Rahier J, Junien C, Nihoul-Fékété C, Robert J, Saudubray J: Clinical features of 52 neonates with hyperinsulinism. N Engl J Med 1999;340:1169–1175.

4 Chigot V, De Lonlay P, Nassogne, M, Laborde K, Delagne V, Fournet J, Ninoul-Fékété C, Saudubray JM, Brunelle F: Pancreatic arterial calcium stimulation in the diagnosis and localization of persistent hyperinsulinemic hypoglycemia of infancy. Pediatr Radiol 2001;31:650–655.

5 Stanley CA, Thornton P, Ganguly A, MacMullen C, Underwood P, Bhatia P, Steinkrauss L, Wanner L, Kaye R, Ruchelli E, Suchi M, Adzick NS: Preoperative evaluation of infants with focal or diffuse congenital hyperinsulinism by intravenous acute insulin response tests and selective pancreatic arterial calcium stimulation. J Clin Endocrinol Metab 2004;89: 288–296.

6 Otonkoski T, Nänto-Salonen K, Seppänen M, Veijola R, Huopio H, Hussain K, Tapanainen Pi, Eskola O, Parkkola R, Ekström K, Guiot Yv, Rahier J, Laakso M, Rintala R, Nuutila P, Minn H: Noninvasive diagnosis of focal hyperinsulinism of infancy with [^{18}F]-DOPA positron emission tomography. Diabetes 2006;55:13–18.

7 Borelli MI, Villar MJ, Orezzoli A, Gagliardino JJ: Presence of DOPA decarboxylase and its localization in adult rat pancreatic islet cells. Diabetes Metab 1997;23:161–163.

8 Mezey E, Eisenhofer G, Harta G, Hansson S, Gould L, Hunyady B, Hoffman BJ: A novel nonneuronal catecholaminergic system: exocrine pancreas synthesizes and releases dopamine. Proc Natl Acad Sci USA 1996;93:10377–10382.

9 de Lonlay P, et al: Congenital hyperinsulinism: pancreatic [^{18}F]fluoro-L-dihydroxyphenylalanine (DOPA) positron emission tomography and immunohistochemistry study of DOPA decarboxylase and insulin secretion. J Clin Endocrinol Metab 2006;91: 933–940.

10 Mohnike K, Blankenstein O, Christensen HT, et al: Proposal for a standardized protocol for ^{18}F-DOPA-PET (PET/CT) in congenital hyperinsulinism. Horm Res 2006;66:40–42.

11 Peranteau WH, Bathaii SM, Pawel B, Hardy O, Alavi A, Stanley CA, Adzick NS: Multiple ectopic lesions of focal islet adenomatosis identified by positron emission tomography scan in an infant with congenital hyperinsulinism. J Pediatr Surg 2007;42:188–192.

12 Suchi M, et al: Congenital hyperinsulinism: intraoperative biopsy interpretation can direct the extent of pancreatectomy. Am J Surg pathol 2004;28:1326–1335.

13 Laje PS, Stanley CA, Palladino AA, Becker SA, Adzick NS: Pancreatic head resection and Roux-en-Y pancreaticojejunostomy for the treatment of the focal form of congenital hyperinsulinism. J Pediatr Surg, in progress.

Lisa J. States, MD
Department of Radiology
The Children's Hospital of Philadelphia
34th Street and Civic Center Boulevard
Philadelphia, PA 19104 (USA)
Tel. +1 215 425 4186, E-Mail states@email.chop.edu

Stanley CA, De León DD (eds): Monogenic Hyperinsulinemic Hypoglycemia Disorders.
Front Diabetes. Basel, Karger, 2012, vol 21, pp 79–86

Role of Incretin Hormones in Hyperinsulinemic Hypoglycemia

Diva D. De León

Division of Endocrinology/Diabetes, The Children's Hospital of Philadelphia, Philadelphia, Pa., USA

Abstract

Incretin hormones play a key role in the regulation of postprandial insulin release. Glucose-dependent insulinotropic polypeptide (GIP) and glucagon-like peptide-1 (GLP-1) account for approximately 90% of the incretin effect, but only GLP-1 has been shown to play a role in the control of fasting glycemia. In addition to its insulinotropic actions, GLP-1 has other glucose-lowering effects including inhibition of glucagon secretion, hepatic glucose production, gastric emptying, and appetite. Studies in mice and pancreatic islets lacking ATP-sensitive potassium (K_{ATP}) channels point to a role of GLP-1 and its receptor in the pathophysiology of K_{ATP} hyperinsulinism (K_{ATP}HI). Particularly, the GLP-1 receptor antagonist exendin-(9–39) inhibits insulin secretion and corrects fasting hypoglycemia in *SUR1*$^{-/-}$ mice, suggesting a potential therapeutic application of this peptide in the treatment of K_{ATP}HI. In addition, early evidence in individuals with postprandial hyperinsulinemic hypoglycemia after gastric surgery suggests that GLP-1 may also play a causal role in this entity. The GLP-1 receptor has been used successfully in the localization of pancreatic insulinomas with radiolabeled peptides. Future studies are needed to examine the potential application of the GLP-1 receptor as a therapeutic target for congenital and acquired forms of hyperinsulinemic hypoglycemia.

Overview of Incretin Hormones

The incretin effect refers to the observation that insulin secretion in response to oral glucose is significantly higher than the response to an isoglycemic intravenous glucose infusion. The recognition of this phenomenon led to the discovery of incretin hormones, which are gut-derived peptides secreted by enteroendocrine cells in response to a meal that make a significant contribution to postprandial insulin release. Two peptides account for approximately 90% of the incretin effect: glucose-dependent insulinotropic polypeptide (GIP) and glucagon-like peptide-1 (GLP-1). GIP is secreted from the intestinal K cells, located predominantly in the duodenum, while GLP-1 is produced by L cells located throughout the small and large intestine, but more abundantly in the ileum and colon [1].

The main stimulus for incretin hormone secretion is the absorption of nutrients (carbohydrates, proteins, fats) in the intestine. Although fasting levels are detectable, their release throughout a 24-hour period largely coincides with meal ingestion. After meal ingestion, secretion of both GIP and GLP-1 increases within 5–15 min. Circulating levels of GIP and GLP-1 decrease rapidly, as both are quickly inactivated in plasma by the enzyme dipeptidyl peptidase IV and by renal clearance. The circulation half-lives of GLP-1 and GIP are 1–2 and 5–7 min, respectively.

GIP and GLP-1 exert their actions in target tissues through specific G protein-coupled receptors. The GIP receptor is predominantly expressed in islet beta-cells and, to a lesser extent, in adipose, bone, and brain tissues. In contrast, the GLP-1 receptor is expressed in the alpha- and beta-cells of the islets and in other tissues, including the central and peripheral nervous system, heart, kidney, lung, and gastrointestinal tract (reviewed in [1]).

The physiological importance of endogenous GIP and GLP-1 for glucose homeostasis has been extensively investigated in studies using receptor antagonists and gene-knockout mice. Both incretins contribute to postprandial glucose regulation, but only GLP-1 is essential for the control of fasting glycemia, as genetic and pharmacologic disruption of GLP-1 receptor signaling leads to fasting hyperglycemia [2–4].

In addition to being a potent stimulator of glucose-dependent insulin release, GLP-1 has other complementary actions, including inhibition of glucagon secretion, hepatic glucose production, gastric emptying, and appetite (reviewed in [5]). In contrast, GIP does not delay gastric emptying [6] nor inhibit glucagon secretion; rather, glucagon may be stimulated by GIP under certain conditions [7]. Importantly, and unlike GIP, the effects of GLP-1 on glucose metabolism are retained in individuals with diabetes [8]. This has led to the development of novel therapeutic products that either enhance endogenous GLP-1 actions or act as agonists of the GLP-1 receptor.

The current premise is that GLP-1 insulinotropic effects are glucose-dependent, but there is evidence that exogenous or endogenous GLP-1 could contribute to overt hypoglycemia by stimulating an exaggerated insulin response and suppressing glucagon. In healthy individuals, paired studies infusing glucose alone or GLP-1 together with glucose at a rate adjusted to achieve comparable glycemia showed glucose levels decreased further after administration of GLP-1 [9]. Administration of pharmacologic doses of GLP-1 and the GLP-1 receptor agonist, exenatide, to islet and whole pancreatic transplant recipients has also been associated with hypoglycemia [10, 11]. Additionally, hypersecretion of endogenous GLP-1, as described in a woman with a GLP-1-secreting tumor, was associated with overt hypoglycemia, which resolved after tumor resection [12]. On the other hand, the clinical use of the GLP-1 receptor agonist exenatide (Byetta) has not been associated with significant hypoglycemia in individuals with diabetes, except when given concomitantly with sulfonylureas.

Incretins in ATP-Sensitive Potassium Channel Hyperinsulinism

A few observations point to a potential role of GLP-1 in the pathophysiology of congenital hyperinsulinism due to inactivating mutations in the ATP-sensitive potassium channels (K_{ATP}HI). First, studies in a GLP-1 secreting cell line (GLUTag) have shown that stimulation by glucose and other nutrients induces plasma membrane depolarization by closure of K_{ATP} channels [13] followed by a rise in cytoplasmic Ca^{2+} concentration [14], suggesting that K_{ATP} channel defects affecting the pancreatic beta-cells may also affect the enteroendocrine L cells. More recently, a different mechanism involving electrogenic substrate entry to the cell through sodium-glucose transporters has been described resulting in K_{ATP} channel independent glucose-stimulation of GLP-1 release [15]. Secondly, although GLP-1 secretion has not been studied in K_{ATP}HI, withdrawal of enteral feedings results in a dramatic reduction of glucose requirements in neonates with severe disease (De León DD, unpubl. data). These observations prompted us to examine the role of GLP-1 signaling in insulin secretion in islets from *SUR1*$^{-/-}$ mice.

In *SUR1*$^{-/-}$ islets, we showed that exendin-(9–39), a GLP-1 receptor antagonist/inverse agonist, decreases basal cellular cAMP levels and insulin secretion [16]. These findings suggest that there is a tonic effect of GLP-1 receptor signaling in these islets. The effects were independent of calcium, as exendin-(9–39) did not affect basal or stimulated cytosolic calcium [16]. The fact that switching off the tonic effect of the GLP-1 receptor on cAMP can completely inhibit insulin secretion in islets lacking K_{ATP} channels despite the continued elevated cellular Ca^{2+} concentration points to a more important role of the amplifying pathway of insulin secretion than previously thought.

In addition, we found that exendin-(9–39) inhibited amino acids-stimulated insulin secretion in *SUR1*$^{-/-}$ islets and in wild-type islets that had been depolarized by high glucose (fig. 1). This suggests that the hypersensitivity to amino acids under depolarized conditions is mediated by GLP-1 receptor signaling. Further, in vivo treatment with exendin-(9–39) decreases the abnormally elevated fasting insulin/glucose ratio in *SUR1*$^{-/-}$ mice and corrects fasting hypoglycemia (fig. 2) [16].

These findings suggest that GLP-1 and its receptor play a role in the pathophysiology of K_{ATP} hyperinsulinism and further studies of the mechanisms involved may prove important for the development of new therapeutic targets for this condition.

Incretins in Acquired Hyperinsulinemic Hypoglycemic

Postprandial hyperinsulinemic hypoglycemia, also known as 'late dumping syndrome', is a severe complication of surgical procedures affecting nutrient delivery to the gastrointestinal tract in both children and adults. In children, postprandial

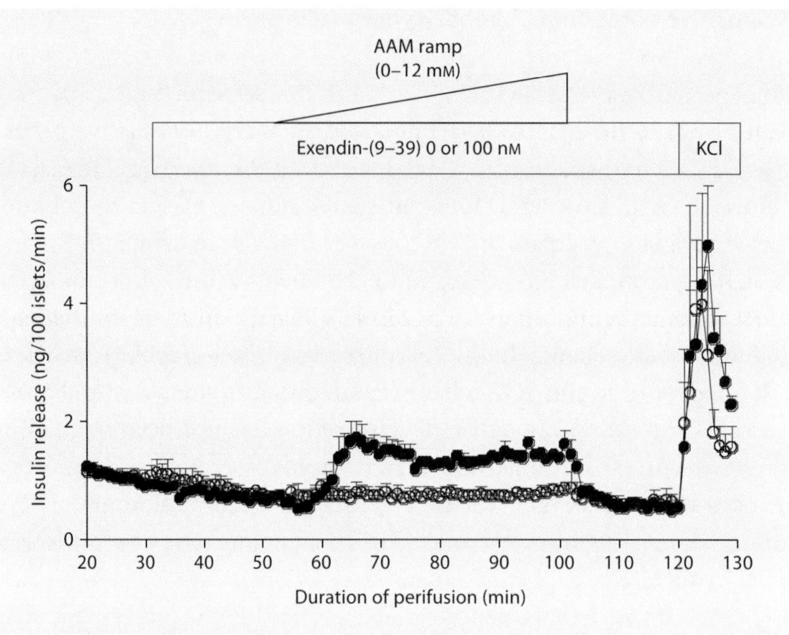

Fig. 1. Effect of the GLP-1 receptor antagonist exendin-(9–39) on insulin secretion in *SUR1*$^{-/-}$ mouse islets. Insulin secretion in response to a ramp of a physiologic mixture of amino acids in the presence (open circles) or absence (black circles) of exendin-(9–39) at a concentration of 100 nM. Reproduced with permission from [16].

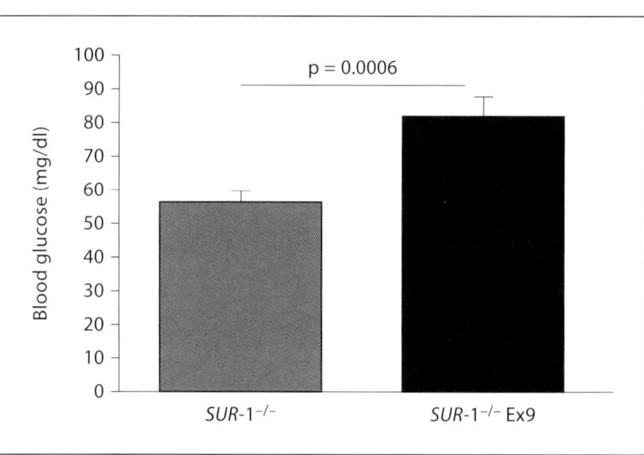

Fig. 2. Effect of the GLP-1 receptor antagonist exendin-(9–39) on *SUR1*$^{-/-}$ mice. Mice were treated with a continuous subcutaneous infusion of exendin-(9–39) at 150 pmol/kg/min or vehicle over 2 weeks. Fasting blood glucose in *SUR1*$^{-/-}$ mice during vehicle (gray) or exendin-(9–39) infusion (black). Reproduced with permission from [16].

hyperinsulinemic hypoglycemia is a frequent complication of Nissen fundoplication and other fundoplasty surgeries to treat severe gastroesophageal reflux. We estimate that one fourth of the children undergoing fundoplasty develop postprandial hypoglycemia [17]. In adults, postprandial hyperinsulinemic hypoglycemia is seen after gastrectomy and after Roux-en-Y gastric bypass bariatric surgery [9, 18, 19]. It is a matter of controversy as to whether this complication is frequent but not appropriately recognized, or a truly rare complication. A large study estimated that the risk of hypoglycemia or hypoglycemia-related conditions leading to hospitalization after Roux-en-Y is approximately 1% [20]. In contrast, there was no increase in hypoglycemia-related conditions after other bariatric surgeries such as banding procedures or vertical banding gastroplasty.

While the specific pathophysiologic mediators of hyperinsulinemic hypoglycemia after gastric surgery remain controversial, food intake in these individuals results in rapid elevations of plasma glucose, insulin, and glucagon with subsequent development of hypoglycemia during the later postprandial period (fig. 3a, b). An exaggerated secretion of GLP-1 in individuals with postprandial hyperinsulinemic hypoglycemia has been implicated in the pathophysiology of this condition (fig. 3c) [21, 22]. It remains controversial whether increased insulin secretion in this syndrome is due to: (1) observed increases in GLP-1 secretion, (2) altered responsiveness to GLP-1, or (3) cell-autonomous insulin secretion. Despite initial reports suggesting that expansion of beta-cell mass was involved in the pathogenesis of hyperinsulinemic hypoglycemia after gastric bypass [19, 23], others have refuted that theory [24]. Insulin response to intravenous glucose is normal, making it unlikely that the hyperinsulinemia following a meal is due to either a morphological or functional change in the endocrine pancreas [25]. Furthermore, in hyperinsulinemic hypoglycemia after gastric bypass, the metabolic abnormalities resolve when food is administered to the remnant stomach and allowed to pass through the native gastrointestinal tract rather than delivered through the bypassed tract [26]. These findings are consistent with an alteration in the GLP-1 response to a meal resulting in an exaggerated insulin response, rather than a beta-cell autonomous defect.

Diagnostic and Therapeutic Applications

G protein-coupled peptide hormone receptors play an increasing role in imaging and targeted therapy for neuroendocrine tumors. Overexpression of a specific receptor on tumor cells permits diagnostic (receptor-targeted scintigraphic tumor imaging) and therapeutic procedures using radiolabeled peptide analogs. The somatostatin receptors are one of the oldest examples of the application of this approach. These receptors are expressed in high density on neuroendocrine tumors and the use of somatostatin receptor scintigraphy is an integral part of the diagnostic procedures in patients with these types of tumors. The GLP-1 receptor is a new candidate for this approach.

Several tumors have been shown to express the GLP-1 receptor in high density in vitro, e.g. insulinomas, and at lower density, e.g. gastrinomas, pheochromocytomas,

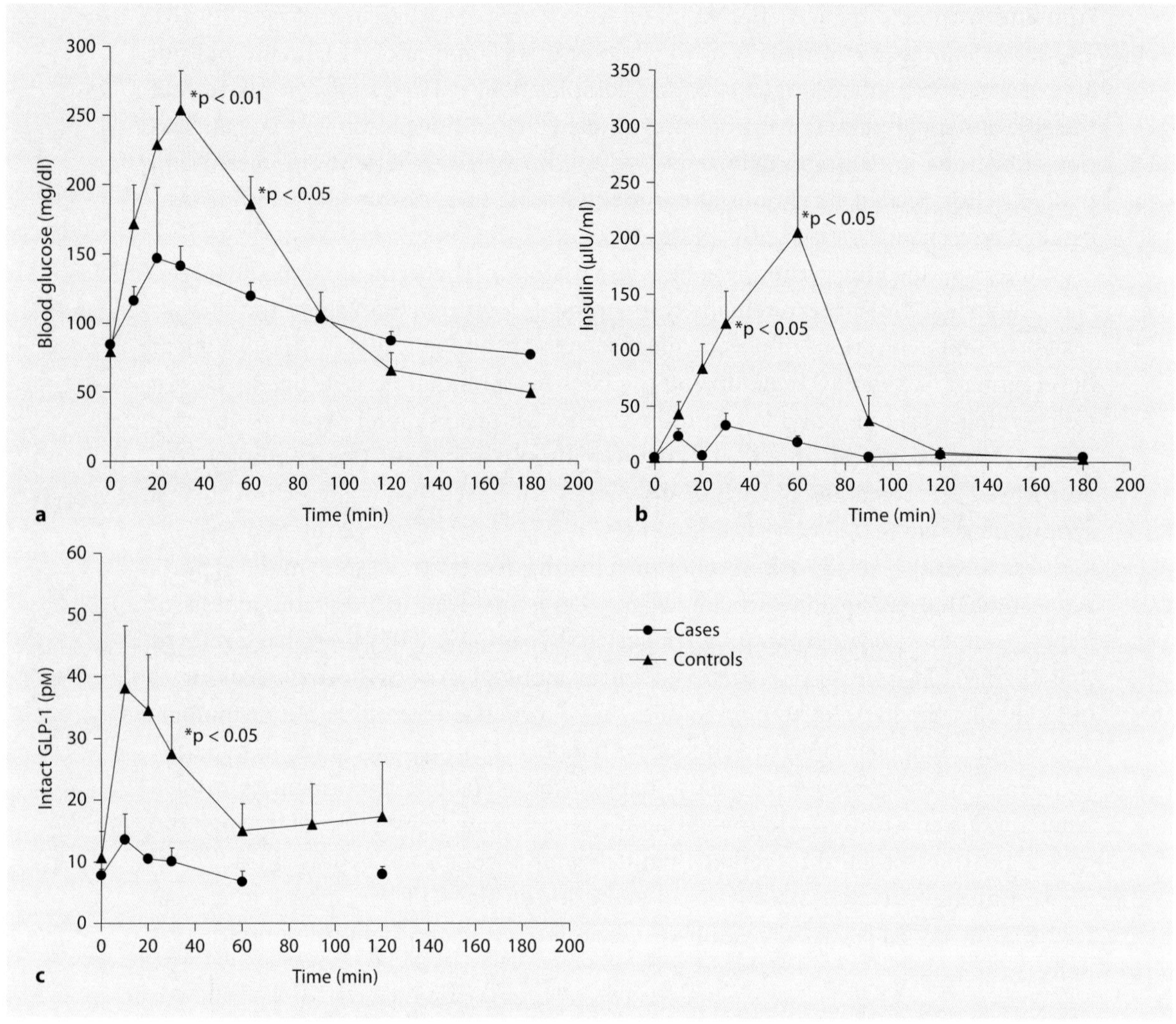

Fig. 3. Response to an oral glucose tolerance test in children with hyperinsulinemic hypoglycemia after Nissen fundoplication. **a** Mean blood glucose ± SEM in cases (solid triangles) and controls (solid circles) following oral glucose tolerance test (OGTT). **b** Mean plasma insulin ± SEM in cases and controls following OGTT. **c** Mean intact plasma GLP-1 ± SEM in cases and controls following OGTT. Reproduced with permission from [21].

paragangliomas, and medullary thyroid carcinomas. Because of the importance of preoperative localization of insulinomas and the poor performance of other imaging modalities, GLP-1 receptor scintigraphy provides an innovative approach to diagnosis. ^{111}In-DOTA-exendin-4 or ^{111}IN-DPTA-exendin-4 has successfully localized pancreatic and extrapancreatic insulinomas [27]. In addition, intraoperative localization with a gamma probe has been highly effective for in situ localization and successful tumor resection.

Future Directions

The recognition of the importance of incretin actions on the control of glucose metabolism has proven very useful in the development of new targets for the treatment of diabetes mellitus aimed at restoring incretin effects. New evidence suggests that the GLP-1 receptor may also be a useful diagnostic and therapeutic target for the management of individuals both with congenital K_{ATP}HI and with postgastric surgery acquired hyperinsulinemic hypoglycemia.

References

1 Girard J: The incretins: from the concept to their use in the treatment of type 2 diabetes. Part A: incretins: concept and physiological functions. Diabetes Metab 2008;34:550–559.

2 Hansotia T, Drucker DJ: GIP and GLP-1 as incretin hormones: lessons from single and double incretin receptor knockout mice. Regul Pept 2005;128: 125–134.

3 Edwards CM, Todd JF, Mahmoudi M, Wang Z, Wang RM, Ghatei MA, Bloom SR: Glucagon-like peptide 1 has a physiological role in the control of postprandial glucose in humans: studies with the antagonist exendin 9–39. Diabetes 1999;48: 86–93.

4 D'Alessio DA, Vogel R, Prigeon R, Laschansky E, Koerker D, Eng J, Ensinck JW: Elimination of the action of glucagon-like peptide 1 causes an impairment of glucose tolerance after nutrient ingestion by healthy baboons. J Clin Invest 1996;97: 133–138.

5 Nauck MA: Unraveling the science of incretin biology. Am J Med 2009;122:S3–S10.

6 Meier JJ, Goetze O, Anstipp J, Hagemann D, Holst JJ, Schmidt WE, Gallwitz B, Nauck MA: Gastric inhibitory polypeptide does not inhibit gastric emptying in humans. Am J Physiol Endocrinol Metab 2004;286:E621–E625.

7 Baggio LL, Drucker DJ: Biology of incretins: GLP-1 and GIP. Gastroenterology 2007;132:2131–2157.

8 Nauck MA, Heimesaat MM, Orskov C, Holst JJ, Ebert R, Creutzfeldt W: Preserved incretin activity of glucagon-like peptide 1 [7–36 amide] but not of synthetic human gastric inhibitory polypeptide in patients with type-2 diabetes mellitus. J Clin Invest 1993;91:301–307.

9 Toft-Nielsen M, Madsbad S, Holst JJ: Exaggerated secretion of glucagon-like peptide-1 (GLP-1) could cause reactive hypoglycaemia. Diabetologia 1998;41: 1180–1186.

10 Froud T, Faradji RN, Pileggi A, Messinger S, Baidal DA, Ponte GM, Cure PE, Monroy K, Mendez A, Selvaggi G, Ricordi C, Alejandro R: The use of exenatide in islet transplant recipients with chronic allograft dysfunction: safety, efficacy, and metabolic effects. Transplantation 2008;86:36–45.

11 Rickels MR, Naji A: Reactive hypoglycaemia following GLP-1 infusion in pancreas transplant recipients. Diabetes Obes Metab 2010;12:731–733.

12 Todd JF, Stanley SA, Roufosse CA, Bishop AE, Khoo B, Bloom SR, Meeran K: A tumour that secretes glucagon-like peptide-1 and somatostatin in a patient with reactive hypoglycaemia and diabetes. Lancet 2003;361:228–230.

13 Reimann F, Gribble FM: Glucose-sensing in glucagon-like peptide-1-secreting cells. Diabetes 2002;51:2757–2763.

14 Sidhu SS, Thompson DG, Warhurst G, Case RM, Benson RS: Fatty acid-induced cholecystokinin secretion and chagnes in intracellular Ca^{2+} in two enteroendocrine cell lines, STC-1 and GLUTag. J Physiol 2000;528:165–176.

15 Gribble FM, Williams L, Simpson AK, Reimann F: A novel glucose-sensing mechanism contributing to glucagon-like peptide-1 secretion from the GLUTag cell line. Diabetes 2003;52:1147–1154.

16 De Leon DD, Li C, Delson MI, Matschinsky FM, Stanley CA, Stoffers DA: Exendin-(9–39) corrects fasting hypoglycemia in SUR-1-/- mice by lowering cAMP in pancreatic beta-cells and inhibiting insulin secretion. J Biol Chem 2008;283:25786–25793.

17 Calabria AC, Gallagher PR, Simmons R, Blinman T, De Leon DD: Postoperative surveillance and detection of postprandial hypoglycemia after fundoplasty in children. J Pediatr 2011;159:597–601.

18 Gebhard B, Holst JJ, Biegelmayer C, Miholic J: Postprandial GLP-1, norepinephrine, and reactive hypoglycemia in dumping syndrome. Dig Dis Sci 2001;46:1915–1923.

19 Service GJ, Thompson GB, Service FJ, Andrews JC, Collazo-Clavell ML, Lloyd RV: Hyperinsulinemic hypoglycemia with nesidioblastosis after gastric-bypass surgery. N Engl J Med 2005;353:249–254.
20 Marsk R, Jonas E, Rasmussen F, Naslund E: Nationwide cohort study of post-gastric bypass hypoglycaemia including 5,040 patients undergoing surgery for obesity in 1986–2006 in Sweden. Diabetologia 2010;53:2307–2311.
21 Palladino AA, Sayed S, Levitt Katz LE, Gallagher PR, De Leon DD: Increased glucagon-like peptide-1 secretion and postprandial hypoglycemia in children after Nissen fundoplication. J Clin Endocrinol Metab 2009;94:39–44.
22 Goldfine AB, Mun EC, Devine E, Bernier R, Baz-Hecht M, Jones DB, Schneider BE, Holst JJ, Patti ME: Patients with neuroglycopenia after gastric bypass surgery have exaggerated incretin and insulin secretory responses to a mixed meal. J Clin Endocrinol Metab 2007;92:4678–4685.
23 Patti ME, McMahon G, Mun EC, Bitton A, Holst JJ, Goldsmith J, Hanto DW, Callery M, Arky R, Nose V, Bonner-Weir S, Goldfine AB: Severe hypoglycaemia post-gastric bypass requiring partial pancreatectomy: evidence for inappropriate insulin secretion and pancreatic islet hyperplasia. Diabetologia 2005;48:2236–2240.
24 Meier JJ, Butler AE, Galasso R, Butler PC: Hyperinsulinemic hypoglycemia after gastric bypass surgery is not accompanied by islet hyperplasia or increased beta-cell turnover. Diabetes Care 2006;29:1554–1559.
25 Kim SH, Abbasi F, Lamendola C, Reaven GM, McLaughlin T: Glucose-stimulated insulin secretion in gastric bypass patients with hypoglycemic syndrome: no evidence for inappropriate pancreatic beta-cell function. Obes Surg 2010;20:1110–1116.
26 McLaughlin T, Peck M, Holst J, Deacon C: Reversible hyperinsulinemic hypoglycemia after gastric bypass: a consequence of altered nutrient delivery. J Clin Endocrinol Metab 2010;95:1851–1855.
27 Christ E, Wild D, Forrer F, Brandle M, Sahli R, Clerici T, Gloor B, Martius F, Maecke H, Reubi JC: Glucagon-like peptide-1 receptor imaging for localization of insulinomas. J Clin Endocrinol Metab 2009;94:4398–4405.

Diva D. De León, MD
Division of Endocrinology/Diabetes
The Children's Hospital of Philadelphia
34th Street and Civic Center Boulevard
Philadelphia, PA 19104 (USA)
Tel. +1 215 590 3420, E-Mail deleon@email.chop.edu

Stanley CA, De León DD (eds): Monogenic Hyperinsulinemic Hypoglycemia Disorders.
Front Diabetes. Basel, Karger, 2012, vol 21, pp 87–99

Glutamate Dehydrogenase: Structure, Regulation, and Its Role in Insulin Homeostasis

Thomas James Smith

Donald Danforth Plant Science Center, Saint Louis, Mo., USA

Abstract

This chapter reviews the structure and allosteric regulation of glutamate dehydrogenase (GDH). For decades, it was known that mammalian GDH was regulated by a wide array of metabolites, but the reason for such regulation was not at all clear. The demonstration that hyperinsulinism/hyperammonemia (HHS) is caused by the loss of some of this regulation, for the first time, demonstrated that GDH regulation was essential for insulin homeostasis. Presented here are the atomic details for this complex network of allosteric regulation and how such information can lead to development of pharmaceutical agents that might not only be useful in treating HHS, but may also have utility as anticancer agents.

Glutamate dehydrogenase (GDH) is found in all organisms and catalyzes the reversible oxidative deamination of L-glutamate to 2-oxoglutarate using NAD^+ and/or $NADP^+$ as the coenzyme(s) [1]. GDH is a homohexameric enzyme with subunits comprised of approximately 500 residues in animals. While the chemical details of the enzymatic reaction have been tightly conserved through the epochs, only GDH from animal sources is allosterically regulated by a wide array of metabolites. Structural studies have shown that GDH is a highly dynamic enzyme and that allosteric regulation is likely mediated by control of conformational changes that occur during catalysis. While this complex network of allosteric regulation has been known for decades, only recently has the metabolic role for allosteric control of GDH been suggested by the finding that the hyperinsulinism/hyperammonemia syndrome (HHS) is due to the loss of GTP inhibition. Patients with HHS have increased beta-cell responsiveness to leucine and susceptibility to hypoglycemia following high-protein meals [2]. We have identified several lead compounds that inhibit the HHS form of GDH and show promise in controlling this disease.

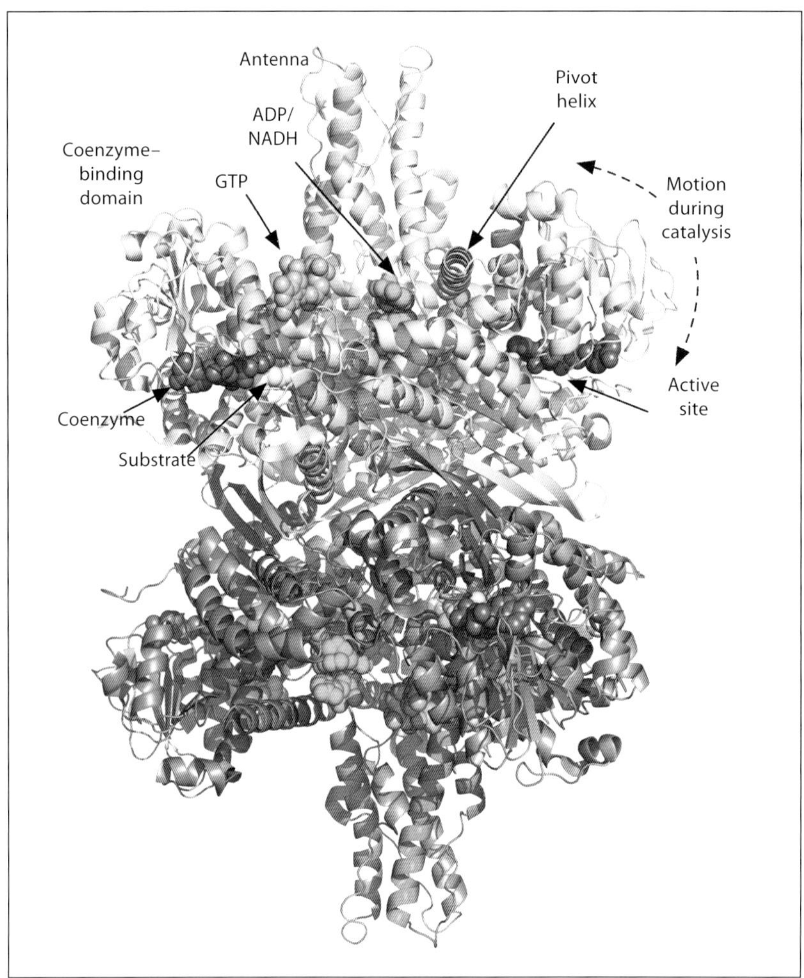

Fig. 1. Structure of mammalian GDH. Shown here is a ribbon diagram of the homohexamer of GDH. Noted are the locations of the various substrate and allosteric ligand binding sites.

Structure of Animal Glutamate Dehydrogenase

The structure of GDH (fig. 1) is essentially two trimers of subunits stacked directly on top of each other with each subunit being composed of at least three domains [3–6]. The bottom domain makes extensive contacts with a subunit from the other trimer. Resting on top of this domain is the 'NAD-binding domain' that has the conserved nucleotide-binding motif. Animal GDH has a long protrusion, 'antenna', rising above the NAD-binding domain that is not found in bacteria, plants, fungi, and the vast majority of protists. The antenna from each subunit lies immediately behind the adjacent counter-clockwise neighbor within the trimer. Since these intertwined antennae are only found in the forms of GDH that are allosterically regulated by numerous ligands, it is reasonable to speculate that it plays an important role in regulation.

Glutamate Dehydrogenase Dynamics

From the structures of GDH with and without active site ligands, it is possible to observe the opening and closing of the active site cleft and some of the large conformational changes that occur throughout the hexamer during each catalytic cycle [3–6]. The substrate binds to the deep recesses of the cleft between the coenzyme-binding domain and the lower domain. The coenzyme binds along the coenzyme-binding domain surface of the cleft. Upon binding, the coenzyme-binding domain rotates by approximately 18° to firmly close down upon the substrate and coenzyme. As the catalytic cleft closes, the base of each of the long ascending helices in the antenna appears to rotate out in a counter-clockwise manner to push against the 'pivot' helix of the adjacent subunit. There is a short helix in the descending loop of the antenna that becomes distended and shorter as the mouth closes in a manner akin to an extending spring. The 'pivot helix' rotates in a counter-clockwise manner along the helical axes as well as counter-clockwise around the trimer threefold axis. Finally, the entire hexamer seems to compress as the mouth closes. The three pairs of subunits that sit on top of each other move as a rigid unit towards each other, compressing the cavity at the core of the hexamer. Therefore, it is quite clear that the GDH active site cleft does not open and close in isolation, but rather this motion involves the entire hexamer.

Allosteric Regulation of Glutamate Dehydrogenase

GTP/ATP Inhibition

GTP, and to a much lesser extent ATP, is a potent inhibitor of GDH (fig. 2). This inhibition represents a feedback mechanism that dampens GDH oxidative deamination when the TCA cycle is highly active. It is logical that GTP is used to communicate this GDH regulation rather than ATP, as most of the ATP in the mitochondria is produced from oxidative phosphorylation that is driven by the potential across the mitochondrial membrane created by NADH oxidation. Therefore, the number of ATP molecules generated from one turn of the TCA cycle can vary between 1 and 29. In contrast, one GTP is generated per turn of the TCA cycle and there is a slow mitochondria/cytoplasm exchange rate. Therefore, the GTP/GDP ratio within the mitochondria is a much better metric of TCA cycle activity than the ATP/ADP ratio.

GTP binds at the base of the antenna (fig. 1), wedged between the NAD-binding domain and the pivot helix [3, 4]. This binding site is only available for GTP binding when the catalytic cleft is closed. Therefore, it is likely that GTP binding to the 'closed' conformation makes it more difficult for the 'mouth' to open and release product. This is entirely consistent with the finding that GTP inhibits the reaction by slowing down product release and concomitantly increasing the affinity of substrate and coenzyme [7]. The majority of the interactions between GTP and GDH are via the gamma-phosphate moiety and explains why, in terms of inhibition, GTP>>GDP>GMP [8].

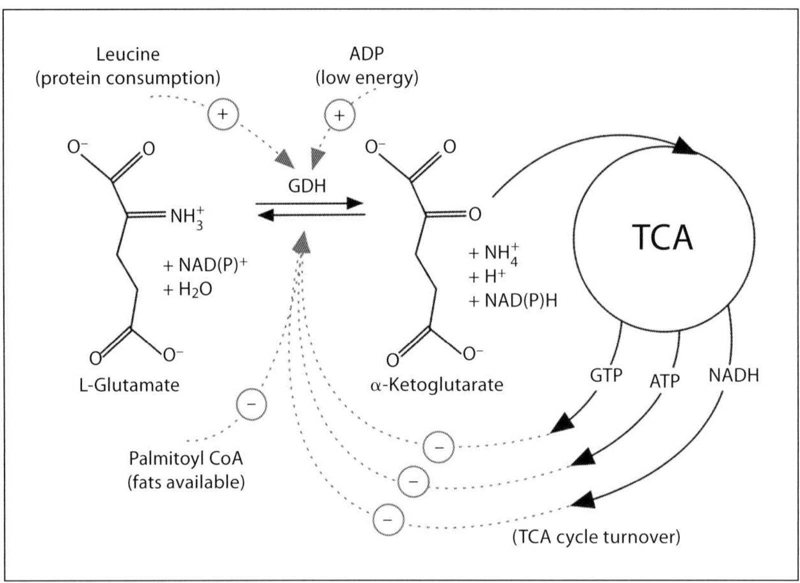

Fig. 2. Schematic of the allosteric regulation of GDH.

NADH Inhibition

NADH has been shown to bind to a second site on GDH, inhibiting the reaction directly and is agonistic with the inhibitor, GTP. In the presence of glutamate and/or GTP, NADH binds more tightly and the stoichiometry increases from 1 to 2 per subunit [9]. This second coenzyme site strongly favors NADH over NADPH with Kd of 57 and 700 μM, respectively, suggesting that NAD(H) is the more pertinent coenzyme with regard to allosteric regulation. This also suggests that this type of regulation is tied to catabolism since NADPH is involved in anabolic reactions in the cell while NADH is generated by the TCA cycle.

However, the possible in vivo role of NADH inhibition is less clear. In mammalian mitochondria the concentrations of NAD(H) and NADP(H) are approximately 0.5–2.0 mM [10]. However, activity of the transhydrogenase transfers much of the reductive power of NADH to NADPH. The mitochondrial NADH/NAD^+ ratio was estimated to be approximately 0.2 and the NADPH/$NADP^+$ ratio was approximately 200 [11]. These results suggest that the range of NADH concentration is approximately 0.083–0.33 mM. NADH inhibition is observed at concentrations above 0.2 mM (e.g. see [12]), but only reaches approximately 50% inhibition at 1 mM NADH. Therefore, if NADH inhibition is physiologically relevant, it seems more likely that its purpose is to synergistically enhance GTP inhibition. It may be that high flux through the TCA cycle would generate elevated NADH and GTP levels that, together, act to keep GDH in a tonic state.

The second NADH site lies directly behind the pivot helix and overlaps with the ADP-binding site [4, 6]. The adenosine-ribose moiety of NADH exactly matched that of ADP. While it seems to be a paradox that an inhibitor, NADH, and activator, ADP, bind to the same site, the nicotinamide moiety of NADH binds down between the adjacent subunits and perhaps has an inhibitory effect on the conformational changes associated with catalytic turnover.

ADP Activation

While the actions of ADP on GDH activity are complex, it essentially acts in a manner opposite to GTP. In the oxidative deamination reaction, ADP activates at high pH, but inhibits at low pH with either NAD^+ or $NADP^+$ as the coenzyme. In the reductive amination reaction, ADP is a potent activator at low pH and low substrate concentration. At pH 6.0, high concentrations of alpha-KG and NADH, but not NADPH, inhibit the reaction. This substrate inhibition is alleviated by ADP [13]. Therefore, while GTP and glutamate bind synergistically with NADH to inhibit GDH, ADP activates the reaction by decreasing the affinity of the enzyme for a coenzyme at the active site. Therefore, under conditions where product release is the rate-limiting step (i.e. substrate inhibition), ADP activates by facilitating catalytic turnover. Since substrate (2-oxoglutarate) inhibition in the reductive amination reaction is only observed using NADH as coenzyme, this inhibition may be due to NADH binding to the second coenzyme site. Further, it has been suggested that ADP activation under these conditions may be due to ADP displacement of NADH from the second allosteric site [8].

ADP binds behind the NAD-binding domain and immediately under the pivot helix [6]. This interaction might facilitate the rotation of the NAD-binding domain and the release of product [6]. To test this, R459 (R463 in human GDH) was mutated to an alanine and this led to a loss in ADP activation. This suggests that ADP activates the reaction by 'pulling' on the back of the NAD-binding domain to help open the active site cleft and facilitating product release.

The physiological role of ADP activation is easily understood; when the energy level of the mitochondria is low and ADP levels are high, the catabolism of glutamate is facilitated for energy production.

Fatty Acid Regulation

GDH is strongly inhibited by palmitoyl-CoA, with an ED_{50} of approximately 30 nM [14, 15]. This inhibition is allosteric in that ADP and leucine abrogate palmitoyl-CoA effects and there is likely only one binding site per subunit [14]. With this high binding affinity, GDH can successfully compete with the other mitochondrial proteins for palmitoyl-CoA. This pattern of regulation suggests that the catabolism of amino acids via GDH is downregulated when there are sufficient levels of fatty acids in the mitochondrion. When the mitochondrion has been depleted of fatty acids and its energy state is low (i.e. high ADP levels), only then will amino acids be catabolized. The binding site for palmitoyl-CoA is unknown at this time.

Leucine Activation

Leucine, as well as some other monocarboxylic acids, has been shown to activate mammalian GDH by facilitating coenzyme release in a manner similar to ADP, but probably not via the same binding site [16]. Since leucine is a weak substrate for GDH, one binding site is the active site. It is unclear whether there is a second allosteric leucine-binding site, and a possible location for it is not known.

The choice of leucine as a regulator is likely not accidental since leucine is the most abundant amino acid in protein (10%). Leucine levels, therefore, provide a good metric of protein abundance. For this reason, leucine serves as an effective signal to GDH that there has been pulse of free amino acids from protein digestion.

Together, these allosteric regulators appear to use GDH to establish a priority in the mitochondria for catabolism (fig. 2). If fats (e.g. palmitoyl-CoA) are available, or if the TCA cycle is churning away and making GTP, ATP, and NADH, then GDH is kept in a tonic state. Only if there is a bolus of amino acids, as sensed by an elevated leucine concentration, and/or if the mitochondrion is in a low-energy state, as per high ADP concentrations, will GDH be released from its turgor and catabolism of amino acids will be allowed. Therefore, GDH allosteric regulation seems to infer that amino acid catabolism will occur mainly when other carbon sources have been depleted.

Evolution of Glutamate Dehydrogenase Allostery

Animal GDH contains an internal 48-residue insert (the antenna; fig. 1), compared to GDH from the other kingdoms, and is allosterically regulated by a wide array of metabolites. It is not at all clear, however, when and why the antenna evolved and whether it was linked to the complex pattern of allostery in animal GDH. Tetrahymena GDH (tGDH) likely represents an evolutionary missing link since it too has this approximate 48-residue insert that forms the antenna in animal GDH. Like mammalian GDH, tGDH is activated by ADP and inhibited by palmitoyl-CoA [17]. However, like bacterial GDH, tGDH is coenzyme specific [NAD(H)] and is not regulated by GTP or leucine. Therefore, with regard to allosteric regulation, tGDH is indeed an evolutionary 'missing link' between bacterial and animal GDH.

To directly address the role of the antenna on allosteric regulation, a number of hybrid forms of GDH were analyzed (table 1). From structural studies, it was clear that the antenna was not directly involved in ADP or GTP binding [3, 4, 6]. However, when the antenna on human GDH was replaced by the short loop found in bacterial GDH, the enzyme lost GTP, ADP, and palmitoyl-CoA regulation [17]. When the ciliate antenna was spliced onto human GDH, this hybrid enzyme had a fully functional repertoire of mammalian allostery. This demonstrated that the antenna is essential for communicating allosteric regulation by GTP and ADP while not being directly involved in their binding. Evolutionarily, this also demonstrated that the primitive

Table 1. Allosteric regulation of human, bacterial, and tGDH antenna hybrids

	Human GDH	Human GDH minus antenna	tGDH	Human GDH + tGDH
GTP inhibition	+	–	–	+
Palmitoyl-CoA inhibition	+	–	+	+
ADP activation	+	–	+	+
Leucine activation	+	+	–	+

antenna in ciliate GDH is capable of transmitting the GTP inhibitory signal, but GTP regulation was apparently not needed in the ciliates.

This suggests that GDH allostery evolved in at least a two-step process. The first evolutionary step may have been due to the changing functions of the cellular organelles as the ciliates branched off from the other kingdoms. In the other eukaryotic organisms, all fatty acid oxidation occurs in the peroxisomes [18]. In the ciliates, fatty acid oxidation is shared between the peroxisomes and the mitochondria [19]. Eventually, all medium- and long-chain fatty oxidation moved into the mitochondria in animals. Therefore, it appears that GDH regulation evolved in response to fatty acid and amino acid oxidation being brought into the same subcellular compartment.

The second step of evolution was to add leucine and GTP allostery as animals needed even more sophisticated and rapid-response regulation of GDH activity. As a likely response to the growing complexity of multiorgan animals, two very important regulators, leucine and GTP, were added to the allosteric regulatory repertoire. In the pancreas, GDH needs to be activated when amino acids (protein) are ingested to promote insulin secretion and appropriate anabolic effects on peripheral tissues. In the glucose-fed state, triphosphate levels are high and GDH needs to be inhibited to redirect amino acids into glutamine synthesis in order to amplify insulin release. In the liver, GDH needs to be suppressed when other fuels, such as fatty acids, are available; however, it needs to be increased when surplus amino acids are oxidized. To this end, mammals added layers of regulation onto ciliate GDH to include leucine activation and GTP inhibition.

Possible Therapeutics for Glutamate Dehydrogenase-Mediated Insulin Disorders

As discussed in other chapters, HHS is caused by loss of GTP regulation of GDH [20–22]. This disease causes multiorgan pathology (fig. 3), hypersecretion of insulin following high-protein meals [2], elevation of serum ammonium concentration likely due to enhanced glutamate oxidation and impaired urea synthesis, and effects

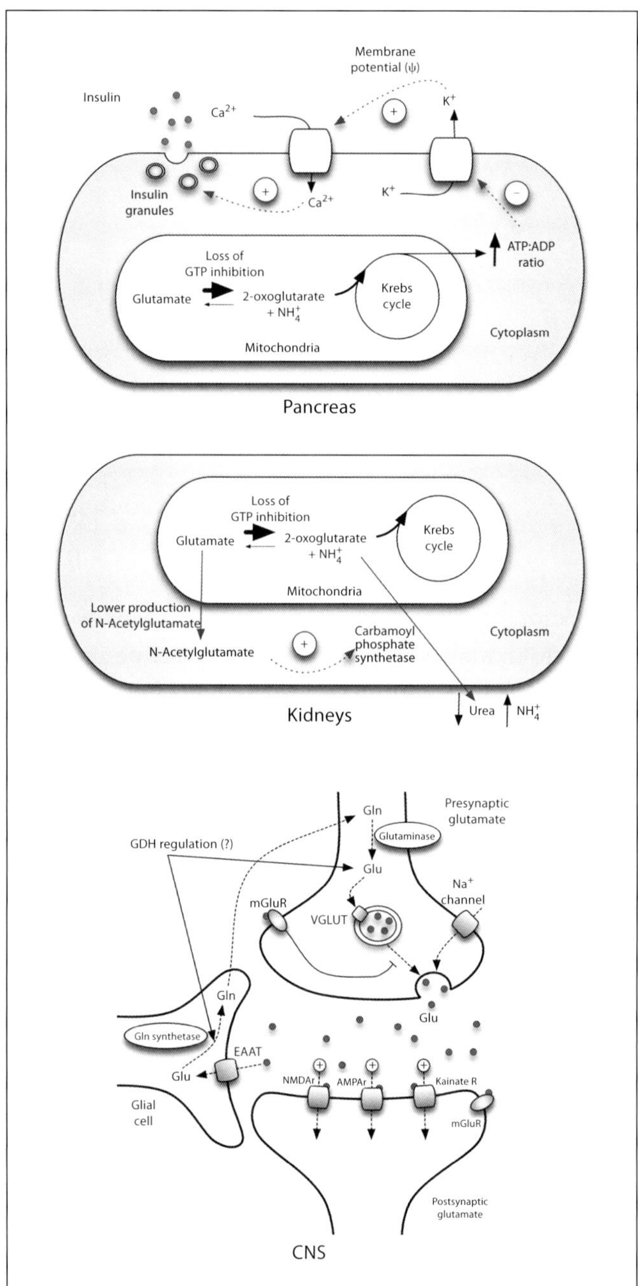

Fig. 3. Summary of the multi-organ pathology of HHS. The top figure shows how hyperactive GDH stimulates insulin secretion from the pancreas. The middle figure shows how HHS disrupts the production of urea in the kidneys and the bottom figure shows how the dysregulated form of HHS GDH may cause central nervous system (CNS) pathology.

on the central nervous system as indicated by a high correlation between HHS and childhood-onset epilepsy, learning disabilities, and seizures [23]. The current treatment for HHS is to pharmaceutically control insulin secretion (e.g. diazoxide, a potassium channel activator), but this does not address the serum ammonium and

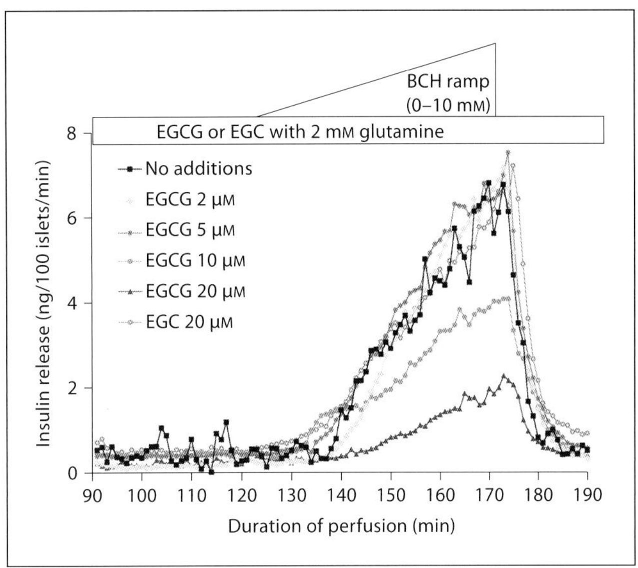

Fig. 4. Effects of EGCG on GDH-mediated stimulation of insulin secretion. In this assay, the beta-cells were run down prior to the administration of glutamine and polyphenols (or buffer). Under these conditions, catabolism of glutamate via GDH is the main carbon source for the cells. When the leucine analog BCH is added, GDH is stimulated, ATP is generated, and the beta-cells secrete insulin. As shown here, EGCG but not epigallocatechin (EGC) is able to block this GDH-stimulated insulin secretion in a dose-dependent manner.

central nervous system pathologies. To directly target the hyperactive form of GDH rather than just control the hypersecretion of insulin, a high throughput search of GDH inhibitors was performed, leading to two bioactive compounds found in green tea.

Green tea is a significant source of a type of flavonoids called catechins, which include epigallocatechin gallate (EGCG), epigallocatechin, epicatechin gallate (ECG), and epicatechin. One 200-ml cup of green tea supplies 140, 65, 28, and 17 mg of these polyphenols, respectively. Of the four major catechins found in green tea, only two showed inhibitory activity against GDH: ECG and EGCG. EGCG and ECG allosterically inhibit purified animal GDH in vitro with a nanomolar ED_{50}. Since epicatechin or epigallocatechin were not active against GDH, but have the same antioxidant activity as ECG and EGCG, the antioxidant property of these catechins cannot be relevant to GDH inhibition. EGCG inhibition is noncompetitive and, similar to GTP inhibition, is abrogated by leucine, BCH, and ADP. As with GTP inhibition and ADP activation [17], EGCG does not inhibit the 'antenna-less' form of GDH, and thus provides further evidence that EGCG is an allosteric inhibitor. Most importantly, EGCG inhibits HHS GDH mutants as effectively as wild-type [24], making it a possible therapeutic lead compound.

The next step was to ascertain whether EGCG could inhibit GDH in tissue (fig. 4). GDH plays a major role in leucine-stimulated insulin secretion by controlling glutaminolysis [25, 26]. Therefore, EGCG was tested on pancreatic beta-cells using the perifusion assay [24]. EGCG, but not epigallocatechin, blocked the GDH-mediated stimulation of insulin secretion by the beta-cells, but did not have any effect on insulin secretion, glucose oxidation, or cellular respiration during glucose stimulation where GDH is known to not play a major role in the regulation of insulin secretion. Therefore, EGCG is indeed a specific inhibitor of GDH both in vitro and in situ, and ongoing studies are evaluating whether it is similarly active in vivo.

Other Applications of Glutamate Dehydrogenase Inhibitors

More recent studies on glioblastoma cells have demonstrated that EGCG inhibition of GDH might have even broader utility than just with HHS. Increased glucose and glutamine utilization are hallmarks of tumor metabolism [27]. The phosphatidylinositol 3′-kinase/Akt pathway is enhanced in many human tumors and upregulates glucose uptake and utilization [28]. c-Myc, on the other hand, upregulates glutamine utilization by increasing cell surface transporters and enzymes [29]. At least in vitro, the enhanced utilization of one of these carbon sources also makes the cells sensitive to its withdrawal [30]. Using our results on EGCG, it was demonstrated that EGCG sensitizes glioblastoma cells to glucose withdrawal and to inhibitors of Akt signaling and glycolysis [31]. Indeed, the addition of EGCG mirrored the effects of knocking out GDH in the tissue. Therefore, these results suggest that anticancer therapy that combines GDH inhibitors with those that inhibit glucose utilization could be very effective in treating tumors.

Subsequent work also demonstrated EGCG inhibition of GDH activity may be useful in treating the tuberous sclerosis complex (TSC) disorder [32]. The TSC disorder is characterized by benign tumors due to the loss of either TSC1 or TSC2 and the subsequent hyperactivation of the mammalian target of rapamycin. Inhibitors of mammalian target of rapamycin can decrease the size of TSC-associated tumors, but only in a cytostatic manner. The TSC1/$2^{-/-}$ cells are hypersensitive to glucose deprivation and highly dependent on GDH-mediated catabolism of glutamine. Nearly all of the TSC1/$2^{-/-}$ cells that were deprived of glucose and given rapamycin died upon administration of EGCG. As expected, EGCG effects were reversed if GDH-mediated oxidation of glutamate was circumvented by the addition of 2-oxoglutarate, pyruvate, or aminooxyacetate. This is an exciting result since attempts to make glutamine analogs have only yielded toxic compounds.

Other Novel Inhibitors of Glutamate Dehydrogenase

High-throughput screening was used to find additional compounds that might have better efficacy and/or pharmacokinetics than EGCG/ECG [33, 34], resulting in the identification of small hydrophobic compounds: bithionol, hexachlorophene, GW5074, and diethylstilbestrol. Structural studies demonstrated that these compounds bind to subunit interfaces in the enzyme that are critical for conformational transitions [34]. HCP binds deep in the core of the enzyme and forms a ring in the inner cavity of the hexamer. The majority of the interactions between HCP and GDH are hydrophobic and form a 'chain link' of aromatic stacking interactions. Bithionol and GW5074 bind halfway between the core and the exterior of the hexamer. Unlike HCP, all six drug molecules are associated with separate subunits and form pairs that are related by the hexameric twofold axes. The binding environments of these two drugs are nearly identical. They both form dimers and interact with hydrophobic residues and the aliphatic portions of the polar and charged side chains of residues.

All three of these compounds bind to interfaces between the subunits, distal to the active site, that expand and contract as the catalytic mouth opens and closes [34]. This is very much the same theme as we observed with the naturally occurring allosteric regulators – regulation via modulation of protein dynamics. Interestingly, the original form of GDH (i.e. bacterial) apparently found it kinetically advantageous to undergo these sweeping conformational changes during each catalytic event. Such large conformational changes open up a number of pockets and clefts in the protein where ligands can bind to affect catalytic turnover. Therefore, it appears that the original design for GDH yielded a very mobile enzyme that evolution took advantage of for subsequent allosteric regulation. Similarly, we too can take advantage of this complex network of conformational changes to create allosteric inhibitors without resorting to substrate/coenzyme analogs that are likely to be toxic.

Conclusions

GDH may have initially evolved these large conformational changes to improve catalytic efficiency [35]. This complex ballet of motion creates numerous sites on the protein where ligands can bind and modulate catalytic activity. Through this allosteric regulation, new functions and roles for GDH were created for GDH rather than needing to create entirely new gene products to accommodate the changing needs of the cell (e.g. linkage between amino acid catabolism and insulin secretion). While it seems that GDH regulation is overly complex for an enzyme involved in such a mundane chemical reaction, it is in fact remarkable that a single enzyme can control levels of glutamate in the central nervous system, ureagenesis in the liver, and insulin secretion in the pancreas. The findings that EGCG can effectively control GDH activity in tissue are very promising, but its low absorption and rapid catabolism in vivo remain problematic. Ongoing studies are using this panel of new allosteric inhibitors as scaffolds for further drug design that will hopefully lead to therapeutics that can directly control GDH activity in HHS.

References

1 Hudson RC, Daniel RM: L-Glutamate dehydrogenases: distribution, properties and mechanism. Comp Biochem Physiol 1993;106B:767–792.
2 Hsu BY, Kelly A, Thornton PS, Greenberg CR, Dilling LA, Stanley CA: Protein-sensitive and fasting hypoglycemia in children with the hyperinsulinism/hyperammonemia syndrome. J Pediatr 2001; 138:383–389.
3 Peterson PE, Smith TJ: The structure of bovine glutamate dehydrogenase provides insights into the mechanism of allostery. Structure Fold Des 1999;7: 769–782.
4 Smith TJ, Peterson PE, Schmidt T, Fang J, Stanley C: Structures of bovine glutamate dehydrogenase complexes elucidate the mechanism of purine regulation. J Mol Biol 2001;307:707–720.
5 Smith TJ, Schmidt T, Fang J, Wu J, Siuzdak G, Stanley CA: The structure of apo human glutamate dehydrogenase details subunit communication and allostery. J Mol Biol 2002;318:765–777.
6 Banerjee S, Schmidt T, Fang J, Stanley CA, Smith TJ: Structural studies on ADP activation of mammalian glutamate dehydrogenase and the evolution of regulation. Biochemistry 2003;42:3446–3456.
7 Frieden C: Different structural forms of reversibly dissociated glutamic dehydrogenase: relation between enzymatic activity and molecular weight. Biochem Biophys Res Comm 1963;10:410–415.
8 Frieden C: Glutamate dehydrogenase VI. Survey of purine nucleotides and other effects on the enzyme from various sources. J Biol Chem 1965;240:2028–2037.
9 Koberstein R, Sund H: The influence of ADP, GTP and L-glutamate on the binding of the reduced coenzyme to beef-liver glutamate dehydrogenase. Eur J Biochem 1973;36:545–552.
10 Lenartowicz E: A complex effect of arsenite on the formation of alpha-ketoglutarate in rate liver mitochondria. Arch Biochem Biophys 1990;283:388–396.
11 Hoek JB, Rydström J: Physiological roles of nicotinamide nucleotide transhydrogenase. Biochem J 1988;254:1–10.
12 Batra SP, Colman RF: Isolation and identification of cysteinyl peptide labeled by 6-[(4-bromo-2, 3-dioxobutyl)thio]-6-deaminoadenosine 5′-diphosphate in the reduced diphosphopyridine nucleotide inhibitory site of glutamate dehydrogenase. Biochemistry 1986; 25:3508–3515.
13 Bailey JS, Bell ET, Bell JE: Regulation of bovine glutamate dehydrogenase. J Biol Chem 1982; 257:5579–5583.
14 Fahien LA, Kmiotek E: Regulation of glutamate dehydrogenase by palmitoyl-coenzyme A. Arch Biochem Biophys 1981;212:247–253.
15 Fang J, Macmullen C, Smith TJ, Stanley CA: Expression, purification, and characterization of human glutamate dehydrogenase (GDH) regulatory mutations associated with a dominantly-expressed congenital hyperinsulinism/hyperammonemia syndrome. Biochem J 2001;363:81–87.
16 Prough RA, Culver JM, Fisher HF: The mechanism of activation of glutamate dehydrogenase-catalyzed reactions by two different, cooperatively bound activators. J Biol Chem 1973;248:8528–8533.
17 Allen A, Kwagh J, Fang J, Stanley CA, Smith TJ: Evolution of glutamate dehydrogenase regulation of insulin homeostasis is an example of molecular exaptation. Biochemistry 2004;43:14431–14443.
18 Gerhardt B: Fatty acid degradation in plants. Prog Lipid Res 1992;31:417–446.
19 Muller M, Hogg JF, De Duve C: Distribution of tricarboxylic acid cycle enzymes and glyoxylate cycle enzymes between mitochondria and peroxisomes in Tetrahymena pyriformis. J Biol Chem 1968;243: 5385–5395.
20 Stanley CA, Lieu YK, Hsu BY, Burlina AB, Greenberg CR, Hopwood NJ, Perlman K, Rich BH, Zammarchi E, Poncz M: Hyperinsulinism and hyperammonemia in infants with regulatory mutations of the glutamate dehydrogenase gene. N Engl J Med 1998;338:1352–1357.
21 Stanley CA, Fang J, Kutyna K, Hsu BYL, Ming JE, Glaser B, Poncz M: Molecular basis and characterization of the hyperinsulinism/hyperammonemia syndrome of the glutamate dehydrogenase gene. Diabetes 2000;49:667–673.
22 MacMullen C, Fang J, Hsu BYL, Kelly A, de Lonlay-Debeney P, Saudubray JM, Ganguly A, Smith TJ, Stanley CA: The Hyperinsulinism/hyperammonemia Contributing Investigators: Hyperinsulinism/hyperammonemia syndrome in children with regulatory mutations in the inhibitory guanosine triphosphate-binding domain of glutamate dehydrogenase. J Clin Endocrinol Metab 2001;86:1782–1787.
23 Bahi-Buisson N, Roze E, Dionisi C, Escande F, Valayannopoulos V, Feillet F, Heinrichs C: Neurological aspects of hyperinsulinism-hyperammonaemia syndrome. Dev Med Child Neurol 2008;50: 945–949.
24 Li C, Allen A, Kwagh K, Doliba NM, Qin W, Najafi H, Collins HW, Matschinsky FM, Stanley CA, Smith TJ: Green tea polyphenols modulate insulin secretion by inhibiting glutamate dehydrogenase. J Biol Chem 2006;281:10214–10221.

25 Li C, Buettger C, Kwagh J, Matter A, Daihkin Y, Nissiam I, Collins HW, Yudkoff M, Stanley CA, Matschinsky FM: A signaling role of glutamine in insulin secretion. J Biol Chem 2004;279:13393–13401.

26 Li C, Najafi H, Daikhin Y, Nissim I, Collins HW, Yudkoff M, Matschinsky FM, Stanley CA: Regulation of leucine stimulated insulin secretion and glutamine metabolism in isolated rat islets. J Biol Chem 2003;278:2853–2858.

27 Kim JW, Dang CV: Cancer's molecular sweet tooth and the Warburg effect. Cancer Res 2006;66: 8927–8930.

28 Elstrom RL, Bauer DE, Buzzai M, Karnauskas R, Harris MH, Plas DR, Zhuang H, Cinalli RM, Alavi A, Rudin CM, Thompson CB: Akt stimulates aerobic glycolysis in cancer cells. Cancer Res 2004;64: 3892–3899.

29 Wise DR, DeBerardinis RJ, Mancuso A, Sayed N, Zhang XY, Pfeiffer HK, Nissim I, Daikhin E, Yudkoff M, McMahon SB, Thompson CB: Myc regulates a transcriptional program that stimulates mitochondrial glutaminolysis and leads to glutamine addiction. Proc Natl Acad Sci USA 2008;105: 18782–18787.

30 Buzzai M, Bauer DE, Jones RG, Deberardinis RJ, Hatzivassiliou G, Elstrom RL, Thompson CB: The glucose dependence of Akt-transformed cells can be reversed by pharmacologic activation of fatty acid β-oxidation. Oncogene 2005;24:4165–4173.

31 Yang C, Sudderth J, Dang T, Bachoo RG, McDonald JG, DeBerardinis RJ: Glioblastoma cells require glutamate dehydrogenase to survive impairments of glucose metabolism or Akt signaling. Cancer Res 2009;69:7986–7993.

32 Choo AY, Kim SG, Vander Heiden MG, Mahoney SJ, Vu H, Yoon S-O, Cantley LC, Blenis J: Glucose addiction of TSC null cells is caused by failed mTORC1-dependent balancing of metabolic demand with supply. Molecular Cell 2010;38:487–499.

33 Li M, Allen A, Smith TJ: High throughput screening reveals several new classes of glutamate dehydrogenase inhibitors. Biochemistry 2007;46:15089–15102.

34 Li M, Smith CJ, Walker MT, Smith TJ: Novel inhibitors complexed with glutamate dehydrogenase: allosteric regulation by control of protein dynamics. J Biol Chem 2009;284:22988–23000.

35 Smith TJ, Stanley CA: Untangling the glutamate dehydrogenase allosteric nightmare. Trends Biochem Sci 2008;33:557–564.

Thomas James Smith, PhD
Donald Danforth Plant Science Center
975 North Warson Road
Saint Louis, MO 63132 (USA)
Tel. +1 314 587 1451, E-Mail tsmith@danforthcenter.org

Stanley CA, De León DD (eds): Monogenic Hyperinsulinemic Hypoglycemia Disorders.
Front Diabetes. Basel, Karger, 2012, vol 21, pp 100–111

Congenital Hyperinsulinism Due to Activating Mutations of Glutamate Dehydrogenase: The Hyperinsulinism/Hyperammonemia Syndrome

Andrea Kelly · Andrew Palladino · Charles A. Stanley

Division of Endocrinology/Diabetes, The Children's Hospital of Philadelphia, Philadelphia, Pa., USA

Abstract

Activating mutations of glutamate dehydrogenase (GDH) were first demonstrated in 1998 to be the cause of hyperinsulinism (HI) in children with an unusual phenotype of hyperinsulinemic hypoglycemia combined with persistent hyperammonemia (HA). These children are commonly not diagnosed at birth and not until late in the first year of life. The disease-causing mutations are heterozygous missense amino acid substitutions of GLUD1 on 10q23.3 that increase GDH enzyme activity by impairing allosteric inhibition by GTP. De novo mutations account for 80% of the cases, the remainder showing a pattern of dominant transmission. Mutated residues affect either sites of interaction with GTP or with the antenna region of GDH. The HI/HA syndrome is one of the most common genetic causes of diazoxide-responsive HI. Tissues involved by the enzyme defect include beta-cells, kidney, and brain. Patients with HI-HA show increased sensitivity to leucine stimulation of insulin release and to protein-induced hypoglycemia, but not to other secretagogues such as glucose. HA appears to be due to increased renal ammonia production and is not associated with the usual symptoms of ammonia toxicity. Recent observations indicate that the activating mutations of GDH also impact on central nervous system function, including increased risks of developmental delay, behavior problems, and absence seizure disorder.

Congenital hyperinsulinism (HI) due to activating mutations of glutamate dehydrogenase (GDH) is the second most common of the genetic forms of HI and the most common form of the disorder that responds to treatment with diazoxide. As described in the chapter by Stanley and Matschinsky [pp. 1–6], the discovery of GDH-HI closely followed the recognition of mutations in the ATP-sensitive potassium (K_{ATP}) channel subunits and in glucokinase as genetic causes of HI. The first cases were identified as a consequence of having a very peculiar clinical phenotype that combined recurrent

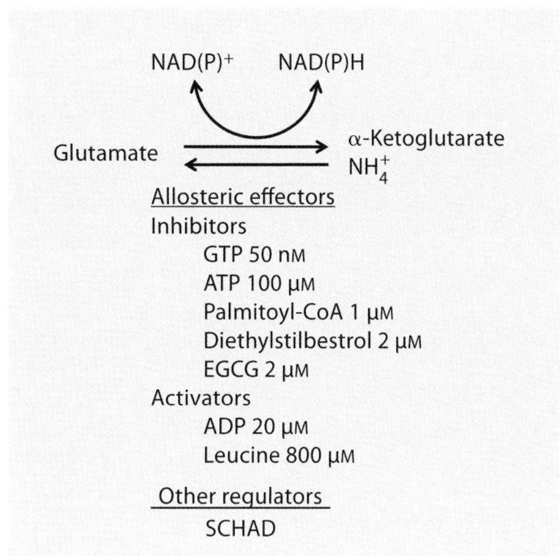

Fig. 1. GDH enzymatic reaction and allosteric activators and inhibitors: half-maximal concentrations for inhibition or activation.

episodes of hyperinsulinemic hypoglycemia with persistent elevations of plasma concentrations of ammonia: the hyperinsulinism/hyperammonemia (HI/HA) syndrome. The unusual nature of this combination suggested GDH as a candidate site for the genetic locus of the disorder, as described below, and has generated novel insights into the role of amino acids in regulating insulin secretion and into the biochemistry of GDH itself, which are described further in the chapters by Smith [pp. 87–99], Li et al. [pp. 112–124], Carobbio et al. [pp. 125–136], and Molven et al. [pp. 137–145].

Identification of Glutamate Dehydrogenase as a Candidate Locus for the Hyperinsulinism/Hyperammonemia Syndrome

The unusual combination of HI plus HA suggested that the defect in insulin regulation in the HI/HA syndrome must involve amino acid metabolism at some step involved in the pathway of amino acid-stimulated insulin secretion. As described in the chapter by Stanley and Matschinsky [pp. 1–6], amino acids were first recognized in the 1950s and 1960s as being of equal importance to glucose in regulating insulin secretion in the 1950s and 1960s, thanks to observations of protein and leucine-sensitive hypoglycemia in children with congenital HI. One potential mechanism of amino acid-stimulated insulin secretion which had been proposed was an allosteric activation of GDH by leucine. As shown in figure 1, the GDH reaction is highly regulated by a large number of allosteric effectors, the most potent being GTP, which inhibits GDH with an ED50 of approximately 50 nM. Kibbey et al. [1] pointed out that mitochondrial GTP is generated by a GTP-dependent isoenzyme of succinyl-CoA synthase so that GTP inhibition of GDH provides a way of tightly linking negative regulation of the enzyme to the rate of TCA cycle turnover. Leucine is a positive allosteric effector of GDH, and in the early 1980s both leucine and its nonmetabolizable analog, BCH (2-aminobicyclo-[2,2,1]-heptane-2-carboxylic acid), were reported to stimulate insulin release from isolated islets [2]. Although the GDH reaction is formally reversible, an activation of GDH in the direction of oxidative deamination of glutamate could explain increased insulin release by generating alpha-ketoglutarate to produce an elevation of the ATP/ADP ratio, thus stimulating insulin secretion as shown in the figure in the chapter by Stanley and Matschinsky [pp. 1–6]. At the same time, since GDH expression is restricted to pancreatic islets, liver, kidney, and brain, an increase in glutamate oxidation in one of the latter tissues might also be able to explain the persistent elevation of plasma ammonia concentrations. Thus, it was attractive to hypothesize that GDH was mutated in the HI/HA syndrome to become more active, but only if it were also assumed that the GDH reaction was functionally not reversible, and was instead poised to run in the oxidative deamination direction upon allosteric activation or loss of allosteric inhibition [3].

The chapter by Li et al. [pp. 112–124] describes studies confirming that GDH operates essentially exclusively in the oxidative deamination direction in pancreatic islets, which supports the above hypothesis for GDH and the HI/HA syndrome. Direct evidence for the origin of HA in the syndrome has recently been provided by studies in rats using the leucine analog, BCH, to stimulate GDH activity. These studies show that BCH specifically activates renal ammoniagenesis, demonstrating that the kidney and not the liver, as originally suggested, is the source of the HA in the HI/HA syndrome [4].

Demonstration that Activating Mutations in *GLUD1* Cause the Hyperinsulinism/Hyperammonemia Syndrome

To test the hypothesis that GDH was the genetic locus for the HI/HA syndrome, *GLUD1* was sequenced in affected patients and GDH kinetics were studied in patient lymphoblasts. Heterozygous missense mutations were found in all patients. As shown in figure 2, these mutations affected either the inhibitory GTP-binding site itself or the nearby antenna loop of the enzyme which communicates between adjacent enzyme subunits [3, 5, 6] (see Smith [this vol., pp. 87–99] for a detailed discussion of the structure and function of GDH).

As shown in table 1, the effect of all these HI/HA mutations was primarily to markedly impair the inhibitory allosteric effect of GTP on GDH enzyme activity. Basal GDH activity and enzyme responsiveness to other positive and negative allosteric effectors were not changed (including ADP, leucine, palmitoyl-CoA, diethylstilbesterol). Sensitivity to inhibition by ATP was reduced in parallel with the effect on GTP, although ATP may not be a particularly relevant effector since its inhibitory potency is about 1,000-fold lower than that of GTP. Note that the GTP IC50s of the mutants ranged from about twofold to about tenfold higher than normal, although there was not an obvious clinical difference between these defects in terms

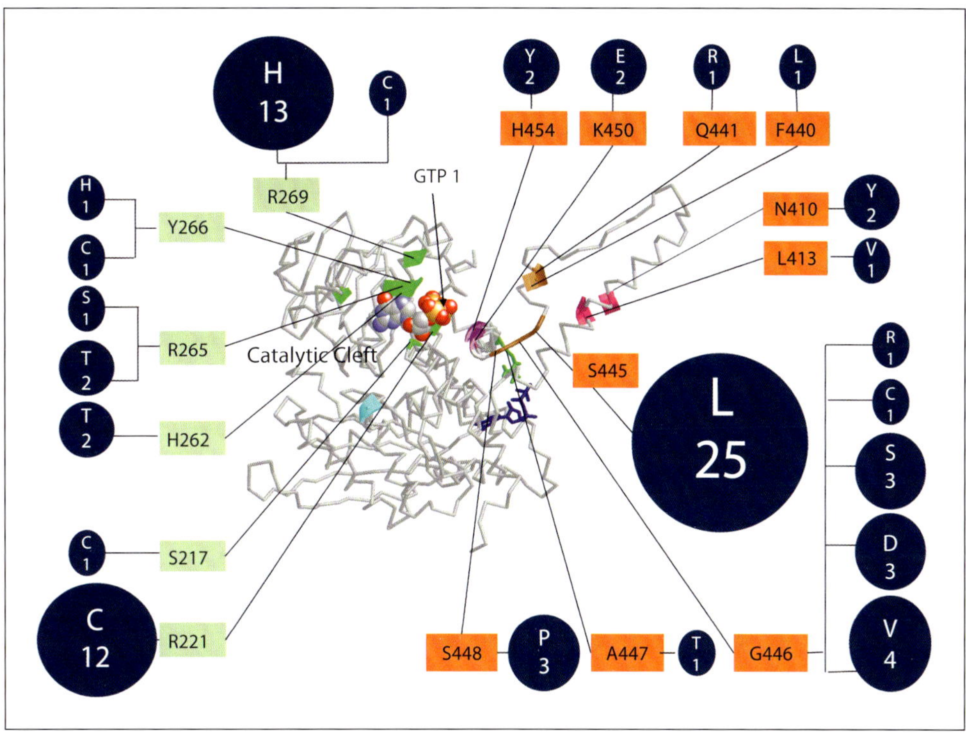

Fig. 2. Location of GDH mutations in 84 probands with HI/HA syndrome. Number of affected for each mutation is shown; orange residues indicate exons 11 and 12 mutations, green residues indicate exons 6 and 7 mutations. Inhibitory GTP shown as space-filling structure; activating ADP shown as purple stick structure.

of hypoglycemia or degree of hyperammonemia. For some of the HI/HA mutations, studies were also done with the mutant forms of GDH expressed in vitro. As shown in table 1, these studies demonstrated that sensitivity to GTP was profoundly impaired in two examples of purified mutant GDH (S448P and H454Y; the chapter by Li et al. [pp. 112–124] describes the alterations in insulin secretion observed in isolated mouse islets expressing the human H454Y GDH transgene).

Additional regulators of GDH have yet to be fully explored in HI/HA. The sirtuin (silent information regulator protein) SIRT4 has mitochondrial ADP-ribosyltransferase activity and suppresses GDH activity [7] (see Carobbio et al. [this vol., pp. 125–136]). Additional inhibitory regulators of GDH include palmitoyl-CoA and diethylstilbestrol, although the binding sites for these compounds are not known. Epigallocatechin gallate, a polyphenol in green tea, inhibits both wild-type and HI/HA mutant forms of GDH. In perifused islet studies, epigallocatechin gallate blocks GDH-mediated insulin secretion, suggesting a potential pharmaceutical therapy that directly targets the cause of the HI/HA syndrome [8] (see Smith [this vol., pp. 87–99]).

Table 1. Half-maximal concentration for GTP inhibition of GDH in HI/HA patient lymphoblasts and expressed S448P and H454Y mutations [5, 27]

Mutation	Basal activity nmol/min/mg	GTP IC50 nM
S217C	14	110
R221C	23	250
R265T	17	73
R269C	13	61
R269H	19	73
P440L	22	190
Q441R	22	94
S445L	28	280
G446R	21	300
G446D	23	480
S448P	10	290
K450E	19	230
H454Y	19	280
Normal (n = 7, m ± SD)	22±2.3	48±17
Pure S448P	19	3,100
Pure H454Y	74	210,000
Normal	84±9.5	42±12

Recently, the enzyme short-chain 3-hydroxyacyl-CoA dehydrogenase (SCHAD), encoded by *HADH,* was identified as an additional inhibitor of GDH [9]. This novel protein-protein interaction was uncovered following identification of mutations in *HADH* in a form of protein-sensitive HI in which HA is absent, SCHAD-HI (see the chapters by Molven et al. [pp. 137–145] and Li et al. [pp. 112–124]). In knockout mice with SCHAD deficiency, loss of inhibitory regulation of GDH by 3-hydroxyacyl-CoA dehydrogenase produces islets that are very similar to islets expressing an HI/HA mutant transgene in that they display increased sensitivity to leucine as well as to an amino acid mixture [9].

Clinical Features of the Hyperinsulinism/Hyperammonemia Syndrome

To date, nearly 100 probands with the HI/HA syndrome have been identified with mutations of GDH. As shown in figure 2, a total of 23 different disease-causing *GLUD1* mutations have been identified. In approximately 70% of the cases, the mutations were de novo [10]. This high proportion of de novo mutations has also been observed in other dominant forms of HI, associated with glucokinase or K_{ATP} mutations (see the chapters by De León and Stanley [pp. 18–29] and Sayed et al. [pp. 146–157]).

Table 2. Acute insulin responses in the HI/HA syndrome vs. $K_{ATP}HI$ (μU/ml)

	Calcium	Leucine	Glucose	Tolbutamide
HI/HA	–4.2±4.0 (8)	73±56 (4)	117±60 (16)	30±7.4 (16)
$K_{ATP}HI$	22±14 (8)	4.7±5.0 (4)	14±11 (10)	0.7±2.8 (10)
Normals	0.1±1.9 (8)	2±11 (4)	42±29 (10)	53±38 (10)

Values are reported as means ± SD, with values in parentheses representing the number of subjects tested.

Among the 30% of HI/HA cases that were familial, a clear autosomal dominant pattern of inheritance was evident. In a few cases with clinical features of the HI/HA syndrome, no mutations of GDH were detected in peripheral blood DNA and the disease appears to have been caused by mosaicism for a postzygotic mutation.

The clinical phenotype of HI/HA is dominated by hypoglycemia due to HI. Based on a series of 44 patients, birth weight is usually normal (in contrast to $K_{ATP}HI$ and glucokinase HI in which large-for-gestational age birth weight is common) [5, 6]. Hypoglycemia is usually not recognized at birth and is recognized around 4–12 months of age. Plasma levels of ammonia are elevated 3–5 times above the normal range to approximately 58–150 μM. HA is not associated with the typical symptoms of ammonia toxicity seen in the urea cycle enzyme deficiencies. As discussed later, children with HI/HA have a greater than expected risk of developmental delay, behavior problems, and seizures. Affected children have protein-sensitive hypoglycemia in addition to fasting hypoglycemia. Diazoxide in doses of approximately 10 mg/kg/day is very effective in preventing both types of hypoglycemia (see below).

Abnormalities of Insulin Secretion in Children with *GLUD1* Mutations

Given the role of GDH as the target for leucine-stimulated insulin secretion and the reports from the 1960s of increased insulin levels in children with leucine-sensitive hypoglycemia [11, 12], we were interested to see whether HI/HA was associated with hypersensitivity to leucine and whether this leucine-sensitivity was specific to this form of HI. Table 2 compares the acute insulin responses to a variety of insulin secretagogues of children with HI/HA and children with the more common form of recessive $K_{ATP}HI$ (see De León and Stanley [this vol., pp. 18–29]) [13, 14]. The HI/HA children display a dramatic increase in insulin following an intravenous bolus of leucine, whereas the $K_{ATP}HI$ patients show little or no response. The HI/HA patients do not respond to calcium stimulation (unlike $K_{ATP}HI$) and respond to glucose and tolbutamide similar to normals. As shown in figure 3, the hypersensitivity to leucine can be ameliorated by raising plasma glucose concentrations, presumably because

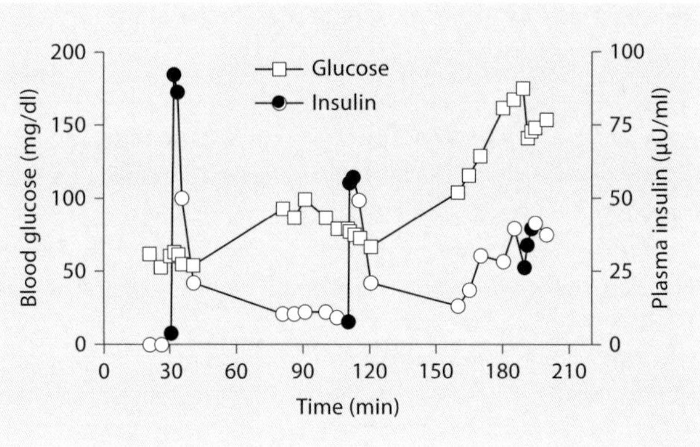

Fig. 3. Glucose suppression of acute insulin response to leucine in HI/HA. Blood glucose (open squares) and insulin (closed circles) responses to an intravenous bolus of leucine (15 mg/kg). Robust insulin secretion occurred in response to leucine at normal blood glucose. At higher glucose levels, the acute insulin response to leucine is inhibited.

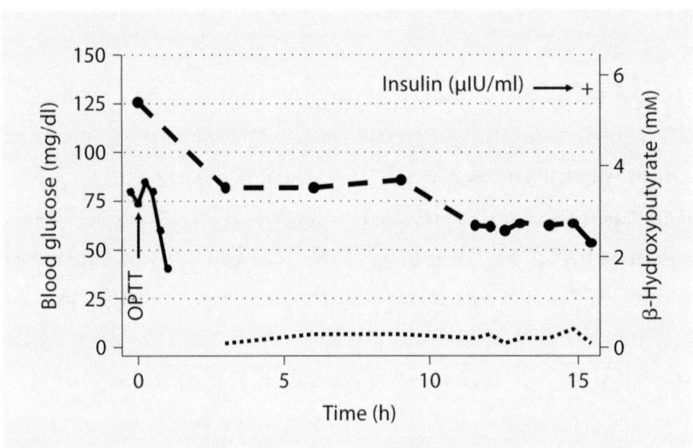

Fig. 4. Fasting and protein-sensitive hypoglycemia in HI/HA. Blood glucose concentrations during fasting (dashed line) and following a protein meal (solid line) in a 5-year-old girl with HI/HA. She was able to fast for 15 h before the blood glucose fell below 60 mg/dl; note the suppression of plasma beta-hydroxybutyrate concentrations (dotted line) throughout the fast and the inappropriately elevated insulin concentration (+) when the fast was terminated for symptoms at a blood glucose of 54 mg/dl. In contrast, blood glucose rapidly dropped to 40 mg/dl within 1 h after protein ingestion.

the increase in beta-cell phosphate potential induced by high glucose suppresses the overactivity of GDH. The chapter by Li et al. [pp. 112–124] describes further details of the mechanisms of dysregulation of insulin secretion in isolated islets from mice expressing one of the HI/HA mutants.

We also asked whether the activation of GDH enzymatic activity in HI/HA would reproduce the protein-sensitive hypoglycemia originally described by Cochrane et al. [11]. Figure 4 shows the responses of a girl with HI/HA to a protein load and to a prolonged period of fasting. Plasma glucose declined only gradually with fasting to reach a value of 50 mg/dl after 15 h (note that ketogenesis remained inappropriately

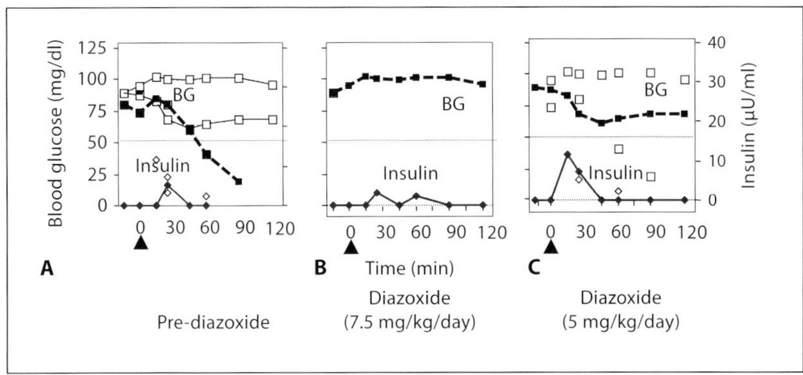

Fig. 5. Effect of diazoxide treatment in HI/HA. Blood glucose (dashed line) and plasma insulin (solid line) responses to a protein drink in the same child from figure 4. Prior to diazoxide, protein triggers hypoglycemia (panel A). Adequate diazoxide treatment prevented protein-induced hypoglycemia (panel B). After the child outgrew the diazoxide dose, protein-sensitivity reappears (panel C).

suppressed and insulin inappropriately elevated at the time of hypoglycemia). In contrast, plasma glucose fell precipitously after the protein meal to a hypoglycemic value in less than 1 h (as described in the chapters by De León and Stanley [pp. 18–29] and Li et al. [pp. 112–124], patients with K_{ATP}HI also have protein-induced hypoglycemia, although the mechanism does not involve leucine activation of GDH). As shown in figure 5, protein sensitivity in the HI/HA syndrome responds well to adequate doses of diazoxide.

Glutamate Dehydrogenase and Ammonia Metabolism

Given the importance of the liver in ammonia metabolism, the source of hyperammonemia in HI/HA was initially presumed to be of hepatic origin. Excessive GDH activity was hypothesized to simultaneously enhance hepatic ammonia production while compromising ureagenesis through depletion of hepatic glutamate, the substrate for N-acetylglutamate. N-acetylglutamate is a required allosteric activator of carbamoyl phosphate synthetase, the enzyme responsible for the rate-controlling first step in ammonia detoxification. However, because hepatic GDH has been reported to be highly active in both directions, a further increase in GDH activity would only be expected to bring the reaction closer to equilibrium [15]. An alternative, renal mechanism for the HA of HI/HA has thus been proposed. Treberg et al. [4] examined the effect of systemic activation of GDH on ammonia metabolism using BCH, a nonmetabolizable analog of the GDH allosteric activator leucine. Rats treated with BCH demonstrated increased circulating ammonia concentrations. Measurements of arteriovenous ammonia differences eliminated the liver, intestine, and skeletal muscle as the sources of HA and suggested that the kidney was the major contributor. BCH increased the rate of ammoniagenesis from glutamine by 40% in isolated renal cortical tubules and doubled ammonia flux through GDH in renal mitochondria respiring on glutamine. Flux through glutaminase was unaffected while flux through glutamate-oxaloacetate transaminase decreased. These results implicate activation of renal GDH, *not* hepatic GDH, in the HA of HI/HA. HA is thought to be absent in patients with SCHAD-HI, possibly because the ratio of HADH to GDH is higher in islets than in kidney [9].

Hyperammonemia in Hyperinsulinism/Hyperammonemia

A unique clinical feature of gain-of-function mutations in *GLUD1* is persistent HA. Despite the presence of high ammonia levels, patients with HI/HA appear to be asymptomatic: classic signs of either acute or chronic ammonia intoxication, as occur in children with urea cycle disorders, are not evident [16]. HA in patients with *GLUD1* mutations occur in both the fed and fasted states and is unaffected by blood glucose concentrations or protein intake. In 14 patients with HI/HA, following a standard oral protein tolerance test, plasma ammonia rose only slightly more than in controls (delta 22 ± 45 μM vs. 10 ± 1 μM in controls) [17]. In addition, plasma amino acid concentrations are normal in the HI/HA syndrome and plasma glutamine elevations that characterize other hyperammonemic states are absent [18]. Treatment of HI/HA patients with standard therapies for HA (arginine, benzoate) or the carbamoyl synthetase 1 activator N-carbamoyl-glutamate (used in treatment of N-acetylglutamate synthase deficiency) does not impact plasma ammonia levels.

Central Nervous System Manifestations of Hyperinsulinism/Hyperammonemia

GDH is highly expressed in brain, more so in astrocytes than neurons. Despite this high expression, central nervous system manifestations, beyond those directly attributable to hypoglycemia, are not initially evident in individuals with HI/HA. Moreover, symptoms of either acute or chronic hyperammonemia – lethargy, headaches, coma, and encephalopathy – are lacking in patients. EEGs do not show evidence of metabolic encephalopathy, such as slowing, disorganization, or triphasic waves, and cerebral edema is absent [19, 20].

Stanley [16] originally proposed that enhanced GDH oxidation in the brain could prevent glutamine accumulation and account for the dearth of hyperammonemic symptoms in HI/HA. Amination of glutamate by glutamine synthetase in astrocytes is the primary mechanism for central nervous system ammonia 'detoxification'. Glutamine can then be shuttled to neurons and either reconverted to glutamate, the major excitatory neurotransmitter, or converted to the major inhibitory neurotransmitter, GABA, by glutamic acid decarboxylase. Accumulation of glutamine by astrocytes may lead to cerebral edema [21]. In the setting of hyperammonemia, enhanced glutamate amination in astrocytes, glutamate deficits, and alterations in intracellular compartmentalization of glutamate may occur and may compromise mitochondrial energy metabolism.

Over the past several years, three separate groups have observed that individuals with HI/HA are at special risk for nonhypoglycemic seizures, mental retardation, and behavior disorders [19, 20, 22]. In the first report, atypical absence seizures were described in 6 children and young adults with HI/HA in the absence of hypoglycemia [20]. The EEG patterns were consistent with generalized epilepsy and were unlike the seizures that result from previous hypoglycemic brain injury; these usually have a focal mechanism of onset and may be associated with focal or multifocal interictal epileptiform and nonspecific EEG abnormalities.

In 22 children and adults with HI/HA, Bahi-Buisson et al. [19] identified not only atypical absence seizures, but generalized tonic-clonic seizures, focal motor seizures, dystonia, and other pyramidal signs occurring in the absence of concomitant hypoglycemia. Learning disabilities were also common. Interictal EEGs were abnormal in 12 of 14 patients with epilepsy and included generalized spike and wave discharges in 8 patients and sleep-activated photosensitive discharges in 2. The remaining 8 patients without epilepsy had normal EEGs. The occurrence of epilepsy was not related to plasma ammonium concentration. Unlike the original Raizen study, the subsequent two series reported increased frequency of seizures with *GLUD1* mutations occurring in exons 6 and 7 versus those in exons 10, 11, and 12 [19, 22]. The reason for any difference in seizure risk is not obvious, since amino acids in both areas contact the inhibitory GTP of GDH, although the residues of exons 10 and 11 lie in the antenna region of the enzyme (fig. 2). Larger series of patients will need to be examined before this speculation can be confirmed.

The mechanisms of the central nervous system disorder in HI/HA are not known. Although both HA and hypoglycemia are known causes of brain injury, these do not explain the generalized epilepsy of HI/HA. A direct central nervous system effect of the activating mutation of GDH is an attractive mechanism, given that GDH is highly expressed in the brain. For example, excessive GDH activity could deplete glutamate and alter intracellular compartmentalization of glutamate or create imbalances in the neurotransmitters, glutamate, and GABA. Alterations in the glutamate/GABA ratio are epileptogenic in other models: (1) inhibition of the reconversion of glutamine to glutamate leads to GABA and glutamate loss, thereby increasing cellular excitability; (2) inhibition of glutamate conversion to glutamine generates seizures [23]; and (3) GABA receptor subunit gene mutations are responsible for monogenic forms of epilepsy [24, 25]. An additional complication is that *GLUD2*, an intronless form of GDH that is not allosterically regulated by GTP, is expressed in the human (not rat or other species) brain [26].

Conclusion

Disturbances in regulatory control of GDH via *GLUD1* mutations that interrupt normal GTP inhibition or *HADH* mutations that impair 3-hydroxyacyl-CoA dehydrogenase inhibition of GDH are now recognized to cause congenital HI. The clinical phenotype of protein sensitivity has inspired a re-examination of amino acid-stimulated insulin secretion, a field that has lain dormant for nearly 20 years. The findings of epilepsy and of HA in the absence of typical toxicity symptoms in patients with *GLUD1* mutations provide additional stimulus for examining the role of activating mutations of GDH upon the central nervous system.

Acknowledgements

This work was supported in part by grants from the NIH: R37-DK056268 (C.A.S.), R01-DK053012 (C.A.S.), T32 DK-063688 (A.P.), DK-19525, and UL1-RR024134.

References

1 Kibbey RG, Pongratz RL, Romanelli AJ, Wollheim CB, Cline GW, Shulman GI: Mitochondrial GTP regulates glucose-stimulated insulin secretion. Cell Metab 2007;5:253–264.

2 Sener A, Malaisse WJ: L-leucine and a nonmetabolized analogue activate pancreatic islet glutamate dehydrogenase. Nature 1980;288:187–189.

3 Stanley CA, Lieu YK, Hsu BY, Burlina AB, Greenberg CR, Hopwood NJ, Perlman K, Rich BH, Zammarchi E, Poncz M: Hyperinsulinism and hyperammonemia in infants with regulatory mutations of the glutamate dehydrogenase gene. N Engl J Med 1998;338:1352–1357.

4 Treberg JR, Clow KA, Greene KA, Brosnan ME, Brosnan JT: Systemic activation of glutamate dehydrogenase increases renal ammoniagenesis: implications for the hyperinsulinism/hyperammonemia syndrome. Am J Physiol Endocrinol Metab 2010;298:E1219–E1225.

5 Stanley CA, Fang J, Kutyna K, Hsu BY, Ming JE, Glaser B, Poncz M: Molecular basis and characterization of the hyperinsulinism/hyperammonemia syndrome: predominance of mutations in exons 11 and 12 of the glutamate dehydrogenase gene. HI/HA Contributing Investigators. Diabetes 2000;49:667–673.

6 MacMullen C, Fang J, Hsu BYL, Kelly A, de Lonlay-Debeney P, Saudubray JM, Ganguly A, Smith TJ, Stanley CA: Hyperinsulinism/hyperammonemia syndrome in children with regulatory mutations in the inhibitory GTP binding domain of glutamate dehydrogenase. J Clin Endocrinol Metab 2001;86:1782–1787.

7 Haigis MC, Mostoslavsky R, Haigis KM, Fahie K, Christodoulou DC, Murphy AJ, Valenzuela DM, Yancopoulos GD, Karow M, Blander G, Wolberger C, Prolla TA, Weindruch R, Alt FW, Guarente L: SIRT4 inhibits glutamate dehydrogenase and opposes the effects of calorie restriction in pancreatic beta cells. Cell 2006;126:941–954.

8 Li C, Allen A, Kwagh J, Doliba NM, Qin W, Najafi H, Collins HW, Matschinsky FM, Stanley CA, Smith TJ: Green tea polyphenols modulate insulin secretion by inhibiting glutamate dehydrogenase. J Biol Chem 2006;281:10214–10221.

9 Li C, Chen P, Palladino A, Narayan S, Russell LK, Sayed S, Xiong G, Chen J, Stokes D, Butt YM, Jones PM, Collins HW, Cohen NA, Cohen AS, Nissim I, Smith TJ, Strauss AW, Matschinsky FM, Bennett MJ, Stanley CA: Mechanism of hyperinsulinism in short-chain 3-hydroxyacyl-CoA dehydrogenase deficiency involves activation of glutamate dehydrogenase. J Biol Chem 2010;285:31806–31818.

10 Stanley CA: Two genetic forms of hyperinsulinemic hypoglycemia caused by dysregulation of glutamate dehydrogenase. Neurochem Int 2011;59:465–472.

11 Cochrane WA, Payne WW, Simpkiss MJ, Woolf LI: Familial hypoglycemia precipitated by amino acids. J Clin Invest 1956;35:411–422.
12 McQuarrie I: Idiopathic spontaneously occurring hypoglycemia in infants. Clinical significance of problem and treatment. AMA Am J Dis Child 1954; 87:399–428.
13 Kelly A, Ng D, Ferry RJ Jr, Grimberg A, Koo-McCoy S, Thornton PS, Stanley CA: Acute insulin responses to leucine in children with the hyperinsulinism/hyperammonemia syndrome. J Clin Endocrinol Metab 2001;86:3724–3728.
14 Magge SN, Shyng SL, MacMullen C, Steinkrauss L, Ganguly A, Katz LE, Stanley CA: Familial leucine-sensitive hypoglycemia of infancy due to a dominant mutation of the beta-cell sulfonylurea receptor. J Clin Endocrinol Metab 2004;89:4450–4456.
15 Treberg JR, Brosnan ME, Watford M, Brosnan JT: On the reversibility of glutamate dehydrogenase and the source of hyperammonemia in the hyperinsulinism/hyperammonemia syndrome. Adv Enzyme Regul 2010;50:34–43.
16 Stanley CA: Hyperinsulinism/hyperammonemia syndrome: insights into the regulatory role of glutamate dehydrogenase in ammonia metabolism. Mol Genet Metab 2004;81(suppl 1):S45–S51.
17 Hsu BY, Kelly A, Thornton PS, Greenberg CR, Dilling LA, Stanley CA: Protein-sensitive and fasting hypoglycemia in children with the hyperinsulinism/hyperammonemia syndrome. J Pediatr 2001; 138:383–389.
18 Weinzimer SA, Stanley CA, Berry GT, Yudkoff M, Tuchman M, Thornton PS: A syndrome of congenital hyperinsulinism and hyperammonemia. J Pediatr 1997;130:661–664.
19 Bahi-Buisson N, Roze E, Dionisi C, Escande F, Valayannopoulos V, Feillet F, Heinrichs C, Chadefaux-Vekemans B, Dan B, de Lonlay P: Neurological aspects of hyperinsulinism-hyperammonaemia syndrome. Dev Med Child Neurol 2008;50:945–949.
20 Raizen DM, Brooks-Kayal A, Steinkrauss L, Tennekoon GI, Stanley CA, Kelly A: Central nervous system hyperexcitability associated with glutamate dehydrogenase gain of function mutations. J Pediatr 2005;146:388–394.
21 Hertz L, Kala G: Energy metabolism in brain cells: effects of elevated ammonia concentrations. Metab Brain Dis 2007;22:199–218.
22 Kapoor RR, Flanagan SE, Fulton P, Chakrapani A, Chadefaux B, Ben-Omran T, Banerjee I, Shield JP, Ellard S, Hussain K: Hyperinsulinism-hyperammonaemia syndrome: novel mutations in the GLUD1 gene and genotype-phenotype correlations. Eur J Endocrinol 2009;161:731–735.
23 Pan JW, Williamson A, Cavus I, Hetherington HP, Zaveri H, Petroff OA, Spencer DD: Neurometabolism in human epilepsy. Epilepsia 2008;49(suppl 3):31–41.
24 Cossette P, Liu L, Brisebois K, Dong H, Lortie A, Vanasse M, Saint-Hilaire JM, Carmant L, Verner A, Lu WY, Wang YT, Rouleau GA: Mutation of GABRA1 in an autosomal dominant form of juvenile myoclonic epilepsy. Nat Genet 2002;31:184–189.
25 Wallace RH, Marini C, Petrou S, Harkin LA, Bowser DN, Panchal RG, Williams DA, Sutherland GR, Mulley JC, Scheffer IE, Berkovic SF: Mutant GABA(A) receptor gamma2-subunit in childhood absence epilepsy and febrile seizures. Nat Genet 2001;28:49–52.
26 Plaitakis A, Metaxari M, Shashidharan P: Nerve tissue-specific (GLUD2) and housekeeping (GLUD1) human glutamate dehydrogenases are regulated by distinct allosteric mechanisms: implications for biologic function. J Neurochem 2000;75: 1862–1869.
27 Fang J, Hsu BY, MacMullen CM, Poncz M, Smith TJ, Stanley CA: Expression, purification and characterization of human glutamate dehydrogenase (GDH) allosteric regulatory mutations. Biochem J 2002;363:81–87.

Dr. Andrea Kelly
Division of Endocrinology/Diabetes
The Children's Hospital of Philadelphia
34th Street and Civic Center Boulevard
Philadelphia, PA 19104 (USA)
Tel. +1 215 590 3420, E-Mail kellya@email.chop.edu

Stanley CA, De León DD (eds): Monogenic Hyperinsulinemic Hypoglycemia Disorders.
Front Diabetes. Basel, Karger, 2012, vol 21, pp 112–124

Amino Acid-Stimulated Insulin Secretion: The Role of the Glutamine-Glutamate-Alpha-Ketoglutarate Axis

Changhong Li[a] · Franz M. Matschinsky[b] · Charles A. Stanley[a]

[a]Division of Endocrinology/Diabetes, The Children's Hospital of Philadelphia, and [b]Institute for Diabetes, Obesity and Metabolism, University of Pennsylvania School of Medicine, Philadelphia, Pa., USA

Abstract

The role of amino acids in the regulation of insulin secretion has received relatively little attention because of the clinical and basic science focus on glucose and, more recently, on fatty acids as the essential determinants of this process. However, early clinical observation in 1950s and recent genetic studies of protein-sensitive hypoglycemia in children with congenital hyperinsulinism have highlighted the important role of amino acids in pancreatic beta-cell physiology and pathophysiology. Mouse models of three of these disorders have been investigated to elucidate the mechanisms of amino acid-stimulated insulin secretion (AASIS), including activating mutations of glutamate dehydrogenase (GDH), inactivating mutations of the ATP-sensitive potassium channel [sulfonylurea receptor 1 (SUR1) and Kir 6.2], and inactivating mutations of short-chain 3-hydroxyacyl-CoA dehydrogenase (SCHAD). This chapter describes the effects of these mutations on pathways of AASIS, particularly on the steps of glutamine oxidation [glutamine → glutamate → alpha-ketoglutarate(KG)] and of glutamine synthesis (glutamate → glutamine): the Q → E → alpha-KG axis. The results confirm that leucine-stimulated insulin secretion (LSIS) acts via GDH to drive flux from Q → E → alpha-KG in GDH hyperinsulinism. A similar mechanism applies in SCHAD hyperinsulinism, apparently due to the loss of an inhibitory protein-protein interaction of SCHAD on GDH. In contrast, AASIS in SUR1 hyperinsulinism appears to act via glutamine amplification of distal cAMP-dependent steps in insulin release. These mechanisms responsible for protein-sensitive hypoglycemia in genetic disorders of insulin secretion are likely also relevant to normal regulation of insulin secretion, where insulin responsiveness is required to protein meals (via the Q → E → alpha-KG sequence) and is enhanced when protein is added to carbohydrate meals (via alpha-KG → E → Q).

The importance of amino acids as regulators of insulin secretion was first appreciated in 1955 when Cochrane et al. [1] described familial protein-sensitive hypoglycemia. In these families, affected children developed a worsening of hypoglycemia when placed on a high-protein diet. The hypoglycemic effect of protein was reproduced by specific individual amino acids, most notably by the essential amino acid leucine, the most abundant essential amino acid in dietary protein. Subsequent studies by Yalow and Berson [2], employing their newly discovered insulin radioimmunoassay, showed that the hypoglycemia induced by leucine in susceptible individuals was due to exaggerated insulin release [3].

In vitro studies have confirmed the importance of amino acid-stimulated insulin secretion (AASIS). Experiments in the isolated perfused rat pancreas in the early 1970s confirmed that many individual amino acids can stimulate insulin release, but most are able to do so only in the presence of glucose [4]. These glucose-dependent amino acids include complete mixtures of all 20 amino acids, as well as certain individual amino acids including alanine, asparagine, glycine, glutamate, phenylalanine, and tryptophan [5–8]. Arginine is often cited as an example of ASSIS; however, the effect of arginine is not specific and does not reflect the metabolism of arginine, but rather its action as a zwitterion to cause membrane depolarization. Leucine is a notable exception to the rule that glucose is required for AASIS since the stimulatory effect of leucine in perfused rat pancreas is abolished in the presence of glucose [9]. Insulin release can also be stimulated by the nonmetabolizable analog of leucine, 2-aminobicyclo-(2,2,1)heptane-2-carboxylic acid (BCH), indicating that, unlike glucose, the effect of leucine does not depend on its utilization as a substrate for oxidation. In 1980s, Sener and Malaisse [10] showed that leucine and BCH act to trigger insulin secretion by allosterically stimulating glutamate dehydrogenase (GDH) activity.

Key evidence of the essential role of amino acids in regulation of insulin secretion has come from clinical disorders associated with hypoglycemia in children. In 1998, gain-of-function mutations of GDH were identified in children with a dominant form of hyperinsulinism (HI; the hyperinsulinism/hyperammonemia syndrome) and implicated this enzyme as a key mediator of leucine-stimulated insulin secretion (LSIS) [11] (see Kelly et al. [this vol., pp. 100–111]). In the most common form of genetic HI, due to inactivating mutations of the ATP-sensitive potassium (K_{ATP}) channel, patients have protein-sensitive hypoglycemia, but are not hypersensitive to leucine (see De León and Stanley [this vol., pp. 18–29]). A third form of genetic HI due to inactivating mutations of short-chain 3-hydroxyacyl-CoA dehydrogenase (SCHAD) also shows hypersensitivity to AASIS which appears to result from activation of GDH [12] (see Molven et al. [this vol., pp. 137–145]). These discoveries of the role of GDH and glutamine in insulin secretion have drawn attention to the glutamine-glutamate-alpha-ketoglutarate (KG) sequence as a critical axis for mediating the effects of amino acids in regulation of insulin secretion. The goal of this chapter is to describe how amino acid- and glucose-stimulated insulin secretion is modulated by this axis in the three mouse models of congenital HI.

Amino Acid-Stimulated Insulin Secretion in Normal Humans and Isolated Islets

Studies of insulin secretion using isolated perifused mouse and rat islets illustrate the main features of AASIS in normals. A mixture of amino acids at physiologic

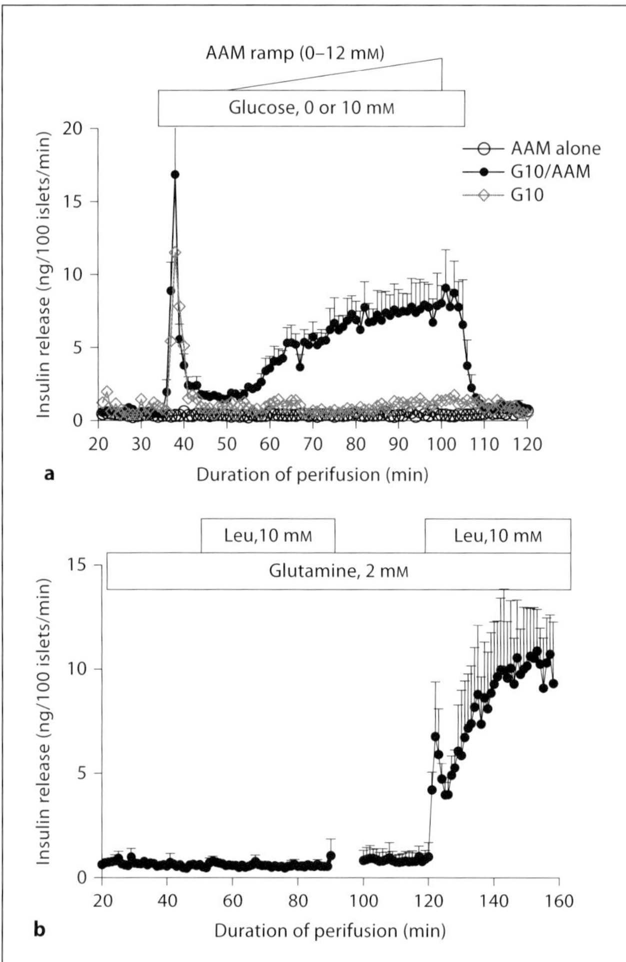

Fig. 1. Amino acid- and leucine-stimulated insulin secretion in normal islets. **a** An amino acid mixture alone fails to stimulate insulin secretion in perifused mouse islets, but potentiates the second phase of insulin secretion stimulated by 10 mM glucose. **b** leucine stimulates insulin secretion in rat islets only after a 120-min period of 'run down'. Means ± SEM, n = 3.

concentrations does not elicit an insulin response, but can potentiate the response to glucose-stimulated insulin secretion (GSIS; fig. 1a). As discussed later, this effect of amino acids may be almost entirely accounted for by glutamine alone. Leucine stimulates insulin release in rat islets with a background of 2 mM glutamine to provide a substrate for the GDH reaction, but only after the islets have undergone a 'run down' period prior to stimulation (fig. 1b). Thus, amino acids can potentiate insulin release once the triggering mechanism has been activated (e.g. by GSIS), but leucine, specifically, can also be a trigger for insulin release, provided the inhibition of GDH by a high phosphate potential does not interfere. Mouse islets are more sensitive than rat islets to the 'run down' phenomenon and respond to leucine stimulation almost immediately. In normal humans, amino acids also potentiate the insulin response to glucose, which is the basis for using a combination of amino acids and glucose for testing maximal insulin secretory responsiveness. Administration of oral amino acids can stimulate insulin release in normal children and adults, but with little or no change in plasma glucose concentrations, presumably due to the counter-balancing effect of glucagon release.

H454Y Human Glutamate Dehydrogenase Transgenic Mice: Flux from Q → E → α-KG Triggers Insulin Secretion

In order to examine how GDH gain-of-function mutations lead to hypersecretion of insulin in children with the hyperinsulinism/hyperammonemia syndrome, transgenic mice were generated using the rat insulin promoter to express the disease-causing H454Y gain-of-function mutation of human GDH specifically in beta-cells [13]. GDH enzymatic activity in islets from the transgenic mice showed a rightward shift in the GTP inhibition curve, confirming the presence of the mutant huGDH. Random and fasting blood glucose levels were consistently lower in transgenic animals.

Isolated islets from H454Y human GDH transgenic mice showed increased sensitivity to LSIS compared to wild-type (WT) controls. Transgenic islets were also sensitive to AASIS or to stimulation by glutamine alone, whereas control mouse islets were unresponsive (fig. 2a). The maximum AASIS by transgenic islets was similar to that achieved by glutamine alone, suggesting that glutamine was responsible for most of the effect of the mixture of amino acids. Both glutamine and an amino acid mixture stimulated an increase in the ATP/ADP ratio in the transgenic islets, but not in the controls. Inhibition of phosphate-dependent glutaminase (PDG; the step upstream of GDH) by 6-diazo-5-oxo-L-norleucine (DON), completely abolished transgenic islet responsiveness to glutamine stimulation. These observations indicated that the H454Y gain-of-function mutation of GDH stimulates insulin release by increased oxidative flux through the enzyme via the Q → E → alpha-KG axis.

Since the GDH reaction is reversible and it had been suggested that the rise in islet glutamate which accompanies GSIS was due to reductive amination of alpha-KG via GDH (see Carobbio et al. [this vol., pp. 125–136]), questions arise about what is the direction of flux through GDH that is responsible for HI associated with GDH activating mutations. To directly examine the effects of the H454Y GDH mutation on flux through the Q → E → alpha-KG axis, stable isotope studies were carried out using [2-^{15}N]-glutamine to trace its conversion to [2-^{15}N]-glutamate via PDG and subsequently to [^{15}N]-ammonia via deamination of glutamate in the GDH reaction. In the presence of 10 mM [2-^{15}N]-glutamine, basal insulin secretion, total ammonia production, [^{15}N]-ammonia enrichment, and flux through GDH and PDG were all greater in islets from H454Y transgenic mice compared with normal mouse islets (see table 1). In control islets, activation of GDH with 10 mM leucine induced an increase of insulin release, accompanied by increased rates of ammonia production and a threefold stimulation of flux through GDH that were similar to the basal rates seen in unstimulated

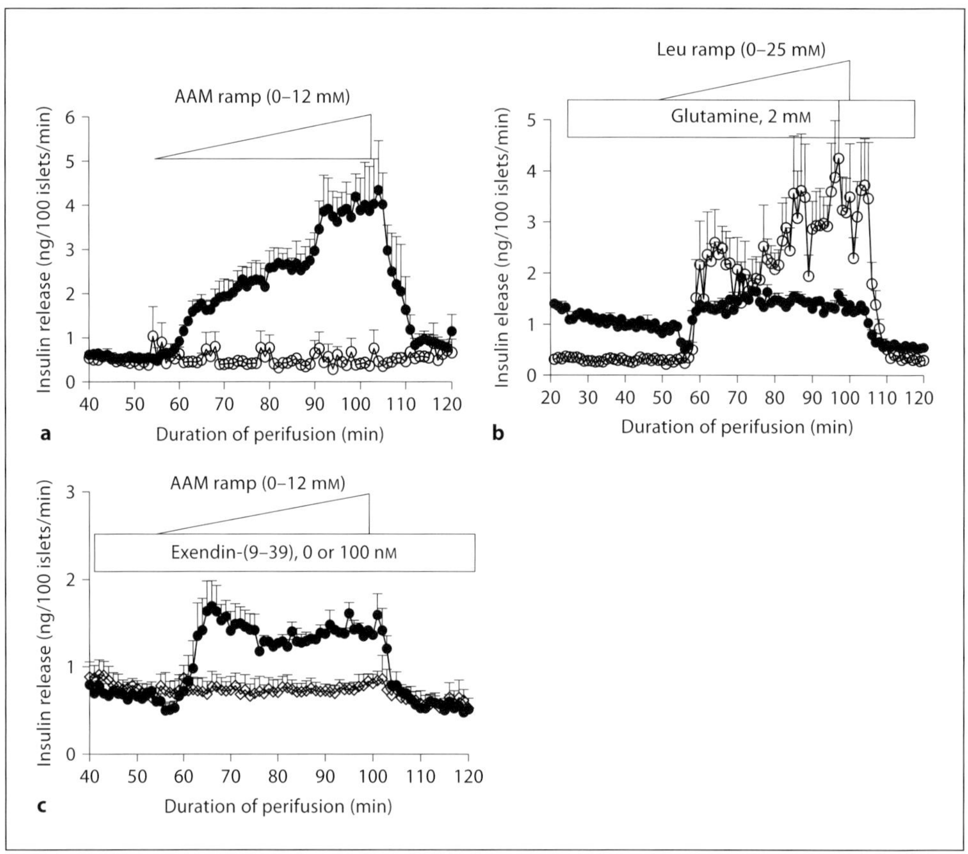

Fig. 2. AASIS and LSIS in H454Y huGDH-TG and SUR1-KO mouse islets. **a** Amino acids stimulate insulin secretion in GDH-TG (filled circles), but not in control islets (open circles). **b** Leucine stimulates insulin release in control (open circles), but not in SUR1-KO islets (filled circles). **c** Amino acids stimulate insulin release by SUR1-KO (filled circles); this response is blocked by exendin-(9–39), a GLP-1 receptor antagonist (open diamonds). Means ± SEM, n = 3.

transgenic islets. Leucine slightly increased rates of insulin secretion and ammonia production in transgenic islets, reaching approximately the same levels as in leucine-stimulated control islets, suggesting that these values were close to maximal. Of note, in both normal and transgenic islets, glucose almost completely inhibited ammonia production, ^{15}N-enrichment of ammonia, PDG flux, and GDH flux; leucine was unable to override this inhibitory effect of glucose. This inhibitory effect of glucose on LSIS is also seen in GDH-HI patients (see Kelly et al. [this vol., pp. 100–111]) [14], and presumably reflects the elevation of the phosphate potential generated during glucose oxidation and its strong inhibitory effect on GDH. Efforts to measure the rate of reverse flux through GDH using [^{15}N]-ammonia in both transgenic and control islets indicated that even during GSIS when islet glutamate levels increase, the production of glutamate via reductive amination via GDH is less than 1% of flux in the oxidative direction.

Table 1. Insulin secretion and fluxes of GDH and PDG in islets from H454Y huGDH transgenic mice (n = 3)

	Insulin secretion µg/1,000 islets/h		GDH flux nmol/1,000 islets/h		PDG flux nmol/1,000 islets/h	
	WT	TG	WT	TG	WT	TG
Control	0.3±0.0	1.4±0.4[5]	13±1.2	25±2.1[5]	44±7	87±8[5]
Leu 10	3.7±0.6[1]	3.0±0.2[2]	36±0.8[2]	44±4.9	61±8	49±10
G 25	2.9±0.8[1]	2.3±0.1	14±7.7	4±1.2[2]	28±5	50±8
Leu 10/G 25	3.2±0.2[1]	2.5±0.1	9±4.6[3]	14±1.7[3]	17±8[4]	15±4[1]

Data are means ± SE.

[1] $p < 0.01$ compared with control (10 mM of [2-^{15}N]-glutamine).

[2] $p < 0.05$ compared with control (10 mM of [2-^{15}N]-glutamine).

[3] $p < 0.01$ compared with Leu 10.

[4] $p < 0.05$ compared with Leu 10.

[5] $p < 0.05$ compared with normal mouse islets.

Studies in isolated H554Y human GDH transgenic islets showed that the abnormalities in AASIS can be acutely reversed by inhibition with EGCG, a green tea polyphenol which is a potent inhibitor of GDH enzymatic activity (see the chapter by Smith [pp. 87–99] on GDH structure and function).

In conclusion, these studies show that stimulation of insulin release either by leucine activation of GDH in normals or by GDH activating mutations in the hyperinsulinism/hyperammonemia syndrome is associated with increased oxidative deamination of glutamate via GDH. The results suggest that, in pancreatic islet beta-cells, GDH functions almost exclusively in the oxidative direction of E → alpha-KG (as it also appears to do in kidney and brain, but possibly not in liver) [15]. This is probably essential so that modulation of GDH by allosteric effectors, such as leucine, can generate an increase in high-energy phosphate potential to 'trigger' the release of insulin.

Short-Chain 3-Hydroxyacyl-CoA Dehydrogenase Knockout Mice: Novel Regulation of Glutamate Dehydrogenase by Protein-Protein Interaction

Recently, several children have been described with a recessively inherited form of HI that is associated with deficiency of the mitochondrial fatty acid beta-oxidation enzyme, SCHAD (see Molven et al. [this vol., pp. 137–145]) [16–18]. SCHAD catalyzes the third step in the beta-oxidation cycle for medium- and short chain 3-hydroxy fatty acyl-CoAs (C4–C10). This disease is unusual because while other genetic disorders of mitochondrial fatty acid oxidation cause hypoglycemia, they do not cause HI [19]. An important clue to the mechanism of insulin dysregulation in SCHAD deficiency has been recently provided by the report that affected children are sensitive to protein-induced hypoglycemia [20].

In order to investigate the mechanisms responsible for hypoglycemia in SCHAD deficiency, we studied insulin regulation in islets from SCHAD knockout (KO) mice. These mice have mild hypoglycemia which is not as severe as seen in H545Y human GDH transgenic mice, but slightly more severe than in sulfonylurea receptor 1 (SUR1)-KO mice [13, 21]. In vivo, SCHAD-KO mice showed a rapid decline of blood glucose after receiving amino acids, similar to the protein-induced hypoglycemia seen in patients with SCHAD deficiency. In contrast, responses to glucose tolerance testing in vivo were normal, which suggested that the hypoglycemia phenotype in SCHAD deficiency was unlikely to be caused by increased GSIS.

In isolated islets, there were no differences between SCHAD-KO and WT responses to GSIS, either in the presence or the absence of a medium-chain fatty acid (octanoate) or of a long-chain fatty acid (palmitate). SCHAD-KO islets had normal cytosolic calcium levels, unlike SUR1-KO islets. SCHAD-KO islets showed a brisk AASIS response, whereas WT islets had no response. The threshold for AASIS in KO islets was 2.64 mM, which is similar to but less sensitive than we had found in H454Y human GDH transgenic mouse islets (1.68 mM) [13]. SCHAD-KO islets also had a lower threshold for leucine stimulation of insulin secretion compared to WT islets, suggesting increased sensitivity of GDH to allosteric activation by leucine. Unlike H454Y human GDH transgenic islets, SCHAD-KO islets were not sensitive to stimulation with glutamine alone. Nevertheless, glutamine was the most important of the 20 amino acids, since insulin secretion decreased by 90% in SCHAD-KO islets when glutamine was omitted from the mixture of amino acids. When glutamine and leucine were both removed from the amino acid mixture, KO islets were completely unresponsive, indicating that GDH activation was essential for the release of insulin.

Since the above observations suggested that GDH was being activated in islets lacking SCHAD protein, we examined the possibility of protein-protein interactions between SCHAD and GDH using liver mitochondria from KO and WT mice. Using anti-SCHAD antibody, GDH was coprecipitated with SCHAD in WT mouse liver mitochondria, but not in KO mice, consistent with a GDH-SCHAD protein complex in WT liver mitochondria. When purified His-tagged SCHAD protein was used as bait, GDH was coprecipitated in KO, but not in WT liver extracts, suggesting that free GDH in KO liver mitochondria was readily available to form a protein complex with His-tagged SCHAD protein.

These findings indicated that GDH activation in SCHAD deficiency was due to the loss of a direct protein-protein interaction between the two enzymes. Measurements of enzyme kinetics for GDH in islet homogenates indicated that absence of SCHAD increases the affinity of GDH for alpha-KG, suggesting that the presence of SCHAD affects binding of the carboxyl end of the substrate in the catalytic site. The effect was limited to islet GDH, perhaps reflecting the high levels of SCHAD [22] and, in particular, the high ratio of SCHAD to GDH in this tissue. These results in SCHAD-KO mice suggest that increased metabolic flux from Q → E → alpha-KG is responsible for protein hypersensitivity in SCHAD-HI as well as in GDH-HI. It is interesting to speculate that the inhibitory effect of SCHAD on GDH might be part of a mechanism for reciprocal control of fatty acid and amino acid oxidation.

SUR1-KO Mice: Flux from alpha-KG → E → Q Suggests a Signaling Role of Glutamine in Insulin Secretion

Children with loss of function mutations of K_{ATP} channels are sensitive to protein-induced hypoglycemia [23], but, unlike patients with GDH gain of function mutations, K_{ATP}HI patients have no acute insulin responses to leucine stimulation (De León and Stanley [this vol., pp. 18–29]) [23, 24]. To investigate this apparent paradox, we examined insulin secretion in islets from SUR1-KO mice [25]. SUR-KO islets had no response to either LSIS or to GSIS since the 'triggering' pathway is already maximal, but they do release insulin in response to a mixture of amino acids (fig. 2b, c). Most of the effect of a complete mixture of amino acids could be attributed to glutamine alone, even though glutamine accounted for only a small fraction of the total amino acid mixture. This effect of glutamine on insulin secretion was unlikely to be caused by glutamine oxidation via Q → E → alpha-KG since sensitivity to glutamine was not abolished when glutamine oxidation through PDG was inhibited by DON [25]. Thus, it appeared that glutamine might be exerting effects on the downstream amplification pathways for insulin release, distal to the voltage-gated calcium channel (since SUR1-KO beta-cells have elevated basal cytosolic calcium).

This amplifying effect of glutamine on insulin secretion also occurred in normal control islets under conditions where cytosolic calcium had been elevated by exposure to glyburide or to glucose stimulation [25]. As shown in table 2, islet glutamine content was increased twofold during exposure to 25 mM glucose. When islets were stimulated with 25 mM [U-^{13}C] glucose, over 50% of the glutamine carbon came from glucose. Inhibition of glutamine synthetase by methionine sulfoximine abolished the carbon flux from glutamate to glutamine and reduced the response to GSIS. These results indicate that the metabolic flux from alpha-KG → E → Q (alpha-KG → E via transaminases) might play an important role in normal GSIS insulin secretion [26]. The role of the alpha-KG → E → Q path in GSIS is further illustrated in figure 3a. Inhibition of glutamine synthetase by methionine sulfoximine to block glutamine synthesis, but not its inactive analog buthionine sulfoximine, decreased the response to GSIS. In the presence of methionine sulfoximine to block glutamine

Table 2. Effects of [U-^{13}C]-glucose on insulin secretion and glutamine production in normal mouse islets (n = 3)

	Insulin secretion µg/1,000 islets/h	Glutamine nmol/1,000 islets		^{13}C enrichment *(APE, sum of M+2, +3, +4, +5)*
		content	release	
G, 0	0.2±0.03	0.2±0.02	4.1±0.5	
G, 25	5.4±0.7[1]	0.4±0.04[2]	7.4±0.7[2]	
G, 25/MSO 1 mM	3.5±0.2[3]	NA	NA	
[U-^{13}C]G, 0/AAM 4 mM	0.2±0.0	0.8±0.1		
[U-^{13}C]G, 5/AAM 4 mM	0.5±0.0[4]	1.3±0.0[5]		34±1.2
[U-^{13}C]G, 25/AAM 4 mM	4.5±0.2[4,6]	1.3±0.1[5]		57±1.0[6]
[U-^{13}C]G, 25/AAM 4 mM / MSO 1 mM	4.7±0.4[4,6]	NA		ND

Values are means ± SEM. NA = Data not determined; ND = undetectable.
[1] $p < 0.01$ compared with G, 0.
[2] $p < 0.05$ compared with G, 0.
[3] $p < 0.05$ compared with G, 25.
[4] $p < 0.01$ compared with G, 0/AAM 4 mM.
[5] $p < 0.05$ compared with G, 0/AAM 4 mM.
[6] $p < 0.01$ compared with G, 5/AAM 4.0.

synthesis, GSIS was enhanced in a dose-dependent manner by addition of exogenous glutamine, but could also be enhanced by the addition of DON, which is a nonmetabolizable analog of glutamine. This suggests that the effect of glutamine might be related to activity of a cyclic reaction between glutamine and glutamate or, perhaps more likely, as a direct action of glutamine as an effector distal to the elevation of cytosolic calcium.

Further studies in SUR1-KO mice suggested that the amplifying effect of glutamine may target cAMP-dependent pathways, such as the GLP-1 receptor [21]. AASIS in SUR1-KO islets was accompanied by an increase in cAMP production (fig. 3b). Inhibition of the GLP-1 receptor by its antagonist, exendin-(9–39), decreased baseline cAMP and insulin release, and also blocked the stimulatory effect of amino acids on both cAMP production and insulin secretion (fig. 2c and 3b). This same inhibition of cAMP and diminution of insulin release could be reproduced in control islets during GSIS. The precise mechanism by which glutamine exerts its effects on the amplification pathways of insulin secretion downstream of cytosolic calcium remains to be determined, but it may be important clinically in children with K_{ATP}HI disorders and could also be important in amplifying the stimulation of insulin secretion in normal individuals in response to glucose and other metabolic fuels (see De León [this vol., pp. 79–86]).

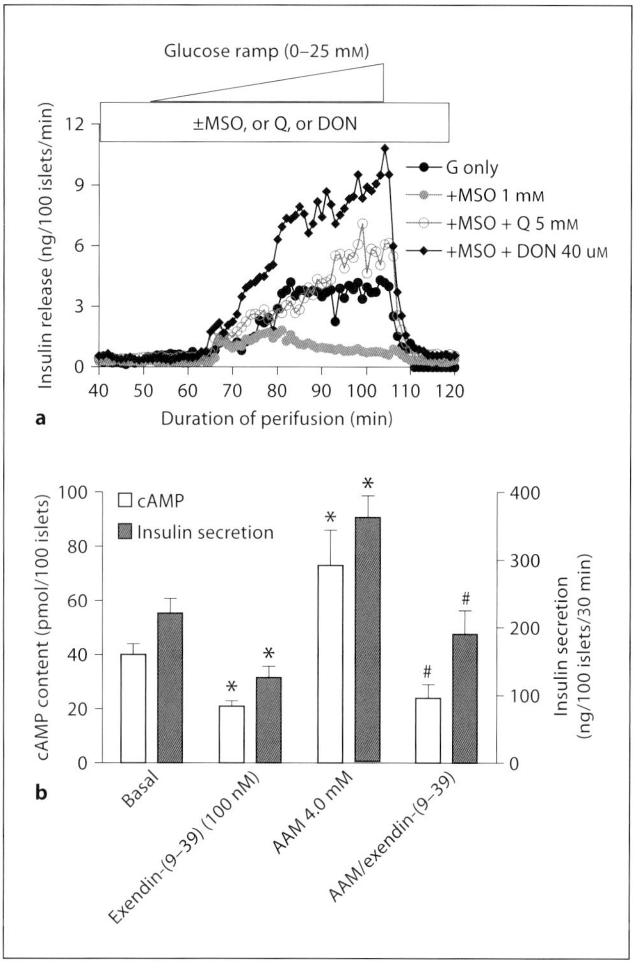

Fig. 3. Effects of PDG and GS inhibitors on GSIS and effects of GLP-1 receptor inhibition on cAMP production in SUR1-KO islets. **a** GSIS in normal control islets is inhibited by 1 mM MSO (inhibitor of GS); this inhibitory effect is reversed by addition of 5 mM glutamine or 40 µM DON (inhibitor of PDG). Means ± SEM, n = 3. **b** Basal and AASIS and cAMP production in batch-incubated SUR1-KO islets are inhibited by exendin-(9–39), an inhibitor of the GLP-1 receptor (compared to basal, *$p < 0.05$; compared to AAM stimulation, #$p < 0.05$; n = 4–8).

Interconnections of Islet Amino Acids and Glucose-Stimulated Insulin Secretion

During GSIS, the levels of the major islet amino acids change, possibly via transamination reactions between glutamate and TCA cycle substrates, such as pyruvate, oxaloacetate, and alpha-KG. For example, increased glucose oxidation during GSIS results in a 50% reduction of intracellular aspartate [13, 25, 26], reflecting the conversion of aspartate to oxaloacetate to form citrate due to faster turnover of the TCA cycle. In contrast, alanine increases by about threefold during GSIS, reflecting production of pyruvate from glycolysis. Islet GABA levels decrease by about 30% during GSIS, reflecting increased activity of the GABA shunt, a beta-cell specific pathway. Interestingly, islet GABA levels are reduced in all three HI mouse models; this may partly reflect the decreased GABA synthesis from glutamate due to downregulation of glutamate decarboxylase expression by elevated cytosolic calcium [12, 13, 26]. Under

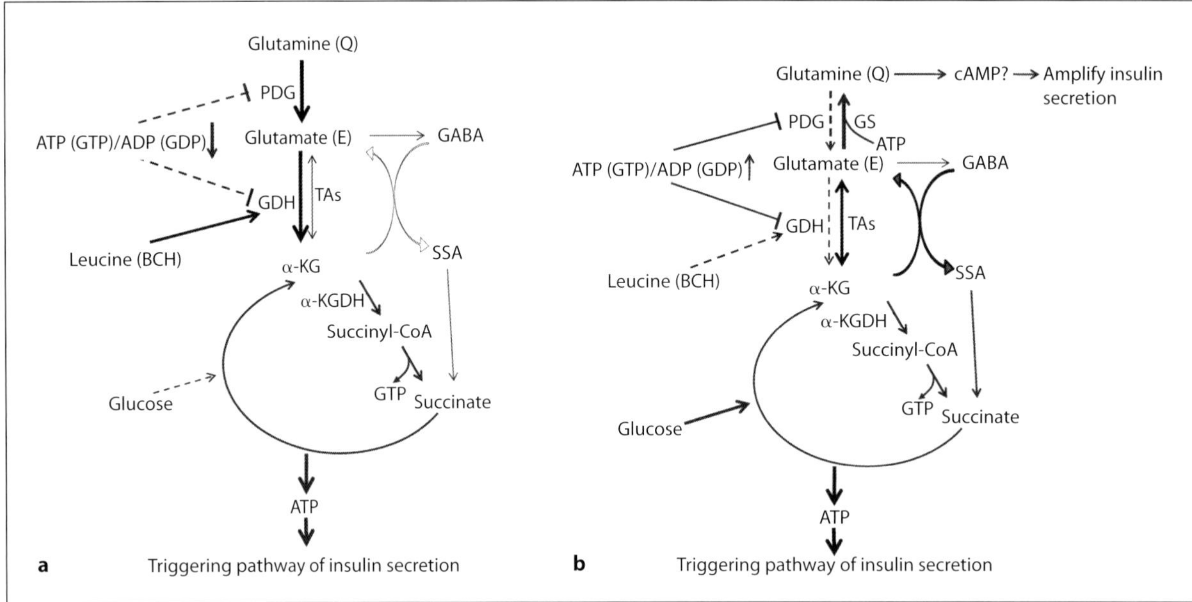

Fig. 4. The Q → E → α-KG axis and insulin secretion: The Q → E → α-KG axis involves three key enzymes, GDH, phosphate-dependent glutaminase (PDG), and glutamine synthetase (GS). The activities of all three enzymes are regulated by changes in the beta-cell phosphate potential. In addition, GDH activity is not only allosterically inhibited by GTP and to a lesser extent by ATP, but is also activated at two other separate allosteric sites by ADP and leucine. **a** Under circumstances where the ratio of ATP vs. ADP plus Pi is low, GDH and PDG are activated while GS is inhibited; metabolic flux from Q to E to α-KG triggers insulin release by generating ATP. **b** In contrast, when phosphate potential is high during glucose oxidation, GDH and PDG are inhibited while GS is activated; glutamine is generated by directing flux from α-KG to E to Q and amplifies insulin release. Note that flux can also occur from α-KG to E via transaminases (TAs).

conditions of GDH activation in GDH-TG and SCHAD-KO islets, aspartate is lowered by 40–60%, reflecting faster rates of amino acid oxidation. In SCHAD-KO islets, maximum insulin responses to leucine require alanine in addition to glutamine, perhaps for feeding into the TCA cycle to ensure complete oxidation of alpha-KG generated via partial activation of GDH. The functional consequences of altered GABA shunt activity and of changes in other islet amino acids in HI models and during GSIS in normal islets remain largely unknown and deserve further investigation since some of these amino acids can have actions as neurotransmitters.

In summary, as shown in figure 4a, activation of GDH, either by leucine in normals or by activating mutations of the enzyme in GDH-HI or the loss of SCHAD inhibition of the enzyme in SCHAD-HI, stimulates insulin release via the Q → E → α-KG axis. Alternatively, when the triggering pathway through K_{ATP} channel has been activated, either by inactivating mutations of SUR1 or Kir6.2 or during GSIS (fig. 4b), and cytosolic calcium is elevated, increased flux of the Q → E → α-KG axis in the direction of α-KG → E → Q can amplify insulin release, possibly via a cAMP-dependent process such as the GLP-1 receptor. Thus, while insulin has well-recognized roles in directing the disposal of amino acids into protein synthesis and controlling their release through protein degradation, genetic HI defects make it clear that amino acids can also control their own fate through their signaling effects on insulin secretion.

Acknowledgements

These studies were supported in part by NIH grants, DK53012 (C.A.S.), DK22122 (F.M.M.), and the Ajinomoto Amino Acid Research Program (C.A.S). Additional support was provided by the Diabetes Research Center of the University of Pennsylvania (DK19525).

References

1 Cochrane WA, Payne WW, Simpkiss MJ, Woolf LI: Familial hypoglycemia precipitated by amino acids. J Clin Invest 1956;35:411–422.

2 Yalow RS, Berson SA: Immunoassay of endogenous plasma insulin in man. J Clin Invest 1960;39:1157–1175.

3 Fajans SS, Floyd JC Jr, Knopf RF, Conn FW: Effect of amino acids and proteins on insulin secretion in man. Recent Prog Horm Res 1967;23:617–662.

4 Pagliara AS, Stillings SN, Hover B, Martin DM, Matschinsky FM: Glucose modulation of amino acid-induced glucagon and insulin release in the isolated perfused rat pancreas. J Clin Invest 1974;54:819–832.

5 Floyd JC Jr, Fajans SS, Conn JW, Knopf RF, Rull J: Stimulation of insulin secretion by amino acids. J Clin Invest 1966;45:1487–1502.

6 Malaisse WJ, Sener A, Carpinelli AR, Anjaneyulu K, Lebrun P, Herchuelz A, Christophe J: The stimulus-secretion coupling of glucose-induced insulin release. XLVI. Physiological role of L-glutamine as a fuel for pancreatic islets. Mol Cell Endocrinol 1980;20:171–189.

7 Sener A, Dunlop ME, Gomis R, Mathias PC, Malaisse-Lagae F, Malaisse WJ: Role of transglutaminase in insulin release. Study with glycine and sarcosine methylesters. Endocrinology 1985;117:237–242.

8 Sener A, Malaisse WJ: The stimulus-secretion coupling of amino acid-induced insulin release. Insulinotropic action of L-alanine. Biochim Biophys Acta 2002;1573:100–104.

9 Matschinsky FM, Brajtburg JK, Stillings S, Ellerman J, Raybaud F, Thurston JH: Factors governing the action of small calorigenic molecules on the islets of langerhans. 8th Midwest Conference on Endocrinology and Metabolism, Columbia, 1972.

10 Sener A, Malaisse WJ: L-leucine and a nonmetabolized analogue activate pancreatic islet glutamate dehydrogenase. Nature 1980;288:187–189.

11 Stanley CA, Lieu YK, Hsu BY, Burlina AB, Greenberg CR, Hopwood NJ, Perlman K, Rich BH, Zammarchi E, Poncz M: Hyperinsulinism and hyperammonemia in infants with regulatory mutations of the glutamate dehydrogenase gene. N Engl J Med 1998;338:1352–1357.

12 Li C, Chen P, Palladino A, Narayan S, Russell LK, Sayed S, Xiong G, Chen J, Stokes D, Butt YM, Jones PM, Collins HW, Cohen NA, Cohen AS, Nissim I, Smith TJ, Strauss AW, Matschinsky FM, Bennett MJ, Stanley CA: Mechanism of hyperinsulinism in short-chain 3-hydroxyacyl-CoA dehydrogenase deficiency involves activation of glutamate dehydrogenase. J Biol Chem 2010;285:31806–31818.

13 Li C, Matter A, Kelly A, Petty TJ, Najafi H, MacMullen C, Daikhin Y, Nissim I, Lazarow A, Kwagh J, Collins HW, Hsu BY, Nissim I, Yudkoff M, Matschinsky FM, Stanley CA: Effects of a GTP-insensitive mutation of glutamate dehydrogenase on insulin secretion in transgenic mice. J Biol Chem 2006;281:15064–15072.

14 Grimberg A, Ferry RJ, Kelly A, Koo-McCoy S, Polonsky K, Glaser B, Permutt A, Aguilar-Bryan L, Stafford D, Thornton PS, Baker L, Stanley CA: Dysregulation of insulin secretion in children with congenital hyperinsulinism due to sulfonylurea receptor mutations. Diabetes 2001;50:322–328.

15 Treberg JR, Clow KA, Greene KA, Brosnan ME, Brosnan JT: Systemic activation of glutamate dehydrogenase increases renal ammoniagenesis: implications for the hyperinsulinism/hyperammonemia syndrome. Am J Physiol Endocrinol Metab 2010;298:E1219–E1225.

16 Hussain K, Clayton PT, Krywawych S, Chatziandreou I, Mills P, Ginbey DW, Geboers AJ, Berger R, van den Berg IE, Eaton S: Hyperinsulinism of infancy associated with a novel splice site mutation in the SCHAD gene. J Pediatr 2005;146:706–708.
17 Molven A, Matre GE, Duran M, Wanders RJ, Rishaug U, Njolstad PR, Jellum E, Sovik O: Familial hyperinsulinemic hypoglycemia caused by a defect in the SCHAD enzyme of mitochondrial fatty acid oxidation. Diabetes 2004;53:221–227.
18 Flanagan SE, Patch AM, Locke JM, Akcay T, Simsek E, Alaei M, Yekta Z, Desai M, Kapoor RR, Hussain K, Ellard S: Genome-wide homozygosity analysis reveals HADH mutations as a common cause of diazoxide-responsive hyperinsulinemic-hypoglycemia in consanguineous pedigrees. J Clin Endocrinol Metab 2011;96:E498–E502.
19 Stanley CA, Bennett MJ, Mayatepek E: Disorders of Mitochondrial Fatty Acid Oxidation and Related Metabolic Pathyways. Heidelberg, Springer, 2006.
20 Kapoor RR, James C, Flanagan SE, Ellard S, Eaton S, Hussain K: 3-Hydroxyacyl-coenzyme A dehydrogenase deficiency and hyperinsulinemic hypoglycemia: characterization of a novel mutation and severe dietary protein sensitivity. J Clin Endocrinol Metab 2009;94:2221–2225.
21 De Leon DD, Li C, Delson MI, Matschinsky FM, Stanley CA, Stoffers DA: Exendin-(9–39) corrects fasting hypoglycemia in SUR-1-/- mice by lowering cAMP in pancreatic beta-cells and inhibiting insulin secretion. J Biol Chem 2008;283:25786–25793.
22 Martens GA, Vervoort A, Van de Casteele M, Stange G, Hellemans K, Van Thi HV, Schuit F, Pipeleers D: Specificity in beta cell expression of L-3-hydroxyacyl-CoA dehydrogenase, short chain, and potential role in down-regulating insulin release. J Biol Chem 2007;282:21134–21144.
23 Fourtner SH, Stanley CA, Kelly A: Protein-sensitive hypoglycemia without leucine sensitivity in hyperinsulinism caused by K(ATP) channel mutations. J Pediatr 2006;149:47–52.
24 Kelly A, Ng D, Ferry RJ Jr, Grimberg A, Koo-McCoy S, Thornton PS, Stanley CA: Acute insulin responses to leucine in children with the hyperinsulinism/hyperammonemia syndrome. J Clin Endocrinol Metab 2001;86:3724–3728.
25 Li C, Buettger C, Kwagh J, Matter A, Daikhin Y, Nissim IB, Collins HW, Yudkoff M, Stanley CA, Matschinsky FM: A signaling role of glutamine in insulin secretion. J Biol Chem 2004;279:13393–13401.
26 Li C, Nissim I, Chen P, Buettger C, Najafi H, Daikhin Y, Nissim I, Collins HW, Yudkoff M, Stanley CA, Matschinsky FM: Elimination of KATP channels in mouse islets results in elevated [U-^{13}C]glucose metabolism, glutaminolysis, and pyruvate cycling but a decreased gamma-aminobutyric acid shunt. J Biol Chem 2008;283:17238–17249.

Changhong Li, MD, PhD
Division of Endocrinology/Diabetes
The Children's Hospital of Philadelphia
34th Street and Civic Center Boulevard
Philadelphia, PA 19104 (USA)
Tel. +1 215 590 5380, E-Mail li@email.chop.edu

Stanley CA, De León DD (eds): Monogenic Hyperinsulinemic Hypoglycemia Disorders.
Front Diabetes. Basel, Karger, 2012, vol 21, pp 125–136

Tissue Specificity of Glutamate Dehydrogenase as Illustrated in Pancreatic Beta-Cells and the Central Nervous System

Stefania Carobbio · Laurène Vetterli · Francesca Frigerio · Melis Karaca · Pierre Maechler

Department of Cell Physiology and Metabolism, Geneva University Medical Centre, Geneva, Switzerland

Abstract

One of the genetic forms of hyperinsulinism highlights the role of glutamate dehydrogenase (GDH) in pancreatic beta-cells. GDH is a mitochondrial enzyme which plays a pivotal role between carbohydrate and protein metabolisms by controlling production and consumption of the messenger molecule glutamate in neuroendocrine cells. GDH activity is controlled by several regulators that confer energy-sensor properties to this enzyme. Moreover, GDH is allosterically regulated by GTP and ADP. GDH is also regulated by ADP-ribosylation, mediated by a member of the energy-sensor family sirtuins, namely SIRT4. In the brain, GDH ensures the cycling of the neurotransmitter glutamate between neurons and astrocytes. GDH also controls ammonia metabolism and detoxification (mainly in the liver and kidney). In pancreatic beta-cells, the importance of GDH as a key enzyme in the regulation of insulin secretion is now well established. Inhibition of GDH activity decreases insulin release, while activating mutations are associated with a hyperinsulinism syndrome. Although GDH enzyme catalyzes the same reaction in every tissue, its function regarding metabolic homeostasis varies greatly according to specific organs. Newly generated mouse models lacking GDH in specific tissues offer an opportunity to decipher organ specificities of GDH regulation.

Glutamate is a multifunctional amino acid that can enter various metabolic pathways according to cellular demand and specificity of tissue function [1]. The mitochondrial enzyme glutamate dehydrogenase (GDH) is closely associated with glutamate metabolism (fig. 1). Besides being a necessary building block for proteins [2], it is also a major neurotransmitter in neuronal and nonneuronal cells [3], a precursor of the tricarboxylic acid (TCA) cycle and metabolic intermediate [2], an intracellular messenger [4], and a key member of ammonia metabolism [5]. Within the mitochondria, different enzymes are directly implicated in the breakdown and generation of glutamate, i.e. GDH, alanine aminotransferase, aspartate aminotransferase,

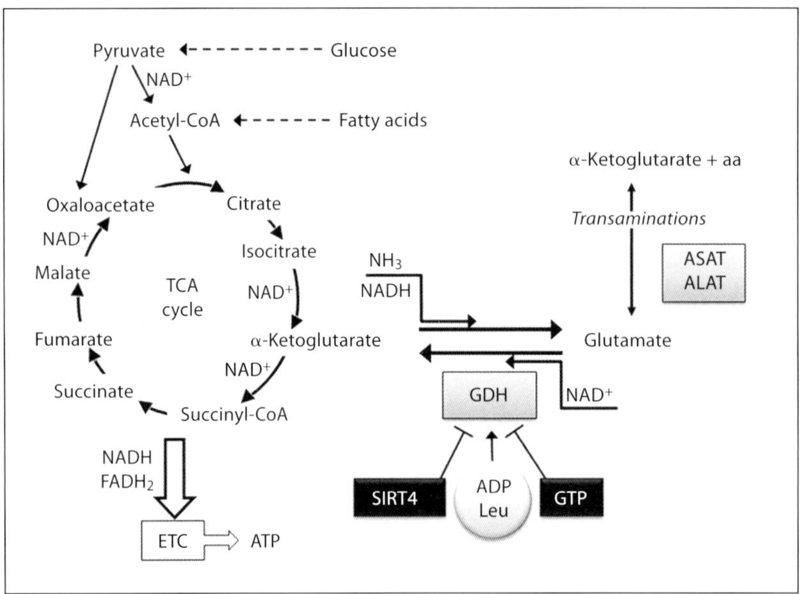

Fig. 1. Simplified scheme depicting major pathways associated with GDH. GDH is activated by ADP and L-leucine (Leu) and inhibited by GTP and SIRT4. Alanine aminotransferase (ALAT) and aspartate aminotransferase (ASAT) also participate in glutamate breakdown and synthesis. Within the mitochondria, NADH is preferentially reoxidized to NAD^+ by complex I of the electron transport chain (ETC) or by GDH.

and glutaminase [6]. However, among these enzymes, only GDH catalyzes reactions resulting in net changes in the amino acid pool by introducing or removing an amino group. Accordingly, GDH contribution to amino acid synthesis and breakdown is not restricted to glutamate (fig. 1).

The metabolic control by hormones and neurotransmitters depends on coordinated usage and storage of nutrients. In this regard, glutamate plays a dual role as it is both a signaling molecule and a metabolite at the frontier between carbohydrate and protein metabolisms. Mitochondria, and the TCA cycle in particular, represent the major metabolic crossroads, enabling fuel oxidation as well as provision of building blocks, or cataplerosis, for lipids and proteins [2]. The glycolytic product pyruvate enters mitochondria and is preferentially oxidized to acetyl-CoA by pyruvate dehydrogenase. Oxaloacetate, produced by malate dehydrogenase or alternatively by the anaplerotic enzyme pyruvate carboxylase, condenses with acetyl-CoA forming citrate, thereby activating the TCA cycle. The fate of the TCA cycle intermediate alpha-ketoglutarate is influenced by the redox state of mitochondria. A low NADH-to-NAD^+ ratio would favor further oxidative decarboxylation to succinyl-CoA as NAD^+ is required as a cofactor for this pathway (fig. 1). Conversely, a high NADH-to-NAD^+ ratio would promote NADH-dependent reductive transamination through GDH, thereby forming glutamate as a cataplerotic product of the TCA cycle [2].

Alternatively, glutamate can originate from glutamine via glutaminase activity and also through transamination reactions catalyzed by aspartate aminotransferase or alanine aminotransferase.

Enzymatic Regulation of Glutamate Dehydrogenase

GDH (EC 1.4.1.3) is encoded by a well-conserved 45-kb gene named *GLUD1*, which is organized into 13 exons [7]. Historically, the GDH from bovine liver has been the most extensively studied [8]. In mammals, this enzyme is a homohexamer located in the mitochondrial matrix. GDH catalyzes the reversible reaction alpha-ketoglutarate + NH_3 + NADH ↔ glutamate + NAD^+ (fig. 1).

GDH is allosterically regulated by leucine, pyridine, adenine, and guanine nucleotides [9, 10]. Each subunit of GDH exhibits specific binding domains: the catalytic domain, the adenine and guanine nucleotide regulatory domains, the reduced coenzyme regulatory domain, and the ADP-ribosylation domain [8, 11]. In most vertebrates, GDH is inhibited by GTP and activated by ADP, but there are differences in the way the enzyme behaves towards the purine nucleoside phosphates [8]. Identification of an unusual hyperinsulinism/hyperammonemia syndrome has been associated with dominant mutations in GDH that cause reduced GTP-mediated inhibition of the enzyme [12].

GDH is also regulated by reversible cysteine-specific ADP-ribosylation in mitochondria. Inactivation of the enzyme is caused by ADP-ribose association, which is suppressed by NAD(P)H. The stoichiometry between incorporated ADP-ribose and GDH subunits suggests that modification of one subunit per catalytically active homohexamer causes the inactivation of the enzyme [11]. SIRT4, a mammalian sirtuin with mitochondrial ADP-ribosyltransferase activity, is a matrix protein and becomes cleaved at amino acid 28 after import into mitochondria [13]. Mitochondrial ADP-ribosyltransferase SIRT4 downregulates GDH activity in pancreatic beta-cells and thereby inhibits insulin secretion [13, 14]. Recently, it has been shown that SIRT4 represses fatty acid oxidation in both hepatocytes and muscle cells [15]. Thus, GDH activity is not only at the intersection of the carbohydrate and protein pathways, but is also associated with lipid metabolism through SIRT4 action. This concept is further substantiated by the recent link established between GDH and a mitochondrial fatty acid beta-oxidation enzyme. Indeed, short-chain 3-hydroxyacyl-CoA dehydrogenase has been proposed to inhibit GDH activity [16].

Glutamate Dehydrogenase Function in Specific Tissues

The enzyme GDH catalyzes the same reaction in every tissue, although the direction of the predominant flux might be tissue-specific and still highly debated. Moreover, the physiological function of GDH regarding metabolic homeostasis varies greatly according to specific organs. In the brain, GDH plays a key role in the recycling of the neurotransmitter glutamate as discussed below [17]. GDH is also of major importance for ammonia detoxification through nitrogen metabolism and urea synthesis in the liver and kidney [1, 5]. It is noteworthy that in vivo GDH activation results in increased plasma ammonia levels contributed by the kidney [18]. This illustrates the importance of GDH-dependent provision of urinary ammonia, thereby facilitating acid excretion [19].

In the liver, the hepatic glutamate pathway is involved in the metabolism of most amino acids through transamination or GDH activity. Quantitatively, the liver is central for nitrogen metabolism, nitrogen being transported from skeletal muscle essentially as glutamine and alanine, especially during periods of active gluconeogenesis [5]. Conversely, the liver can contribute to the clearance of ammonia through generation of glutamate by GDH and then glutamine via glutamine synthetase [20]. GDH-dependent ammoniagenesis is also very active in kidney, in association with acid excretion.

In pancreatic beta-cells, the importance of GDH as a key enzyme in the regulation of insulin secretion was recognized long ago [21]. Inhibition of GDH activity was shown to decrease insulin release [22, 23], while activating mutations have been associated with a hyperinsulinism syndrome [24, 25]. Here, we will focus on two neuroendocrine tissues controlling whole body energy metabolism at different levels: insulin secretion in pancreatic beta-cells and glutamate/glutamine cycling in the central nervous system.

Glutamate Dehydrogenase and Pancreatic Beta-Cell Function

Pancreatic beta-cells function as glycemia sensors and produce corresponding amounts of the hormone insulin, which acts on target tissues to maintain energy homeostasis. Upon nutrient stimulation, elevation of cytosolic Ca^{2+} in the beta-cell is the primary and necessary signal for insulin exocytosis (fig. 2). Then, increasing the magnitude of the secretory response requires amplification of the Ca^{2+} signal involving metabolism-derived additive factors [26]. The importance of GDH as a key enzyme in the control of insulin secretion was highlighted roughly 30 years ago [21]; however, the precise function of GDH in beta-cells remains to be determined. Specifically, GDH might play a role in glucose-induced amplifying pathway through generation of glutamate. Indeed, glutamate has been proposed as an intracellular messenger potentiating Ca^{2+} effects on insulin exocytosis [4, 27–29]. Several mechanisms have been proposed to explain glutamate action, such as uptake by secretory granules [4, 27], an observation correlating with expression of the vesicular glutamate transporters VGLUT1 and VGLUT2 in insulin secreting cells [30]. Once inside the secretory granule, glutamate can induce pH changes as reported in secretory vesicles from pancreatic beta-cells [31] and/or activate metabotropic glutamate receptors mGlu5

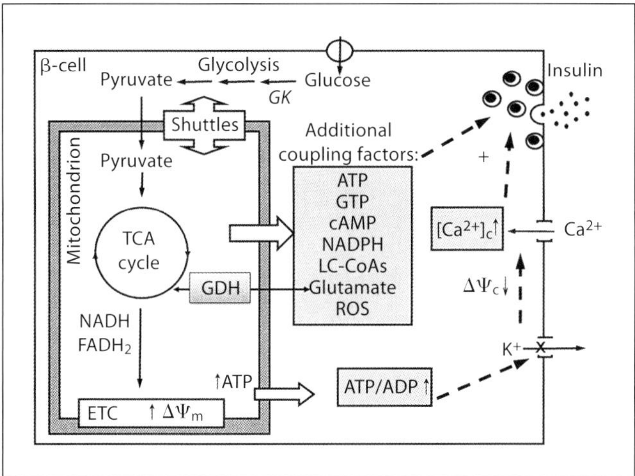

Fig. 2. Model for coupling of glucose metabolism to insulin secretion in the beta-cell. Glucose equilibrates across the plasma membrane and is phosphorylated by glucokinase *(GK)*. Further, glycolysis produces pyruvate, which preferentially enters the mitochondria and is metabolized by the TCA cycle. The TCA cycle generates reducing equivalents transferred by NADH and $FADH_2$ to the electron transport chain (ETC), leading to hyperpolarization of the mitochondrial membrane ($\Delta\Psi_m$) and generation of ATP. ATP is then transferred to the cytosol, raising the ATP/ADP ratio. Subsequently, closure of ATP-sensitive potassium channels depolarizes the cell membrane ($\Delta\Psi_c$). This opens voltage-dependent Ca^{2+} channels, increasing cytosolic Ca^{2+} concentration ($[Ca^{2+}]_c$), which triggers insulin exocytosis. The amplifying pathway of metabolism secretion coupling is contributed by additive signals, such as glutamate that can be generated by GDH.

that have been shown to be expressed in secretory granules [32]. Alternative mechanisms for glutamate action within the beta-cell include activation of acetyl-CoA carboxylase [33] by inhibition of protein phosphatase enzymatic activities [34].

All these proposed mechanisms of action require permissive levels of glutamate to be reached in the cytosolic compartment. Abrogation of GDH specifically in the beta-cells of transgenic mice prevents full development of the secretory response [35], an effect also observed in beta-cells forced to express an enzyme that decarboxylates intracellular glutamate, thereby lowering glucose-induced glutamate levels [28]. Moreover, silencing of the mitochondrial glutamate carrier GC1 inhibits insulin exocytosis evoked by glucose stimulation, an effect rescued by the provision of exogenous glutamate to the cell [29]. Finally, prevention of glutamate release from beta-cells results in concomitant elevations of intracellular glutamate levels and glucose-evoked insulin secretion [36]. Altogether, these experimental approaches strongly indicate that permissive levels of glutamate within the beta-cell are necessary for the full development of glucose-stimulated insulin secretion. Permissive concentrations of glutamate are also required for proper function of the malate-aspartate shuttle, an important player in insulin-secreting cells [37, 38].

About Glutamate Dehydrogenase Flux Direction in Pancreatic Beta-Cells

In addition to glutamate generation, GDH can play a role as an amino acid sensor triggering insulin release upon glutamine stimulation in specific conditions of GDH allosteric activation [39]. These two modes of action each requires opposite directions of GDH reactions. GDH preferential flux direction would be either anaplerotic forming alpha-ketoglutarate from glutamate or, conversely, cataplerotic generating glutamate at the expense of alpha-ketoglutarate. Temporally, these two actions are not mutually exclusive, as specific metabolic states of the cell might dictate one or the other direction. During glucose stimulation, elevation of the mitochondrial NADH-to-NAD^+ ratio should favor NADH-dependent reductive transamination of alpha-ketoglutarate to glutamate. Indeed, such metabolic conditions result in saturated electron transport chain activity. Then, within mitochondria, GDH is the alternative enzyme to complex I activity for NADH reoxidation to NAD^+ (fig. 1). NMR spectroscopy studies performed on insulinoma cells revealed that under glucose stimulation glutamate is generated rather than consumed [40], and that pyruvate dehydrogenase plus pyruvate carboxylase act as the anaplerotic enzymes rather than GDH [41]. Therefore, the flux direction of GDH might primarily depend on the redox and energy state of mitochondria, as well as the provision of specific substrates determining the balance of cataplerosis versus anaplerosis.

GTP-insensitive mutations of GDH might also influence flux direction. In transgenic mouse islets loaded with glutamine, activating mutation of the GDH increases ammonia production at low glucose [42]. In control islets, however, glucose stimulation lowers ammonia production, indicative of a reduced rate of deamination reaction under normal conditions [42]. This illustrates how GDH mutations associated with the hyperinsulinism-hyperammonemia syndrome render islets glutamine sensitive [42].

Increasing Glutamate Dehydrogenase Activity in Pancreatic Beta-Cells

Of note, GDH was investigated in beta-cells mostly by means of amplified activity of the enzyme. Numerous studies have used the GDH allosteric activator L-leucine or its nonmetabolized analogue beta-2-aminobicyclo[2.2.1]heptane-2-carboxylic acid (BCH) to question the role of GDH in the control of insulin secretion [21, 39, 43]. Our group also increased GDH activity by means of overexpression, an approach that we combined with allosteric activation of the enzyme [44].

As mentioned above, some studies investigated activating mutations of GDH that have been associated with a hyperinsulinism syndrome [24, 25]. Reduced GTP-mediated inhibition of the enzyme was associated with most of GDH mutations linked to the hyperinsulinism syndrome [12]. Beta-cells forced to express such mutations become glutamine responsive in terms of insulin secretion, both in cell and mouse models [42, 45]. Unlike glucose, glutamine is not efficiently catabolized to the end-product CO_2 in beta-cells [46]. However, glutamine complete oxidation can be prompted by allosteric activation of GDH, an effect correlating with stimulation of insulin secretion [39]. Alternatively, we have shown that overexpression of GDH in isolated islets promotes glutamine metabolism associated with insulin secretion [44]. It is noteworthy that the secretory pattern of islets isolated from transgenic mice expressing the H454Y GTP-insensitive GDH mutation [42] is similar to the one obtained from islets overexpressing nonmutated GDH [44], i.e. close to normal glucose-stimulated insulin release but unmasked robust glutamine response. Since the GTP-insensitive mutation was artificially expressed under the highly active insulin promoter, it remains to be determined what the respective contributions are of the resulting overexpression versus the activating mutation per se in the secretory responses of the H454Y transgenic islets [42].

Taken together, these gain-of-function approaches demonstrate that amino acids in general, and glutamine in particular, can be turned into secretagogues under pathological or experimental conditions facilitating highly active GDH. However, under such nonphysiological conditions, the secretory response to the primary stimulus of insulin release, namely glucose, is not, or very modestly, modified [16, 42, 44, 45].

Decreasing Glutamate Dehydrogenase Activity in Pancreatic Beta-Cells

In only a limited number of studies was GDH activity reduced in pancreatic islets by the use of inhibitors for which the specificity is questionable [22, 23, 47]. Upon glucose stimulation, GDH inhibition results in both lower insulin release and cellular glutamate levels [47]. Green tea polyphenols inhibit GDH and reduce insulin release when islets are stimulated with glutamine plus BCH, although not upon glucose stimulation [23]. Regarding physiological modulators, it has been shown that the mammalian Sir2 homolog SIRT4 acts in the mitochondria of pancreatic beta-cells to repress the activity of GDH through ADP-ribosylation [14]. SIRT4 downregulates GDH activity and thereby modulates insulin secretion [13, 14]. In particular, we have shown that glucose-stimulated insulin secretion is increased when SIRT4 is downregulated and decreased when overexpressed [13].

It is now clearly established that mutations rendering GDH more active are responsible for a hyperinsulinism syndrome [24]. Mutations producing a less active, or even nonactive, GDH enzyme have not been reported, leaving open the question if such mutations would be either lethal or asymptomatic. An antisense approach used in our laboratory to lower GDH expression in INS-1E beta-cells resulted in reduced GDH activity and inhibition of glucose-evoked insulin release [26]. We recently generated and characterized transgenic mice (named beta-*Glud1*$^{-/-}$) with conditional beta-cell-specific deletion of GDH [35]. The secretory response of beta-*Glud1*$^{-/-}$ has been tested in several ways, revealing similar reductions in the secretory response compared to controls: –49% by islet perifusion, –37% by pancreatic perfusion, –38% during a glucose tolerance test, –55% in the fed state, and –38% upon acute knockout in isolated islets [35]. Thus, data show that GDH accounts for about 40% of glucose-stimulated insulin secretion and that no compensatory mechanisms exist. Generation of ATP upon glucose stimulation is preserved in beta-*Glud1*$^{-/-}$ islets, showing that the partial inhibition of glucose-stimulated insulin secretion is not the consequence of general mitochondrial impairment, but rather specific for glutamate pathway. In beta-*Glud1*$^{-/-}$ mice, the reduced optimal secretory capacity resulted in lower plasma insulin levels in response to both feeding and glucose load, while body weight gain was preserved [35]. Therefore, GDH is essential for the full development of the secretory response in beta-cells, being sensitive in the upper range of physiological glucose concentrations. Interestingly, the beta-*Glud1*$^{-/-}$ mice exhibit normal glycemia, both in the fasting state and upon the glucose tolerance test, despite marked reduction of the secretory capacity evoked at high glucose. This indicates that the maximal potential of insulin production by the beta-cell might not be necessary under a normal energy homeostatic state. Such an assumption is supported by clinical data showing maintenance of glucose tolerance in donors of islets who underwent partial pancreatectomy [48]. However, preservation of normoglycemia, while having half of the full potential for insulin release, might be compromised in conditions requiring increased insulin production, such as obesity-associated insulin resistance or pregnancy [49].

Glutamate Dehydrogenase and Brain Function

In the brain, mitochondrial function is closely associated with glutamate metabolism as this amino acid is the main excitatory neurotransmitter of the central nervous system [50]. In particular, mitochondria regulate energetic status of the brain, utilization of metabolic substrates, and detoxification associated with excess of neurotransmitters.

Glutamate released by activated synapses depolarizes target neurons through specific receptors [51]. Intersynaptic glutamate clearance is mainly operated by astrocytes. Once taken-up by astrocytes, glutamate can be metabolized in several ways, of which either glutamine formation or entry into the TCA cycle are quantitatively the most important (fig. 3). Glutamine, formed by glutamine synthetase in astrocytes, is transported to neurons, transformed back into glutamate by glutaminase, and packed into secretory vesicles to be released as neurotransmitter, thereby completing glutamate cycling (fig. 3). Alternatively, glutamate can undergo oxidative catabolism that is initiated by its conversion into alpha-ketoglutarate. The process is mediated by either GDH or transaminases [52–54]. Complete oxidation of one alpha-ketoglutarate by

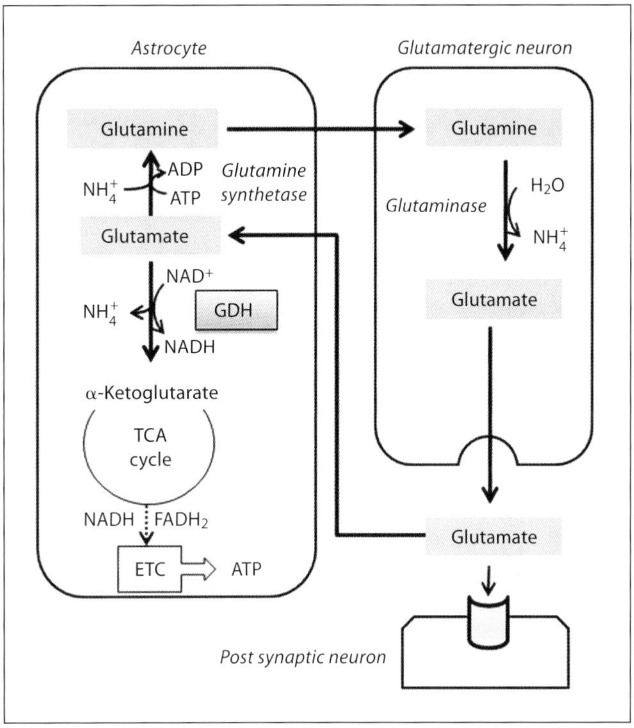

Fig. 3. In the central nervous system, glutamate is the main excitatory neurotransmitter. However, glutamate is also closely associated with brain energy metabolism. Upon glutamatergic transmission, intersynaptic glutamate clearance is achieved mostly by astrocytes. Following its uptake by astrocytes, glutamate may be aminated to glutamine and then recycled back to neurons. Alternatively, glutamate may be deaminated to alpha-ketoglutarate by GDH before further oxidation in the TCA cycle, thereby promoting ATP generation.

the TCA cycle yields about 30 molecules of ATP, which is about 20-fold the ATP required for glutamate uptake.

The relative fluxes through distinct glutamate pathways, i.e. glutamine versus alpha-ketoglutarate formation, can vary according to specific metabolic conditions [53, 55]. Under basal conditions, glutamate taken up by astrocytes is predominantly metabolized via glutamine synthetase rather than via GDH, thereby favoring glutamate cycling [52, 56]. When extracellular glutamate is elevated, the amount of glutamate oxidized through the TCA cycle increases dramatically in a GDH-dependent manner [53, 55]. Indeed, inhibition of transaminase activity does not prevent glutamate oxidation. This suggests that oxidative deamination contributed by GDH is the major route for the entrance of glutamate carbons in the form of alpha-ketoglutarate into the TCA cycle [53]. Ongoing studies using brain-specific *Glud1* null mice indicate that GDH is necessary for glutamate-derived ATP generation in astrocytes [57].

Overall, recent observations highlight GDH as a key enzyme for glutamate metabolism and energy homeostasis within the brain. Astrocytic internalization of glutamate not only participates in the detoxification of the extracellular space, but also supplies energy to brain cells. Neurons and astrocytes are metabolically coupled and tightly related in the regulation of energy balance of the brain.

Conclusion

The mitochondrial enzyme GDH connects several metabolic pathways, thereby playing a key role in the control of energy homeostasis. However, GDH fulfils different functions according to specific tissues. GDH flux direction depends on metabolic parameters such as substrate availability, redox, and energy state of mitochondria. These parameters may be tissue-specific as described in this chapter. Moreover, ADP-ribosylation of GDH mediated by SIRT4 offers another regulatory mechanism that might be tissue-specific, pending different levels of *SIRT4* expression. Activating mutations of GDH have highlighted the importance of regulatory effectors. They may contribute to both flux direction preference and tissue specificity.

Acknowledgements

Current work in our laboratory is supported by the Swiss National Science Foundation, the State of Geneva, and the European Foundation for the Study of Diabetes. The authors are members of the Geneva Programme for Metabolic Disorders.

References

1 Frigerio F, Casimir M, Carobbio S, Maechler P: Tissue specificity of mitochondrial glutamate pathways and the control of metabolic homeostasis. Biochim Biophys Acta 2008;1777:965.

2 Owen OE, Kalhan SC, Hanson RW: The key role of anaplerosis and cataplerosis for citric acid cycle function. J Biol Chem 2002;277:30409.

3 Henn FA, Goldstein MN, Hamberger A: Uptake of the neurotransmitter candidate glutamate by glia. Nature 1974;249:663.

4 Maechler P, Wollheim CB: Mitochondrial glutamate acts as a messenger in glucose-induced insulin exocytosis. Nature 1999;402:685.

5 Brosnan JT: Glutamate, at the interface between amino acid and carbohydrate metabolism. J Nutr 2000;130:988S.

6 Newsholme P, Brennan L, Rubi B, Maechler P: New insights into amino acid metabolism, beta-cell function and diabetes. Clin Sci (Lond) 2005;108:185.

7 Michaelidis TM, Tzimagiorgis G, Moschonas NK, Papamatheakis J: The human glutamate dehydrogenase gene family: gene organization and structural characterization. Genomics 1993;16:150.

8 Hudson RC, Daniel RM: L-glutamate dehydrogenases: distribution, properties and mechanism. Comp Biochem Physiol B 1993;106:767.

9 Fisher HF: L-Glutamate dehydrogenase from bovine liver. Methods Enzymol 1985;113:16.

10 Smith TJ, Peterson PE, Schmidt T, Fang J, Stanley CA: Structures of bovine glutamate dehydrogenase complexes elucidate the mechanism of purine regulation. J Mol Biol 2001;307:707.

11 Herrero-Yraola A, Bakhit SM, Franke P, Weise C, Schweiger M, Jorcke D, Ziegler M: Regulation of glutamate dehydrogenase by reversible ADP-ribosylation in mitochondria. EMBO J 2001;20:2404.

12 Stanley CA, Fang J, Kutyna K, Hsu BY, Ming JE, Glaser B, Poncz M: Molecular basis and characterization of the hyperinsulinism/hyperammonemia syndrome: predominance of mutations in exons 11 and 12 of the glutamate dehydrogenase gene. HI/HA Contributing Investigators. Diabetes 2000;49:667.

13 Ahuja N, Schwer B, Carobbio S, Waltregny D, North BJ, Castronovo V, Maechler P, Verdin E: Regulation of insulin secretion by SIRT4, a mitochondrial ADP-ribosyltransferase. J Biol Chem 2007;282:33583.

14 Haigis MC, Mostoslavsky R, Haigis KM, Fahie K, Christodoulou DC, Murphy AJ, Valenzuela DM, Yancopoulos GD, Karow M, Blander G, Wolberger C, Prolla TA, Weindruch R, Alt FW, Guarente L: SIRT4 inhibits glutamate dehydrogenase and opposes the effects of calorie restriction in pancreatic beta cells. Cell 2006;126:941.

15 Nasrin N, Wu X, Fortier E, Feng Y, Bare OC, Chen S, Ren X, Wu Z, Streeper RS, Bordone L: SIRT4 regulates fatty acid oxidation and mitochondrial gene expression in liver and muscle cells. J Biol Chem 2010;285:31995.
16 Li C, Chen P, Palladino A, Narayan S, Russell LK, Sayed S, Xiong G, Chen J, Stokes D, Butt YM, Jones PM, Collins HW, Cohen NA, Cohen AS, Nissim I, Smith TJ, Strauss AW, Matschinsky FM, Bennett MJ, Stanley CA: Mechanism of hyperinsulinism in short-chain 3-hydroxyacyl-CoA dehydrogenase deficiency involves activation of glutamate dehydrogenase. J Biol Chem 2010;285:31806.
17 Anderson CM, Swanson RA: Astrocyte glutamate transport: review of properties, regulation, and physiological functions. Glia 2000;32:1.
18 Treberg JR, Brosnan ME, Watford M, Brosnan JT: On the reversibility of glutamate dehydrogenase and the source of hyperammonemia in the hyperinsulinism/hyperammonemia syndrome. Adv Enzyme Regul 2010;50:34.
19 Deferrari G, Garibotto G, Robaudo C, Saffioti S, Russo R, Sala MR, Bruzzone M, Tizianello A: Renal ammoniagenesis and interorgan flow of glutamine in chronic metabolic acidosis. Contrib Nephrol. Basel, Karger, 1994;110:144.
20 Cooper AJ, Nieves E, Coleman AE, Filc-DeRicco S, Gelbard AS: Short-term metabolic fate of [13N] ammonia in rat liver in vivo. J Biol Chem 1987; 262:1073.
21 Sener A, Malaisse WJ: L-leucine and a nonmetabolized analogue activate pancreatic islet glutamate dehydrogenase. Nature 1980;288:187.
22 Bryla J, Michalik M, Nelson J, Erecinska M: Regulation of the glutamate dehydrogenase activity in rat islets of Langerhans and its consequence on insulin release. Metabolism 1994;43:1187.
23 Li C, Allen A, Kwagh J, Doliba NM, Qin W, Najafi H, Collins HW, Matschinsky FM, Stanley CA, Smith TJ: Green tea polyphenols modulate insulin secretion by inhibiting glutamate dehydrogenase. J Biol Chem 2006;281:10214.
24 Stanley CA, Lieu YK, Hsu BY, Burlina AB, Greenberg CR, Hopwood NJ, Perlman K, Rich BH, Zammarchi E, Poncz M: Hyperinsulinism and hyperammonemia in infants with regulatory mutations of the glutamate dehydrogenase gene. N Engl J Med 1998;338: 1352.
25 Yorifuji T, Muroi J, Uematsu A, Hiramatsu H, Momoi T: Hyperinsulinism-hyperammonemia syndrome caused by mutant glutamate dehydrogenase accompanied by novel enzyme kinetics. Hum Genet 1999;104:476.
26 Maechler P, Carobbio S, Rubi B: In beta-cells, mitochondria integrate and generate metabolic signals controlling insulin secretion. Int J Biochem Cell Biol 2006;38:696.
27 Hoy M, Maechler P, Efanov AM, Wollheim CB, Berggren PO, Gromada J: Increase in cellular glutamate levels stimulates exocytosis in pancreatic beta-cells. FEBS Lett 2002;531:199.
28 Rubi B, Ishihara H, Hegardt FG, Wollheim CB, Maechler P: GAD65-mediated glutamate decarboxylation reduces glucose-stimulated insulin secretion in pancreatic beta cells. J Biol Chem 2001;276: 36391.
29 Casimir M, Lasorsa FM, Rubi B, Caille D, Palmieri F, Meda P, Maechler P: Mitochondrial glutamate carrier GC1 as a newly identified player in the control of glucose-stimulated insulin secretion. J Biol Chem 2009;284:25004.
30 Bai L, Zhang X, Ghishan FK: Characterization of vesicular glutamate transporter in pancreatic alpha – and beta – cells and its regulation by glucose. Am J Physiol Gastrointest Liver Physiol 2003;284:G808.
31 Eto K, Yamashita T, Hirose K, Tsubamoto Y, Ainscow EK, Rutter GA, Kimura S, Noda M, Iino M, Kadowaki T: Glucose metabolism and glutamate analog acutely alkalinize pH of insulin secretory vesicles of pancreatic beta-cells. Am J Physiol Endocrinol Metab 2003;285:E262.
32 Storto M, Capobianco L, Battaglia G, Molinaro G, Gradini R, Riozzi B, Di Mambro A, Mitchell KJ, Bruno V, Vairetti MP, Rutter GA, Nicoletti F: Insulin secretion is controlled by mGlu5 metabotropic glutamate receptors. Mol Pharmacol 2006;69:1234.
33 Kowluru A, Chen HQ, Modrick LM, Stefanelli C: Activation of acetyl-CoA carboxylase by a glutamate- and magnesium-sensitive protein phosphatase in the islet beta-cell. Diabetes 2001;50:1580.
34 Lehtihet M, Honkanen RE, Sjoholm A: Glutamate inhibits protein phosphatases and promotes insulin exocytosis in pancreatic beta-cells. Biochem Biophys Res Commun 2005;328:601.
35 Carobbio S, Frigerio F, Rubi B, Vetterli L, Bloksgaard M, Gjinovci A, Pournourmohammadi S, Herrera PL, Reith W, Mandrup S, Maechler P: Deletion of glutamate dehydrogenase in beta-cells abolishes part of the insulin secretory response not required for glucose homeostasis. J Biol Chem 2009;284:921.
36 Feldmann N, Del Rio RM, Gjinovci A, Tamarit-Rodriguez J, Wollheim CB, Wiederkehr A: Reduction of plasma membrane glutamate transport potentiates insulin but not glucagon secretion in pancreatic islet cells. Mol Cell Endocrinol 2011; 338:46.

37 Casimir M, Rubi B, Frigerio F, Chaffard G, Maechler P: Silencing of the mitochondrial NADH shuttle component aspartate-glutamate carrier AGC1/Aralar1 in INS-1E cells and rat islets. Biochem J 2009;424:459.

38 Rubi B, del Arco A, Bartley C, Satrustegui J, Maechler P: The malate-aspartate NADH shuttle member Aralar1 determines glucose metabolic fate, mitochondrial activity, and insulin secretion in beta cells. J Biol Chem 2004;279:55659.

39 Sener A, Malaisse-Lagae F, Malaisse WJ: Stimulation of pancreatic islet metabolism and insulin release by a nonmetabolizable amino acid. Proc Natl Acad Sci USA 1981;78:5460.

40 Broca C, Brennan L, Petit P, Newsholme P, Maechler P: Mitochondria-derived glutamate at the interplay between branched-chain amino acid and glucose-induced insulin secretion. FEBS Lett 2003;545:167.

41 Cline GW, Lepine RL, Papas KK, Kibbey RG, Shulman GI: 13C NMR isotopomer analysis of anaplerotic pathways in INS-1 cells. J Biol Chem 2004;279:44370.

42 Li C, Matter A, Kelly A, Petty TJ, Najafi H, MacMullen C, Daikhin Y, Nissim I, Lazarow A, Kwagh J, Collins HW, Hsu BY, Yudkoff M, Matschinsky FM, Stanley CA: Effects of a GTP-insensitive mutation of glutamate dehydrogenase on insulin secretion in transgenic mice. J Biol Chem 2006;281:15064.

43 Fahien LA, MacDonald MJ, Kmiotek EH, Mertz RJ, Fahien CM: Regulation of insulin release by factors that also modify glutamate dehydrogenase. J Biol Chem 1988;263:13610.

44 Carobbio S, Ishihara H, Fernandez-Pascual S, Bartley C, Martin-Del-Rio R, Maechler P: Insulin secretion profiles are modified by overexpression of glutamate dehydrogenase in pancreatic islets. Diabetologia 2004;47:266.

45 Tanizawa Y, Nakai K, Sasaki T, Anno T, Ohta Y, Inoue H, Matsuo K, Koga M, Furukawa S, Oka Y: Unregulated elevation of glutamate dehydrogenase activity induces glutamine-stimulated insulin secretion: identification and characterization of a GLUD1 gene mutation and insulin secretion studies with MIN6 cells overexpressing the mutant glutamate dehydrogenase. Diabetes 2002;51:712.

46 Malaisse WJ, Sener A, Carpinelli AR, Anjaneyulu K, Lebrun P, Herchuelz A, Christophe J: The stimulus-secretion coupling of glucose-induced insulin release. XLVI. Physiological role of L-glutamine as a fuel for pancreatic islets. Mol Cell Endocrinol 1980;20:171.

47 Yang SJ, Huh JW, Kim MJ, Lee WJ, Kim TU, Choi SY, Cho SW: Regulatory effects of 5′-deoxypyridoxal on glutamate dehydrogenase activity and insulin secretion in pancreatic islets. Biochimie 2003;85:581.

48 Matsumoto S, Okitsu T, Iwanaga Y, Noguchi H, Nagata H, Yonekawa Y, Yamada Y, Fukuda K, Tsukiyama K, Suzuki H, Kawasaki Y, Shimodaira M, Matsuoka K, Shibata T, Kasai Y, Maekawa T, Shapiro J, Tanaka K: Insulin independence after living-donor distal pancreatectomy and islet allotransplantation. Lancet 2005;365:1642.

49 Robertson RP, Lanz KJ, Sutherland DE, Seaquist ER: Relationship between diabetes and obesity 9 to 18 years after hemipancreatectomy and transplantation in donors and recipients. Transplantation 2002;73:736.

50 Baudry M, Lynch G: Regulation of glutamate receptors by cations. Nature 1979;282:748.

51 Mayer ML, Westbrook GL, Guthrie PB: Voltage-dependent block by Mg^{2+} of NMDA responses in spinal cord neurones. Nature 1984;309:261.

52 Farinelli SE, Nicklas WJ: Glutamate metabolism in rat cortical astrocyte cultures. J Neurochem 1992;58:1905.

53 Sonnewald U, Westergaard N, Schousboe A: Glutamate transport and metabolism in astrocytes. Glia 1997;21:56.

54 Yu AC, Schousboe A, Hertz L: Metabolic fate of 14C-labeled glutamate in astrocytes in primary cultures. J Neurochem 1982;39:954.

55 McKenna MC, Sonnewald U, Huang X, Stevenson J, Zielke HR: Exogenous glutamate concentration regulates the metabolic fate of glutamate in astrocytes. J Neurochem 1996;66:386.

56 Waniewski RA, Martin DL: Exogenous glutamate is metabolized to glutamine and exported by rat primary astrocyte cultures. J Neurochem 1986;47:304.

57 Frigerio F, Carobbio S, Mlynarik V, Gruetter R, Maechler P: Glucose homeostasis is altered in transgenic mice with brain specific knockout of the mitochondrial enzyme glutamate dehydrogenase. Diabetologia 2008;50:S170.

Pierre Maechler, PhD
Department of Cell Physiology and Metabolism
Geneva University Medical Centre
1, rue Michel-Servet
CH–1211 Geneva 4 (Switzerland)
Tel. +41 22 379 55 54, E-Mail Pierre.Maechler@unige.ch

Stanley CA, De León DD (eds): Monogenic Hyperinsulinemic Hypoglycemia Disorders.
Front Diabetes. Basel, Karger, 2012, vol 21, pp 137–145

The Molecular Genetics and Pathophysiology of Congenital Hyperinsulinism Caused by Short-Chain 3-Hydroxyacyl-CoA Dehydrogenase Deficiency

Anders Molven[a,b] · Geir Helgeland[a,c] · Tone Sandal[a,b] · Pål R. Njølstad[c,d]

[a]The Gade Institute and Departments of [b]Pathology, [c]Clinical Medicine and [d]Pediactrics, Haukeland University Hospital, University of Bergen, Bergen, Norway

Abstract

Deficiency of the metabolic enzyme short-chain 3-hydroxyacyl-CoA (SCHAD) is a rare autosomal recessive form of congenital hyperinsulinism of infancy caused by mutations in the *HADH* gene on chromosome 4q. Most cases reported to date are from ethnicities where consanguineous marriages are relatively frequent. SCHAD-deficient patients have normal or slightly elevated birth weights. Hypoglycemia most often manifests within the first 6 months of life and is diazoxide-sensitive. Although SCHAD participates in the degradation of fatty acids, the patients usually do not present a clinical picture that would suggest a fatty acid oxidation disorder. Metabolic profiling may, however, reveal an increased level of 3-hydroxybutyryl-carnitine in blood and the presence of 3-hydroxyglutaric acid in urine. Recently, it was demonstrated that SCHAD serves to inhibit the activity of glutamate dehydrogenase in the pancreatic beta-cells, a finding that also explains why SCHAD-deficient patients tend to be protein-intolerant.

The Discovery of Short-Chain 3-Hydroxyacyl-CoA Deficiency as a Cause of Congenital Hyperinsulinism of Infancy

Fatty acid oxidation (FAO) is catalyzed by a cyclic series of four enzymatic reactions. After the fatty acids have been activated as acyl-CoA thioesters in the cytosol, they are transported by the carnitine shuttle into the mitochondria, where each oxidative cycle produces acetyl-CoA and a two-carbon shortened acyl-CoA species, which then can be re-fed into the pathway (fig. 1). It is well known that FAO disorders may cause hypoglycemia due to the reduced ability to degrade fatty acids and, therefore,

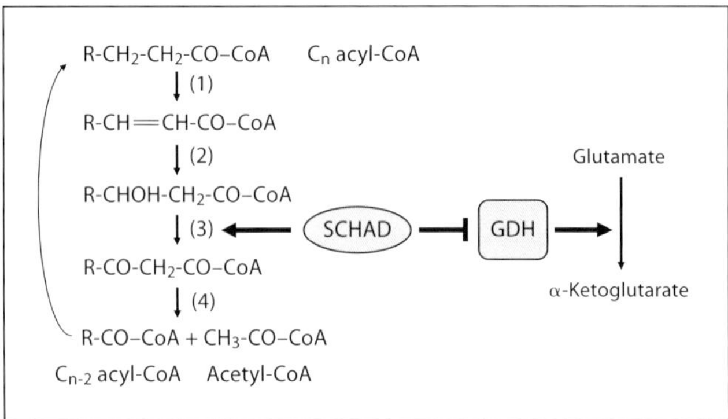

Fig. 1. Functions of the SCHAD enzyme. Fatty acids are oxidized in a cyclic series of four enzymatic reactions where SCHAD catalyzes the third step: dehydrogenation of 3-hydroxyacyl-CoA. The enzyme has a preference for short- and medium-chain (C_4–C_{12}) fatty acids. In pancreatic beta-cells, SCHAD also interacts with and inhibits the activity of glutamate dehydrogenase (GDH).

a limited capacity to mobilize ATP during fasting and metabolic stress. In such situations, the patients will exhibit low insulin levels, appropriately reflecting the inadequate energy state of the body.

Hence, it was very surprising when Clayton et al. [1] in 2001 reported a patient with congenital hyperinsulinism of infancy who had a deleterious mutation in an enzyme of the FAO pathway. This patient presented with episodic hypoglycemic convulsions starting at 4 months of age, and a diagnosis of diazoxide-responsive congenital hyperinsulinism of infancy was established at 19 months of age. Profiling of blood metabolites by mass spectrometry showed a peak of 3-hydroxybutyryl-carnitine, which led Clayton et al. to suspect deficiency of the mitochondrial enzyme short-chain 3-hydroxyacyl-CoA dehydrogenase (SCHAD). This hypothesis was verified by demonstrating reduced short-chain HAD (but not long-chain HAD) activity in the patient's fibroblasts and by finding a homozygous inactivating mutation in *HADH*, the gene that codes for SCHAD [1].

However, the possibility still remained that the patient of Clayton et al. [1] had two genetic defects: one causing SCHAD deficiency and explaining the raised hydroxybutyryl-carnitine level, and the other leading to congenital hyperinsulinism. This option was put to rest when Molven et al. [2] in 2004 reported a consanguineous family with 4 cases of congenital hyperinsulinism of infancy and a mutation in the *HADH* gene. This family had previously been studied by Vidnes and Øyasæter [3], who in 1977 concluded that the severe hypoglycemia was due to glucagon deficiency. Nevertheless, an extensive follow-up of the family demonstrated that its phenotype was consistent with congenital hyperinsulinism of infancy and also excluded already established genetic causes of this disease [4]. Molven et al. [2] then used genome-wide homozygosity mapping to pinpoint the chromosomal region harboring the mutation, identified a disrupted splice site of exon 5 in *HADH*, and subsequently confirmed the genetic finding by demonstrating greatly reduced SCHAD activity and elevated 3-hydroxybutyryl-carnitine levels in patient fibroblasts and blood samples, respectively. Excretion of 3-hydroxyglutaric acid in urine, an observation also mentioned in [1], was attributed to affected metabolism of glutaryl-CoA during catabolic degradation of tryptophan and lysine [2].

Clinical Features of Short-Chain 3-Hydroxyacyl-CoA Dehydrogenase Deficiency

A few SCHAD-deficient patients without mutations in the *HADH* gene have been described [5], but we limit our discussion to those cases where the clinical and enzymatic findings are supported by molecular data. Including the original patients of Clayton et al. [1] and Molven et al. [2], 22 such cases are reported in the literature (table 1).

These patients generally present with hypoketotic hypoglycemia and inappropriately elevated insulin levels, which establish the congenital hyperinsulinism of infancy diagnosis. Free fatty acids are usually within the normal range. A glucose supply of at least 10 mg/kg/min or glucagon infusion is necessary to stabilize the patients. They are responsive to diazoxide, which is the treatment of choice. When an appropriate treatment is not installed, psychomotor retardation or even death may occur [2, 6]. Recently, it was demonstrated that an oral protein load may induce the hyperinsulinemic hypoglycemia, suggesting that the patients are sensitive to amino acids [7].

In several patients, metabolic screening has revealed increased levels of 3-hydroxybutyryl-carnitine in blood and 3-hydroxyglutaric acid in urine (table 1), findings that are consistent with reduced SCHAD enzyme activity. There are examples of *HADH* mutation-positive children with congenital hyperinsulinism of infancy in whom increased levels of metabolites were not reported (table 1). However, it is not known to which extent these patients were screened for metabolic abnormalities.

All patients described so far were born around term, and most had normal or slightly increased birth weights (table 1). Thus, the macrosomia characteristic for congenital hyperinsulinism of infancy caused by mutations in the *HNF4A* or *ABCC8* genes [8, 9] was not seen. Time of disease recognition may vary from immediately after birth to at least 1 year of age, but is usually within the first 6 months of life. Because inheritance is autosomal recessive, most cases have so far been found in ethnicities where consanguineous marriages are common (table 1).

Notably, patients with *HADH* mutations do not exhibit hepatic dysfunction, cardiomyopathy, or skeletal muscle affection – features which are usually recognized in patients suffering from FAO disorders. The exception is the case described by Bennett et al. [10]. This patient presented without congenital hyperinsulinism of infancy, but with a Reye-like syndrome and a metabolic profile suggesting disrupted fatty acid degradation. Moreover, the patient was compound heterozygous for the *HADH* mutations Y226H and D57G. Biochemical analysis showed that the SCHAD

Table 1. Published patients with congenital hyperinsulinism of infancy caused by mutations in the *HADH* gene

Patient	Sex	Consan-guinity	Ethnicity	Gestational age	Birth weight	Disease onset	Diazoxide dose	Glucose	C4-OH	3OH-GA	Mutation	Ref.
				weeks	kg		mg/kg/day	mM	blood	urine		
1	F	no	Indian	38	3.2	4 months	5	1.4	yes	yes	P258L	1
2	M	yes	Pakistani	42	3.8	3 days	150[1]	0.8	yes	yes	IVS4-3delCAGGTC	2
3	F	yes	Pakistani	40	3.9	1.5 h	100[1]	1.6	yes	yes	IVS4-3delCAGGTC	2
4	M	yes	Pakistani	38	3.1	4 months	5	1.9	yes	yes	IVS6-2A>G	21
5	F	no	Caucasian	NA	NA	10 months	NA	3.9	yes	no[2]	D57G, Y226H	10[3]
6	F	yes	Bangladeshi	40	3.5	4 months	5	1.8	yes	yes	M188V	7
7	M	yes	Caucasian	40	3.9	2 months	5.6	0.9	no	no[4]	R236X	22
8	M	yes	Caucasian	38	3.8	8 months	7	0.3-2.8	yes	yes	S196FfsX3	6
9	F	yes	Caucasian	40	3.2	6 months	8	2.0-2.8	yes	yes	S196FfsX3	6
10	M	NA	Caucasian	NA	NA	14 months	8	2.2-2.4	yes	yes	S196FfsX3	6
11	M	no	Caucasian	41	2.7	7 months	9	2.1-2.8	yes	yes	IVS2+1G>A	6
12	M	yes	Turkish	38	2.9	16 weeks	5	< 3	[5]	[5]	K136E	12
13	M	yes	Turkish	40	2.8	16 weeks	2	< 3	[5]	[5]	Q163X	12
14	M	yes	Turkish	40	4.1	2 weeks	10	< 3	[5]	[5]	R236X	12
15	M	yes	Turkish	40	4.4	5 days	10	< 3	[5]	[5]	R236X	12
16	F	no	Turkish	40	4.0	1 week	2.5	< 3	[5]	[5]	R236X	12
17	M	yes	Pakistani	39	3.2	2 days	11	< 3	[5]	[5]	R236X	12
18	F	no	Iranian	40	3.5	12 weeks	15	< 3	[5]	[5]	R236X	12
19	F	no	Iranian	40	3.7	1 day	8	< 3	[5]	[5]	R236X	12
20	M	no	Indian	40	3.0	26 weeks	10	< 3	[5]	[5]	K95SfsX3/ IVS6 + 39C>G	12
21	M	no	Indian	40	4.0	2 days	10	< 3	[5]	[5]	Exon 1 del	12
22	M	no	Indian	40	3.8	24 weeks	10	< 3	[5]	[5]	Exon 1 del	12

C4-OH = Increased level of 3-hydroxybutyrylcarnitine in plasma; 3OH-GA = 3-hydroxyglutaric acid detected in urine; NA = Information not available.

[1] Dose per day, patient weight not reported.

[2] Medium-chain dicarboxylic acids and glutaric acid detected.

[3] The only patient not presenting with hyperinsulinemic hypoglycemia.

[4] Elevated excretion of 3-hydroxybutyric acid in urine.

[5] Metabolic profiling either not performed or reported as normal.

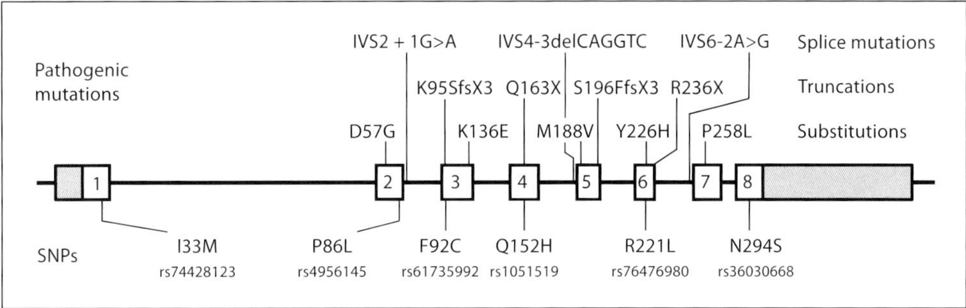

Fig. 2. Schematic overview over the human *HADH* gene based on gene ID 3033 and the reference sequence NM_005327 in the NCBI database (www.ncbi.nlm.nih.gov/gene). Known pathogenic mutations and nonsynonymous single nucleotide polymorphisms (SNPs) are indicated above and below the gene, respectively. In addition, a deletion mutation removing the minimal promoter and exon 1 has been reported [12]. Exons are numbered 1–8 and the untranslated sequence in exons 1 and 8 is shaded. The exons vary from 73 (exon 6) to 937 bp (exon 8) and the introns from 0.9 (intron 7) to 19.7 kb (intron 1) in size.

protein with Y226H had no detectable enzyme activity, whereas D57G had high residual activity with altered cofactor kinetics. Bennett et al. [10] therefore postulated that the biochemical properties of D57G were sufficient to avoid hyperinsulinism, but insufficient to maintain flux through the FAO pathway at times of metabolic stress.

The Molecular Genetics of Short-Chain 3-Hydroxyacyl-CoA Dehydrogenase Deficiency

An outline of the *HADH* gene is shown in figure 2. It is located on chromosome 4q22-q26, and consists of 8 exons [11]. From the consensus coding sequence CCDS3678 (www.ncbi.nlm.nih.gov/gene), the gene is predicted to give rise to a translated protein of 314 amino acid residues. We here refer to the complete open reading frame when numbering the mutations. However, some older publications have not included the N-terminal mitochondrial signal sequence of 12 residues in their nomenclature. There are also alternative *HADH* transcripts described in the databases (e.g. CCDS54790 with an extra in-frame exon between exons 6 and 7), but the biological significance of these transcripts remains to be shown.

The genetic alterations of *HADH* that cause congenital hyperinsulinism of infancy give rise to substitutions of a single amino acid or to truncated protein variants due to frame shifts or disrupted splice sites (fig. 2). A deletion of the minimal promoter and exon 1 has also been noted [12]. Twenty of the 22 reported patients were homozygous for the *HADH* mutation (table 1). In one of the patients described by Flanagan et al. [12], only one mutation was found when analyzing the reference sequence. However, a paternally inherited variant that would result in a missense mutation in one of the alternative *HADH* transcripts was subsequently identified and may explain the disease. Thus, a dominantly inherited form of SCHAD deficiency still remains to be demonstrated.

Some single nucleotide polymorphisms (SNPs) of *HADH* are known to change the SCHAD amino acid sequence. Those nonsynonymous SNPs for which a minimum of population frequency data are available from the SNP database (www.ncbi.nlm.nih.gov/snp) are listed in figure 2. The most common is P86L, which in Asian and European populations has an allele frequency of 0.03–0.10, but may reach a frequency of 0.30–0.40 in some African populations. Van Hove et al. [13] performed an extensive study where they examined the association between four tagging SNPs of the *HADH* gene (including P86L) and type 2 diabetes development. They observed no significant genetic association with disease, enzyme function, or diabetes-related clinical variables. Moreover, *HADH* is so far not among identified risk loci from the numerous genome-wide-association analyses performed for diabetes and related phenotypes [14]. The gene has also not been shown to cause permanent neonatal diabetes or maturity onset diabetes of the young. This is in contrast to many congenital hyperinsulinism of infancy genes, which are also recognized as susceptibility factors for developing type 2 diabetes or have been implicated in monogenic diabetes [14, 15].

The Pathophysiology of Short-Chain 3-Hydroxyacyl-CoA Dehydrogenase Deficiency

When SCHAD deficiency was discovered as a cause of congenital hyperinsulinism of infancy, a satisfactory explanation for the hypersecretion of insulin was lacking. Several theories concerning the mechanism were put forward, mainly focusing on possible effects of disturbed FAO and of metabolites that accumulated in the patients [1, 2].

However, the clinical picture seen in patients with *HADH* mutation is very difficult to reconcile with a FAO defect. In addition, several experimental observations indicate that the SCHAD protein itself might serve some beta-cell-specific function that could be responsible for the phenotype. Firstly, both the SCHAD mRNA and protein are highly expressed in pancreatic beta-cells, whereas mRNAs from other FAO enzymes are expressed at low levels [16]. Secondly, in a mouse model of congenital hyperinsulinism of infancy, the FoxA2 protein functions as a transcriptional activator for both the *Abcc8* and *Kcnj11* genes (encoding subunits of the beta-cell potassium channel) as well as for *Hadh* [17]. Thirdly, when *Hadh* transcription is suppressed in rat insulinoma cells, insulin secretion is stimulated [16, 18, 19] (fig. 3). This stimulation, which can be recapitulated in isolated rat beta-cells by reducing their *Hadh* expression, is not due to increased rate of glucose metabolism or by inhibited FAO [16]. Finally, the metabolites 3-hydroxybutyrate and 3-hydroxyglutaric do not promote insulin secretion [19].

A clue to the disease mechanism was provided by Filling et al. [5], who used the recombinantly expressed SCHAD protein as bait to pull down interacting molecules

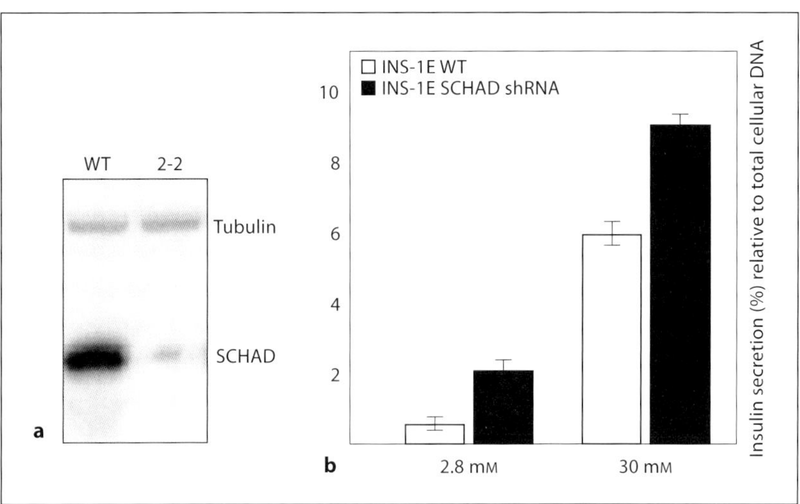

Fig. 3. Reducing SCHAD protein expression in INS-1E rat insulinoma cells stimulates insulin secretion. **a** Western blot showing the SCHAD protein level in cell clone 2-2 compared to wild-type (WT) cells. The expression was reduced by transducing the INS-1E cells with retrovirus that expressed an shRNA construct against rat *Hadh* mRNA. **b** Insulin secretion from clone 2-2 (black bars) is increased at both low (2.8 mM) and high (30 mM) glucose concentration in the growth medium as compared to secretion from WT cells (white bars). Note that the absolute increase in secretion is similar under high and low glucose conditions, suggesting a defect in basal insulin secretion of insulin. Cells were grown in organotypic 3D Matrigel cultures to maintain physiological conditions as much as possible.

from human liver mitochondrial extracts. Two proteins were found to bind to SCHAD, one of them being glutamate dehydrogenase (GDH). As mutations in the GDH-encoding gene *GLUD1* also cause congenital hyperinsulinism of infancy, Filling et al. [5] suggested that there is a link between SCHAD deficiency and the hyperinsulinism/hyperammonemia syndrome. This hypothesis was confirmed when Li et al. [20] published a penetrating analysis of a mouse *Hadh* knock-out model. They showed that *Hadh*$^{-/-}$ mice exhibit protein-sensitive hyperinsulinemic hypoglycemia (see Li et al. [this vol., pp. 112–124]). Similar to the situation in SCHAD-deficient patients, there were increased levels of blood 3-hydroxybutyrylcarnitine and urine 3-hydroxyglutaric acid [20]. Functional analyses suggested activation of GDH activity in islets lacking the SCHAD protein, and immunoprecipitation confirmed the previously reported physical interaction between SCHAD and GDH. Thus, Li et al. [20] concluded that there is an inhibitory protein-protein interaction of SCHAD on GDH (fig. 1) and that the insulin dysregulation observed in SCHAD deficiency is due to a loss of this inhibition, leading to an increase in the sensitivity of the GDH reaction to leucine activation. It might then be predicted that SCHAD-deficient patients will show a disturbance of their ammonium level, and in fact, mild hyperammonemia has been noted in some cases [6, 10].

The picture therefore emerges that SCHAD serves two functions in the body. One is exerted in all or most cells and relates directly to FAO, but may not be absolutely critical for this process. The other function is specific for the pancreatic beta-cell, is involved in the regulation of insulin secretion, and works through an inhibitory effect on the GDH enzyme. This dualistic model explains important clinical observations in SCHAD deficiency: a phenotype very different from that of other FAO disorders, a protein-sensitive hypoglycemia and responsiveness to diazoxide. We therefore recommend that, although SCHAD deficiency is a very rare disease, it should be considered a differential diagnosis for all cases of recessively inherited diazoxide-responsive congenital hyperinsulinism of infancy – also when there is no evidence of abnormal metabolic profile.

Acknowledgements

We are very grateful to Prof. emer. Oddmund Søvik for his long-standing interest in congenital hyperinsulinism of infancy and his valuable contributions to the study of the Norwegian SCHAD family. We also thank Prof. Claes B. Wollheim for providing INS-1E cells and the Helse-Vest Regional Health Authority, Innovest, and the University of Bergen for financial support.

References

1 Clayton PT, Eaton S, Aynsley-Green A, Edginton M, Hussain K, Krywawych S, Datta V, Malingre HE, Berger R, Van Den Berg IE: Hyperinsulinism in short-chain L-3-hydroxyacyl-CoA dehydrogenase deficiency reveals the importance of beta-oxidation in insulin secretion. J Clin Invest 2001;108:457–465.

2 Molven A, Matre GE, Duran M, Wanders RJ, Rishaug U, Njølstad PR, Jellum E, Søvik O: Familial hyperinsulinemic hypoglycemia caused by a defect in the SCHAD enzyme of mitochondrial fatty acid oxidation. Diabetes 2004;53:221–227.

3 Vidnes J, Øyasæter S: Glucagon deficiency causing severe neonatal hypoglycemia in a patient with normal insulin secretion. Pediatr Res 1977;11:943–949.

4 Molven A, Rishaug U, Matre GE, Njølstad PR, Søvik O: Hunting for a hypoglycemia gene: severe neonatal hypoglycemia in a consanguineous family. Am J Med Genet 2002;113:40–46.

5 Filling C, Keller B, Hirschberg D, Marschall HU, Jornvall H, Bennett MJ, Oppermann U: Role of short-chain hydroxyacyl CoA dehydrogenases in SCHAD deficiency. Biochem Biophys Res Commun 2008;368:6–11.

6 Martins E, Cardoso ML, Rodrigues E, Barbot C, Ramos A, Bennett MJ, Teles EL, Vilarinho L: Short-chain 3-hydroxyacyl-CoA dehydrogenase deficiency: the clinical relevance of an early diagnosis and report of four new cases. J Inherit Metab Dis 2011;34:835–842.

7 Kapoor RR, James C, Flanagan SE, Ellard S, Eaton S, Hussain K: 3-Hydroxyacyl-coenzyme A dehydrogenase deficiency and hyperinsulinemic hypoglycemia: characterization of a novel mutation and severe dietary protein sensitivity. J Clin Endocrinol Metab 2009;94:2221–2225.

8 Pearson ER, Boj SF, Steele AM, Barrett T, Stals K, Shield JP, Ellard S, Ferrer J, Hattersley AT: Macrosomia and hyperinsulinaemic hypoglycaemia in patients with heterozygous mutations in the HNF4A gene. PLoS Med 2007;4:e118.

9 Sandal T, Laborie LB, Brusgaard K, Eide SA, Christesen HB, Søvik O, Njølstad PR, Molven A: The spectrum of ABCC8 mutations in Norwegian patients with congenital hyperinsulinism of infancy. Clin Genet 2009;75:440–448.

10 Bennett MJ, Russell LK, Tokunaga C, Narayan SB, Tan L, Seegmiller A, Boriack RL, Strauss AW: Reye-like syndrome resulting from novel missense mutations in mitochondrial medium- and short-chain l-3-hydroxy-acyl-CoA dehydrogenase. Mol Genet Metab 2006;89:74–79.

11 Vredendaal PJ, Van Den Berg IE, Stroobants AK, Van Der AD, Malingre HE, Berger R: Structural organization of the human short-chain L-3-hydroxyacyl-CoA dehydrogenase gene. Mamm Genome 1998;9:763–768.

12 Flanagan SE, Patch AM, Locke JM, Akcay T, Simsek E, Alaei M, Yekta Z, Desai M, Kapoor RR, Hussain K, Ellard S: Genome-wide homozygosity analysis reveals HADH mutations as a common cause of diazoxide-responsive hyperinsulinemic-hypoglycemia in consanguineous pedigrees. J Clin Endocrinol Metab 2011;96:E498–E502.

13 Van Hove EC, Hansen T, Dekker JM, Reiling E, Nijpels G, Jorgensen T, Borch-Johnsen K, Hamid YH, Heine RJ, Pedersen O, Maassen JA, T Hart LM: The HADHSC gene encoding short-chain L-3-hydroxyacyl-CoA dehydrogenase (SCHAD) and type 2 diabetes susceptibility: the DAMAGE study. Diabetes 2006;55:3193–3196.

14 McCarthy MI: Genomics, type 2 diabetes, and obesity. N Engl J Med 2010;363:2339–2350.

15 Molven A, Njølstad PR: Role of molecular genetics in transforming diagnosis of diabetes mellitus. Expert Rev Mol Diagn 2011;11:313–320.

16 Martens GA, Vervoort A, Van De Casteele M, Stange G, Hellemans K, Van Thi HV, Schuit F, Pipeleers D: Specificity in beta cell expression of L-3-hydroxyacyl-CoA dehydrogenase, short chain, and potential role in down-regulating insulin release. J Biol Chem 2007;282:21134–21144.

17 Lantz KA, Vatamaniuk MZ, Brestelli JE, Friedman JR, Matschinsky FM, Kaestner KH: Foxa2 regulates multiple pathways of insulin secretion. J Clin Invest 2004;114:512–520.

18 Hardy OT, Hohmeier HE, Becker TC, Manduchi E, Doliba NM, Gupta RK, White P, Stoeckert CJ Jr, Matschinsky FM, Newgard CB, Kaestner KH: Functional genomics of the beta-cell: short-chain 3-hydroxyacyl-coenzyme A dehydrogenase regulates insulin secretion independent of K+ currents. Mol Endocrinol 2007;21:765–773.

19 Pepin E, Guay C, Delghingaro-Augusto V, Joly E, Madiraju SR, Prentki M: Short-chain 3-hydroxyacyl-CoA dehydrogenase is a negative regulator of insulin secretion in response to fuel and non-fuel stimuli in INS832/13 beta-cells. J Diabetes 2010;2:157–167.

20 Li C, Chen P, Palladino A, Narayan S, Russell LK, Sayed S, Xiong G, Chen J, Stokes D, Butt YM, Jones PM, Collins HW, Cohen NA, Cohen AS, Nissim I, Smith TJ, Strauss AW, Matschinsky FM, Bennett MJ, Stanley CA: Mechanism of hyperinsulinism in short-chain 3-hydroxyacyl-CoA dehydrogenase deficiency involves activation of glutamate dehydrogenase. J Biol Chem 2010;285:31806–31818.

21 Hussain K, Clayton PT, Krywawych S, Chatziandreou I, Mills P, Ginbey DW, Geboers AJ, Berger R, Van Den Berg IE, Eaton S: Hyperinsulinism of infancy associated with a novel splice site mutation in the SCHAD gene. J Pediatr 2005;146:706–708.

22 Di Candia S, Gessi A, Pepe G, Sogno Valin P, Mangano E, Chiumello G, Gianolli L, Proverbio MC, Mora S: Identification of a diffuse form of hyperinsulinemic hypoglycemia by 18-fluoro-L-3,4 dihydroxyphenylalanine positron emission tomography/CT in a patient carrying a novel mutation of the HADH gene. Eur J Endocrinol 2009;160:1019–1023.

Prof. Anders Molven
Section for Pathology
The Gade Institute
Haukeland University Hospital
University of Bergen
NO 5021 Bergen (Norway)
Tel. +47 55 973169 E-Mail anders.molven@gades.uib.no

Stanley CA, De León DD (eds): Monogenic Hyperinsulinemic Hypoglycemia Disorders.
Front Diabetes. Basel, Karger, 2012, vol 21, pp 146–157

Hyperinsulinism Due to Activating Mutations of Glucokinase

Samir Sayed[a] · Franz M. Matschinsky[b] · Charles A. Stanley[a]

[a]Division of Endocrinology/Diabetes, The Children's Hospital of Philadelphia, and [b]Institute for Diabetes, Obesity and Metabolism, University of Pennsylvania School of Medicine, Philadelphia, Pa., USA

Abstract

Glucokinase (GK) initiates glucose oxidation in pancreatic beta-cells and is a critical determinant of the glucose threshold for insulin secretion. Activating mutations of glucokinase were the second form of genetic hyperinsulinism (HI) to be discovered. GK-HI is inherited in an autosomal dominant fashion, but increasing numbers of de novo cases have been detected through genetic mutation analysis. The disease phenotype may include severe neonatal onset HI, but the disorder can go unrecognized until later in life. Patients manifest fasting hypoglycemia, but are not protein- or leucine-sensitive. Most disease-causing missense mutations cluster in the allosteric region of glucokinase near binding sites for GK activators and the inhibitory GK regulatory protein. Mutation expression studies show strong genotype-phenotype relationships; however, in vitro enzyme kinetics correlate poorly with glucose thresholds observed clinically, suggesting that additional factors are involved in controlling glucose levels. This important form of monogenic HI provides a model for the development of GK activating drugs for antidiabetic therapy.

Activating mutations of glucokinase (GK) were first identified as a cause of congenital hyperinsulinemic hypoglycemia (GK-HI) in 1998, shortly after the discovery in 1995 of mutations of the ATP-sensitive potassium (K_{ATP}) channel in children with recessively inherited hyperinsulinism (HI) [1, 2]. The recognition of the GK-HI disorder followed a candidate gene approach, based on the recognition of GK as the key determinant of the glucose threshold for insulin release by beta-cells, In addition, it was already known that inactivating mutations of the enzyme were associated with a dominant form of diabetes [maturity-onset diabetes of the young type 2 (MODY2)]. The first family with GK-HI to be described included affected children and parents, providing the first example of a dominantly inherited form of HI [2]. In this family, the hypoglycemia appeared to respond well to treatment with the K_{ATP} channel agonist, diazoxide. This created an assumption that GK-HI is a mild disorder and easy to manage. Subsequently, it has become apparent that the potent effect of glucokinase on the set-point for beta-cell insulin secretion can be quite difficult to overcome and that control of hypoglycemia in GK-HI can be a serious challenge, similar to controlling hyperglycemia in MODY2 [3–13]. This chapter will review the pathophysiology of GK-HI and the information about the clinical phenotype that has been developed from the relatively small number of additional cases that have been reported over the past 13 years.

Role of Glucokinase in Regulation of Insulin Secretion

The phosphorylation of glucose by GK initiates the pathway of insulin secretion by which glucose metabolism through glycolysis and mitochondrial oxidation generates a high energy phosphate signal to stimulate the release of insulin through plasma membrane K_{ATP} channels, membrane depolarization, and voltage-gated calcium channels (see fig. 1 in the chapter by Stanley and Matschinsky [pp. 1–6]). GK is one of four hexokinase enzymes which phosphorylate sugars, but the enzyme has acquired unique features which make it capable of functioning as the 'glucose sensor' for beta-cells in regulating plasma concentrations of glucose. In contrast to other hexokinases, GK has a much lower affinity for its substrate with half-maximal activity ($S_{0.5}$) at a glucose concentration of 7.6 mM [14]. In addition, the enzyme assumes at least two configurations with different affinities for glucose: a wide-open inactive form with low affinity, a half-closed form with higher affinity, and a closed form that tightly binds glucose as it catalyzes phosphorylation. The effects of varying glucose affinity on GK conformation result in a positive cooperative action of glucose on enzyme activity leading to a sigmoidal activity curve with a Hill number close to 1.7 [14]. Thus, the enzyme activity curve is steep in the range of 5 mM glucose, making GK well suited to tightly control plasma glucose in the normal physiologic range of 70–100 mg/dl (3.9–5.6 mM).

Glucose binding also inhibits enzyme degradation, thus helping to adjust GK activity to ambient glucose levels. Inactivating mutations of GK result in an increase in glucose threshold for insulin release and are associated with a monogenic form of diabetes mellitus, MODY2 [15, 16]. In the liver, but not in pancreas, GK enzyme activity is further controlled by the GK regulatory protein (GKRP), which inhibits the enzyme by binding to an allosteric site in the hinge region of GK (fig. 1) and trapping it in the nucleus [17–20]. Since glucose competes for GKRP binding, this mechanism provides a reserve supply of GK in hepatocytes that can be rapidly recruited in response to glucose ingestion. The GKRP-binding site on GK is also near allosteric sites that bind small molecule GK-activator drugs (under development to treat type 2 diabetes) by increasing beta-cell insulin glucose responsiveness.

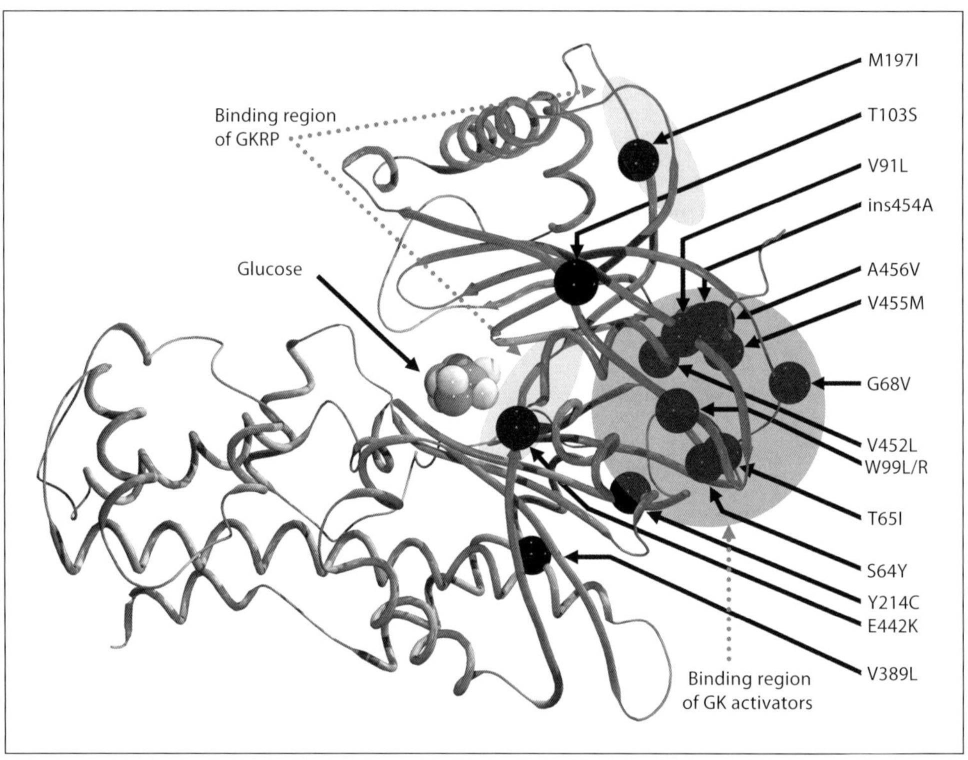

Fig. 1. Location of GK-activating mutations in the closed (active) form of the crystallographic enzyme structure. Also shown are the binding region of the GK activators (large shaded circle) and the suspected binding region of GKRP (smaller shaded ovals).

Clinical Manifestations of Glucokinase Hyperinsulinism Caused by Glucokinase-Activating Mutations

Table 1 summarizes the clinical features of the 38 cases of GK-HI that have been reported in the literature and of the 12 patients with GK-HI who have been seen at the Children's Hospital of Philadelphia (CHOP; including 9 cases not previously reported). As shown in table 1, 10% of the reported cases, and 50% in the CHOP series, are afflicted with GK-HI due to de novo mutations. This high proportion of de novo cases in the CHOP series is also seen in other dominant forms of HI associated with glutamate dehydrogenase (GDH) or K_{ATP} mutations (see the chapters by Kelly et al. [pp. 100–111] and De León and Stanley [pp. 18–29]); the lower de novo rate cases reported in the literature may reflect selection bias toward doing mutation analysis for GK preferentially in familial cases. Two of the CHOP cases have postzygotic mosaicism for GK mutations that were not detected in peripheral blood (proven in one case, suspected in the second). As shown in table 2, large-for-gestational age birth weight is common in GK-HI, as it is in children with K_{ATP}HI, reflecting the growth-promoting effects of

Table 1. Clinical features of GK-HI cases reported and seen at CHOP

	Reported cases[1]	CHOP cases[2]
Total cases	38	12
Probands	15	8
Familial	23	4
De novo	4	6[3]
Age of onset		
Neonatal	8	2
Childhood	9	6
Adolescence	1	1
Adulthood	6	3
Asymptomatic	14	0
Diagnosis		
Undiagnosed	14	2
Diazoxide-controlled	13	7
Surgery	2	3
Diet	9	0

[1] From [2–9] and [11–13].
[2] From [10] and this chapter.
[3] Two with postzygotic mosaicism (one confirmed, one suspected).

Table 2. GK-HI inheritance and birth weight

Inheritance	Birth weight
Maternal (n = 10)	2.93±0.60
Paternal (n = 9)	4.06±0.78
De novo (n = 9)	4.38±0.76

Birth weight in kg (means ± SD). Maternal inheritance vs. paternal inheritance or de novo mutations; $p < 0.005$.

increased fetal insulin secretion. Of note, birth weight is increased when the mutation is de novo or paternal, but not when it is maternal in origin (where the glucose threshold for insulin secretion is the same in the fetus and mother). The effect of the mutation appears to produce a 1- to 1.5-kg increase in birth weight when the fetus, but not the mother, is a carrier. This further illustrates the potent effect of GK on the threshold for insulin secretion as mean birth weight is reduced by approximately 0.5 kg in children with MODY2-inactivating GK mutations when born to normal mothers.

As shown in table 1, hypoglycemia may present in the neonatal period in children with GK-HI, but is often not recognized until later infancy or childhood and, in some

Table 3. Plasma glucose levels and calculated glucose thresholds in GK-HI mutations seen at CHOP (fasting or postabsorptive glucose)

Mutation	Diazoxide responsive	Mean plasma glucose mg/dl (mM)[1]	Calculated glucose threshold, mM
W99L	yes	64±6 (3.6±0.3)	2.2
W99R	yes	N/A	2.8
M197I	yes	63±4.5 (3.5±0.2)[2]	3.5
Y214C	yes	60±9.5 (3.4±0.5)	1.4
V389L	yes	64±5.5 (3.5±0.3)	2.9
V389L	yes	61±6.6 (3.40±0.4)	2.9
V389L	no (surgery)	N/A	2.9
ins454A	no (surgery)	50±6.3 (2.8±0.4)[2]	1.1
ins454A	no (surgery)	60±24 (3.3±1.2)	1.1

[1] Means ± SD.
[2] Postabsorptive.

familial cases, may escape recognition until adulthood. The frequency of cases not detected in infancy or childhood was 55% in the reported cases and 33% in the CHOP series. This contrasts with the recessive form of K_{ATP}HI which almost always presents in the newborn period, but is similar to GDH-HI which is also frequently not recognized at birth. The failure to detect hypoglycemia in carrier individuals with GK-activating mutations is probably due to a combination of factors, such as the common practice of accepting lower glucose levels in newborns, as well as milder symptomatic episodes of hypoglycemia in GK-HI not attracting sufficient attention to be diagnosed [2–5, 7]. The frequency of developmental delay appears to be much lower in GK-HI than in the K_{ATP}HI or GDH-HI groups. Only 2 of the GK-HI cases among the combined CHOP and literature series are reported to have shown evidence of brain injury and developmental delay [6, 10], whereas the frequency of developmental delay in the severe form of K_{ATP}HI ranges from 25 to 40% and may be higher in GDH-HI (see the chapters by Kelly et al. [pp. 100–111] and De León and Stanley [pp. 18–29]).

Diazoxide would seem to be a logical treatment to control hypoglycemia in GK-HI since it inhibits insulin secretion by activating the K_{ATP} channel at a site in the pathway of glucose-stimulated insulin secretion that is downstream of GK (see fig. 1 in the chapter by Stanley and Matschinsky [pp. 1–6]). Unfortunately, as shown in tables 1 and 3, diazoxide has not been entirely effective in many of the GK-HI patients. This frequent failure to respond to diazoxide therapy demonstrates the potent effect of GK-activating mutations to over-ride any effort to raise plasma glucose above the set-point for insulin release. Only 2 of the CHOP cases, shown in table 1, were considered to have good glycemic control on treatment with diazoxide alone: 3 others required near-total pancreatectomy in infancy (including 1 with a proven postzygotic

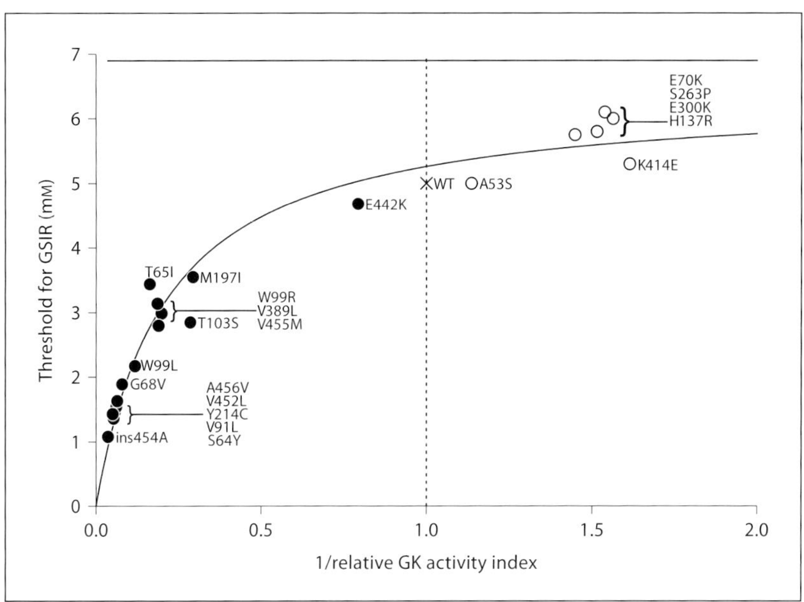

Fig. 2. Calculated thresholds for glucose-stimulated insulin release (GSIR) in activating and inactivating mutations of GK. Thresholds are plotted against the inverse of the mutant enzyme activity index relative to wild-type (WT) enzyme. Because relative expression of the GK forms is affected by enzyme affinity for glucose and the ambient glucose concentration, the wild-type enzyme dominates the estimated threshold for the heterozygous inactivating defects, but the mutant enzyme dominates the threshold for activating mutations. Thus, the threshold for inactivating mutations plateaus at approx. 7 mM, whereas the calculated threshold for severe activating mutations approaches zero as the relative activity increases. For purposes of consistency, all kinetic data in the figure are from the laboratory of F.M. Threshold and activity indexes were calculated per Gloyn et al. [14]. ● = GK-HI mutations; ○ = MODY2 mutations; X = wild-type GK.

mutation). All 3 adolescent patients with GK-HI in the CHOP series found the benefits of diazoxide to be so poor that they chose to stop the drug in favor of treating hypoglycemic symptoms with food. Two of the CHOP cases have required nocturnal continuous intragastric feeding to prevent symptomatic hypoglycemia. Similar poor results with diazoxide treatment have been reported by others, including one severe case with a Y214C mutation and a very low calculated glucose threshold (fig. 2) reported by Cuesta-Munoz's group [6] who had a poor response to diazoxide and required a near-total pancreatectomy. However, one child in the CHOP series carries an identical Y214C mutation and has been well controlled on medication.

In the CHOP series, surgery has also not been very effective in preventing hypoglycemia in GK-HI; most patients have continued to require additional medical management after surgery. This has included continuous intragastric dextrose infusions either overnight or throughout the day. Treatment with octreotide, a somatostatin analog, has been tried in patients with GK-HI, but has been poorly effective in the CHOP series. One of the CHOP cases reported in 1993 showed tachyphylaxis to the insulin suppressive

Table 4. GK-HI: Responses to oral and intravenous insulin secretagogues (insulin, μU/ml; glucose, mg/dl)

	W99L	M197I	V389L	V389L	ins454A	Normal
OGTT, Δ ins/Δ glu	25.3/28		38.9/70	47.5/66		
OPTT, Δ ins/Δ glu		22/–3				10±8/–6±6
Glucose AIR		68.3			69.6	45.8±32.8
Calcium AIR		–3.5				0.1±1.6
Leucine AIR		4.3				1.7±9.5
Cholesterol, mg/dl	166	166			112	108–224
Triglycerides, mg/dl	54.0	150			25.7	35.4–168

Insulin: μU/ml; glucose: mg/dl. OGTT = Oral glucose tolerance test; OPTT = oral protein tolerance test; AIR = acute insulin response.

effect of octreotide, such that the drug had little effect within 1–2 days [1]. This rapid development of unresponsiveness may reflect a combination of the drug downregulating beta-cell plasma membrane somatostatin receptor number, as well as the effect of the lowered glucose threshold for insulin secretion over-riding the effect of octreotide.

Since GK activation in the liver might be expected to increase hepatic glucose metabolism and triglyceride synthesis, it is possible that GK-HI might be associated with hyperlipidemia. For example, it has been reported that a GKRP variant, P466L, which is associated with a diminished ability to inhibit GK, is associated with lower blood glucose concentrations and reduced risk of type 2 diabetes mellitus in obese individuals, but also with increased levels of serum triglycerides [13]. As shown in table 4, the three children with GK-HI followed at CHOP did not appear to have elevated serum triglycerides and their serum cholesterol levels were in the normal range. Serum triglycerides were also not increased in a mouse model with a GK A456V-activating mutation [21]. Diabetes has occurred in a few patients with GK-HI who were treated with surgery, but of the carrier adults, only three are reported to have developed diabetes. Thus, the risk of diabetes does not appear to be increased by the presence of the GK-activating mutation.

Glucokinase Hyperinsulinism Mutations

To date, 15 mutations of GK have been associated with GK-HI (fig. 1). Two families have the A456V mutation, apparently arising independently; one family each has the V455M, T65I, G68V, V91L, E422K, V389L, T103S, or W99R mutations. W99R also occurred in one sporadic case, and a second sporadic case has a W99L mutation. Five other GK-HI mutations occurred in sporadic cases: the Y214C in two unrelated individuals (one reported, one in table 1 at CHOP), and S64Y, V452L, ins454A, and M197I in single cases. As shown in figure 1, most of these mutations are located at either end of a loop of amino acids in the hinge region of GK which includes separate binding regions for GKRP and the various GK-activator drugs. Two of the mutations are more distant, including V389L [13] and M197I [10]. The latter alters a methionine residue that moves in and out of a hydrophobic pocket during the transition between, respectively, the active and inactive forms of the enzyme. Designed mutations of M197 confirm that hydrophobic substitutions favor the active conformation of GK while hydrophilic amino acids cause inactivation [10]. This observation has been further confirmed in a report by Pal and Miller [22]. Based on these two examples, it appears that activating mutations of GK need not be restricted to the allosteric domain, and it seems likely that additional mutation sites may be identified in patients with GK-HI.

Most of the disease-associated GK-HI mutations have been studied by in vitro expression of the mutant protein (usually with a GST-tag for convenience in purification, but similar results have been obtained with the GST-tag cleaved). All of the mutations show reduced glucose $S_{0.5}$ ranging from 1.1 to 4.5 mM (normal 7.6 mM), but only modest changes in k_{cat}. Mutations with greater reductions in glucose $S_{0.5}$ showed lesser responses to activation with a GK-activator drug and less inhibition by GKRP, consistent with greater basal activation, but no alteration in maximal enzyme activity. The net effect of changes in the kinetic properties of GK mutations is illustrated by calculation of the relative activity index compared to a wild-type enzyme and of the glucose threshold based on model computations of the heterozygous state (based on the fact that insulin release begins at 25–30% of maximal wild-type glucose phosphorylation). Figure 2 shows the calculated glucose thresholds for GK mutations expressed in the Matschinsky lab (for consistency). Note that effects of various inactivating (MODY2) mutations of GK are quite similar, raising the glucose threshold only slightly from 5 mM to about 6–7 mM. In contrast, the calculated thresholds for glucose-stimulated insulin release with GK-HI mutations shows a marked variation with genotype, ranging from 4.2 mM to as low as 1.2 mM. This suggests considerable differences in the severity of hypoglycemia among different GK-HI mutations, which might explain why some patients cannot be completely controlled medically on diazoxide treatment. However, as noted below, the calculated glucose thresholds do not predict observed blood glucose levels in patients very well.

Clinical Pathophysiology of Glucokinase Hyperinsulinism

The major pathophysiologic feature of GK-HI is illustrated by the fasting profile obtained in an affected 6-year-old child with a de novo W99L mutation (fig. 3). Prior to diagnosis, he had been thought to be healthy, but, after starting school, was noted to have frequent periods of poor attention and sleepiness that were likely due to hypoglycemia. Hypoglycemia was first recognized after he suffered a hypoglycemic seizure. As shown in figure 3, following a meal, the plasma glucose quickly dropped into the range of 50–60 mg/dl (2.8–3.3 mM) and then remained stable at this level

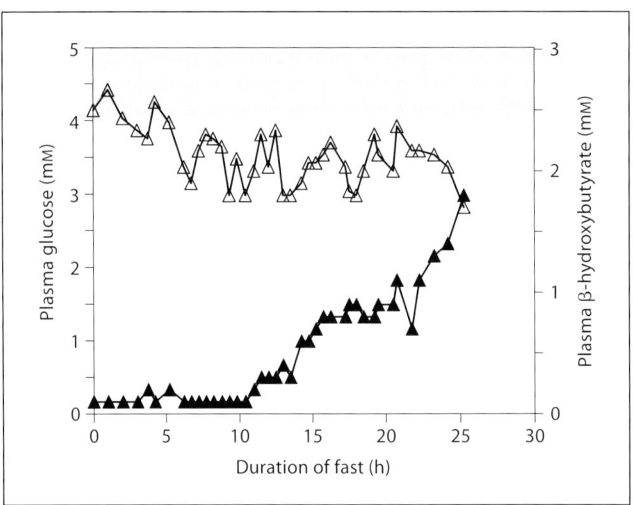

Fig. 3. Plasma glucose and beta-hydroxybutyrate responses to fasting in a 6-year-old boy with a W99L GK-HI mutation. Mean plasma glucose was 64 ± 1 mg/dl. Beta-hydroxybutyrate values increased from 0.1 to 1.8 mM as fasting plasma glucose levels decreased. At the end of the fast, plasma C-peptide was suppressed (0.16 nM, normal 0.26–1.32 nM). The glucose response to glucagon stimulation was 36 mg/dl. Reference normals when fasting: blood glucose <50 mg/dl; beta-hydroxybutyrate >2.5 mM, and glycemic response to glucagon >30 mg/dl. △ = plasma glucose; ▲ = beta-hydroxybutyrate.

for many hours. During this time, the child displayed mild symptoms of hypoglycemia. Plasma beta-hydroxybutyrate remained suppressed, consistent with a failure to appropriately turn off insulin secretion. However, after several hours of low glucose levels, ketogenesis becomes activated, with beta-hydroxybutyrate rising by the end of the test to levels approaching those seen in normal children after prolonged fasting. This pattern of fasting adaptation clearly shows the effect of the GK-activating mutation in lowering the glucose threshold for insulin secretion (in this case, the glucose level at which insulin secretion was suppressed). At the altered set-point, glucose levels remain quite stable, and this probably accounts for the fact that, as in this child, many patients with GK-HI display only mild hypoglycemia and can escape detection for several months or years after birth or even into adulthood.

Table 4 compares the fasting or postabsorptive plasma glucose levels in children with GK-HI seen at CHOP with their calculated glucose thresholds (fig. 2). Although the calculated thresholds ranged from 1.1 to 3.5 mM, the observed glucose levels clustered around 2.8 to 3.5 mM. There was no significant correlation between the calculated glucose thresholds and actual blood glucose concentrations. A similar discrepancy between in vivo plasma glucose levels and calculated glucose threshold has been reported in mice expressing the A456V GK mutation [21]. Neither heterozygous nor homozygous mutant mice are as hypoglycemic as predicted from the kinetics of the expressed enzyme. In vitro studies of isolated islets from these mice show a better correlation of the predicted and actual glucose threshold. The correlations between the predicted and actual glucose levels in vivo and the in vitro glucose threshold in mice are actually closer for an inactivating GK mutation (K414E) than for the activating A456V mutation. These discrepancies with the predicted effects of the activating mutations in both humans and mice may reflect additional factors which are not accounted for by the model calculations, such as counter-regulatory hormone responses.

Table 4 also shows that, in a small number of GK-HI cases, there appears to be a tendency toward greater than normal acute insulin responses to intravenous glucose, but glucose and insulin responses to oral glucose appear to be normal. The acute insulin responses to intravenous leucine or to oral protein tolerance tests appeared to be normal in the few cases of GK-HI examined (table 4), indicating that protein- and leucine-sensitive hypoglycemia (seen in K_{ATP}HI and GDH-HI) are not part of the phenotype of GK-HI.

Islet Histopathology of Glucokinase Hyperinsulinism

Routine pathologic examination of pancreas from the small number of GK-HI cases who have required pancreatectomy or have had postmortem examination have generally been read as showing little or no abnormal features [5, 7, 10]. In a few cases, nuclear enlargement in a small percentage of islets cells has been observed, similar to that seen in pancreas from patients with diffuse HI due to K_{ATP} mutations (see Suchi et al. [this vol., pp. 57–70]), suggesting beta-cell overactivity. Using quantitative morphometry, an increased frequency of large islets has been reported in 2 cases of GK-HI [6, 12], as well as increased markers of beta-cell proliferation and apoptosis. These quantitative morphometric results have been suggested to reflect a regulatory effect of increased beta-cell glucose flux on beta-cell turnover (which might have important implications for the pathogenesis of type 2 diabetes and the effects of GK-activator drugs on beta-cell survival). In mice with the A456V-activating mutation, islet histology was reported as normal [21]. This topic deserves further study, but subtle changes in pancreatic histology may exist in GK-HI that can be helpful in diagnosis.

Impact of the Biochemical Genetics of Glucokinase Hyperinsulinism on Discovery of Glucokinase Activators

Analysis of the GK-HI disorder has had a significant impact on drug discovery programs employing activation of GK as a new means of treating type 3 diabetes mellitus [23–25]. The observation that activating mutations of the enzyme lowers blood glucose, even in patients with only one mutated allele, strongly reinforces the rationale for this strategy by confirming the role of GK as a critical determinant of glucose homeostasis in humans [23–25]. The biochemical genetic analysis of GK-HI and drug discovery efforts on GK activators resulted in a new concept: GK has a distinct allosteric activator region located approximately 20 Å from the substrate-binding site. Mutations of many of the contact amino acids of the drug-binding site were found to be activating and disease-causing (e.g. Y214, V452, V455, and A456), and the majority of the HI-linked GK mutants were found to be located in the very region which is now considered the allosteric activator site of the enzyme. Only two of the GK-HI mutations, M197I and V389L, are not part of this site (fig. 1). Intensive drug discovery efforts by many pharmaceutical companies have resulted in the design of numerous compounds that have GK-activating properties. Several of these have been used in initial clinical trials with type 2 diabetes mellitus patients and were found to be highly effective blood glucose-lowering agents. However, most of the trials were discontinued for undisclosed reasons or due to limited durability or side effects of the drugs. It remains to be seen whether GK activators will gain a place in antidiabetes therapy [25].

Acknowledgements

This work was supported in part by NIH grants RR-024134 (S.S., C.A.S.), R01-DK053012 (C.A.S.), R37-DK056268 (C.A.S.), NIDDK 22122 (F.M.) and NIDDK 19525 (F.M.).

References

1 Thornton PS, Alter CA, Katz LE, Baker L, Stanley CA: Short- and long-term use of octreotide in the treatment of congenital hyperinsulinism. J Pediatr 1993;123:637–643.
2 Glaser B, Kesavan P, Heyman M, Davis E, Cuesta A, Buchs A, Stanley CA, Thornton PS, Permutt MA, Matschinsky FM, Herold KC: Familial hyperinsulinism caused by an activating glucokinase mutation. N Engl J Med 1998;338:226–230.
3 Christesen HB, Jacobsen BB, Odili S, Buettger C, Cuesta-Munoz A, Hansen T, Brusgaard K, Massa O, Magnuson MA, Shiota C, Matschinsky FM, Barbetti F: The second activating glucokinase mutation (A456V): implications for glucose homeostasis and diabetes therapy. Diabetes 2002;51:1240–1246.
4 Dullaart RP, Hoogenberg K, Rouwe CW, Stulp BK: Family with autosomal dominant hyperinsulinism associated with A456V mutation in the glucokinase gene. J Intern Med 2004;255:143–145.
5 Gloyn AL, Noordam K, Willemsen MA, Ellard S, Lam WW, Campbell IW, Midgley P, Shiota C, Buettger C, Magnuson MA, Matschinsky FM, Hattersley AT: Insights into the biochemical and genetic basis of glucokinase activation from naturally occurring hypoglycemia mutations. Diabetes 2003;52:2433–2440.
6 Cuesta-Munoz AL, Huopio H, Otonkoski T, Gomez-Zumaquero JM, Nanto-Salonen K, Rahier J, Lopez-Enriquez S, Garcia-Gimeno MA, Sanz P, Soriguer FC, Laakso M: Severe persistent hyperinsulinemic hypoglycemia due to a de novo glucokinase mutation. Diabetes 2004;53:2164–2168.
7 Wabitsch M, Lahr G, Van de Bunt M, Marchant C, Lindner M, von Puttkamer J, Fenneberg A, Debatin KM, Klein R, Ellard S, Clark A, Gloyn AL: Heterogeneity in disease severity in a family with a novel G68V GCK activating mutation causing persistent hyperinsulinaemic hypoglycaemia of infancy. Diabet Med 2007;24:1393–1399.
8 Christesen HB, Tribble ND, Molven A, Siddiqui J, Sandal T, Brusgaard K, Ellard S, Njølstad PR, Alm J, Jacobson BB, Hussain K, Gloyn AL: Activating glucokinase (GCK) mutations as a cause of medically responsive congenital hyperinsulinism: prevalence in children and characterisation of a novel GCK mutation. Eur J Endocrinol 2008;159:27–34.
9 Meissner T, Marquard J, Cobo-Vuilleumier N, Maringa M, Rodriguez-Bada P, Garcia-Gimeno MA, Baixeras E, Weber J, Olek K, Sanz P, Mayatepek E, Cuesta-Munoz AL: Diagnostic difficulties in glucokinase hyperinsulinism. Horm Metab Res 2009; 41:320–326.

10 Sayed S, Langdon DR, Odili S, Chen P, Buettger C, Schiffman AB, Suchi M, Taub R, Grimsby J, Matschinsky FM, Stanley CA: Extremes of clinical and enzymatic phenotypes in children with hyperinsulinism caused by glucokinase activating mutations. Diabetes 2009;58:1419–1427.
11 Barbetti F, Cobo-Vuilleumier N, Dionisi-Vici C, Toni S, Ciampalini P, Massa O, Rodriguez-Bada P, Colombo C, Lenzi L, Garcia-Gimeno MA, Bermudez-Silva FJ, de Fonseca FR, Banin P, Aledo JC, Baixeras E, Sanz P, Cuesta-Munoz AL: Opposite clinical phenotypes of glucokinase disease: description of a novel activating mutation and contiguous inactivating mutations in human glucokinase (GCK) gene. Mol Endocrinol 2009;23:1983–1989.
12 Kassem S, Bhandari S, Rodríguez-Bada P, Motaghedi R, Heyman M, García-Gimeno A, Cobo-Vuilleumier N, Sanz P, Maclaren NK, Rahier J, Glaser B, Cuesta-Muñoz AL: Large islets, beta-cell proliferation, and a glucokinase mutation. N Engl J Med 2010;362: 1348–1350.
13 Beer NL, van de Bunt M, Colclough K, Lukacs C, Arundel P, Chik C, Grimsby J, Ellard S, Gloyn AL: Discovery of a novel site regulating glucokinase activity following characterisation of a new mutation causing hyperinulinaemic hypoglycaemia in humans. J Biol Chem 2011;286:19118–19126.
14 Gloyn AL, Odili S, Buettger C, Njolstad PR, Shiota C, Magnuson MA, Matschinsky FM: Glucokinase and the regulation of blood sugar; in Matschinsky FM, Magnuson MA (eds): Glucokinase and Glycemic Disease: From Basics to Novel Therapeutics. Basel, Karger, 2004, pp 92–109.
15 Liang Y, Kesavan P, Wang LQ, Niswender K, Tanizawa Y, Permutt MA, Magnuson MA, Matschinsky FM: Variable effects of maturity-onset-diabetes-of-youth (MODY)-associated glucokinase mutations on substrate interactions and stability of the enzyme. Biochem J 1995;309:167–173.
16 Gloyn AL: Glucokinase (GCK) mutations in hyper- and hypoglycemia: maturity-onset diabetes of the young, permanent neonatal diabetes, and hyperinsulinemia of infancy. Hum Mutat 2003;22:353–362.
17 Matschinsky FM: Regulation of pancreatic beta-cell glucokinase: from basics to therapeutics. Diabetes 2002;51(Suppl. 3):S394–S404.
18 van Schaftingen E, Viega da Cunha M: Discovery and role of glucokinase regulatory protein; in Matschinsky FM, Magnuson MA (eds): Glucokinase and Glycemic Disease: From Basics to Novel Therapeutics. Basel, Karger, 2004, pp 193–207.
19 Veiga da Cunha M, Courtois S, Michel A, Gosselain E, and Van Schaftingen E: Amino acid conservation in animal glucokinases: identification of residues implicated in the interaction with the regulatory protein. J Biol Chem 1996;271:6292–6297.
20 Shiota C, Coffey J, Grimsby J, Grippo JF, Magnuson MA. Nuclear import of hepatic glucokinase depends upon glucokinase regulatory protein, whereas export is due to a nuclear export signal sequence in glucokinase. J Biol Chem 1999;274:37125–3713.
21 Pino MF, Kim KA, Shelton KD, Lindner J, Odili S, Li C, Collins HW, Shiota M, Matschinsky FM, Magnuson MA: Glucokinase thermolability and hepatic regulatory protein binding are essential factors for predicting the blood glucose phenotype of missense mutations. J Biol Chem 2007;282:13906–13916.
22 Pal P, Miller BG: Activating mutations in the human glucokinase gene revealed by genetic selection. Biochemistry 2009;48:814–816.
23 Grimsby J, Sarabu R, Corbett WL, Haynes NE, Bizzarro FT, Coffey JW, Guertin KR, Hilliard DW, Kester RF, Mahaney PE: Allosteric activators of glucokinase: potential role in diabetes therapy. Science 2003;301:370–373.
24 Matschinsky FM: Assessing the potential of glucokinase activators in diabetes therapy. Nat Rev Drug Discov 2009;8:399–416.
25 Matschinsky FM, Zelent B, Doliba N, Li C, Vanderkooi JM, Naji A, Sarabu R, Grimsby J: Glucokinase activators for diabetes therapy: May 2010 status report. Diabetes Care 2011;34(Suppl 2): S236–S243.

Charles A. Stanley, MD
Division of Endocrinology/Diabetes
The Children's Hospital of Philadelphia
34th Street and Civic Center Boulevard
Philadelphia, PA 19104 (USA)
Tel. +1 215 590 3420, E-Mail stanleyc@email.chop.edu

Stanley CA, De León DD (eds): Monogenic Hyperinsulinemic Hypoglycemia Disorders.
Front Diabetes. Basel, Karger, 2012, vol 21, pp 158–171

Hyperinsulinism Due to Mutations of Uncoupling Protein 2

Maria del Mar Gonzalez-Barroso[a,e] · Pascale de Lonlay[b,c] · Daniel Ricquier[a,b,d]

[a]Laboratory of Metabolic Biochemistry, Hôpital Necker-Enfants Malades, Assistance Publique Hôpitaux de Paris, [b]Université Paris Descartes, [c]Unit of Metabolism, Department of Pediatrics, Hôpital Necker-Enfants Malades, and [d]Institut Cochin, CNRS and INSERM, Paris, France; [e]Centro de Investigaciones Biologicas, CSIC, Madrid, Spain

Abstract

Glucose-stimulated insulin secretion by pancreatic beta-cells is a highly complex process. Mitochondria play a critical role in the control of this pathway mainly by modulating ATP supply. Reactive oxygen species have also been proposed as metabolic signals in glucose-induced insulin secretion. A partial uncoupling of mitochondrial substrate oxidation from ATP synthesis would decrease insulin secretion. The mitochondrial uncoupling protein UCP2 was firstly considered as a regulator of ATP production in beta-cells by uncoupling oxidative phosphorylation. The mitochondrial proton transporter responsible for heat production by brown adipocyte mitochondria is evolutionarily related to UCP1. Genetic, physiological, and pathological studies suggest that UCP2 is a negative regulator of insulin secretion in rodents and humans. We identified loss-of-function mutations in the *UCP2* gene in 2 young patients with congenital hyperinsulinism, making *UCP2* a candidate gene for this disease. Functional studies of the mutants confirmed this hypothesis. It has been proposed that UCP2 could attenuate insulin secretion through a dual role in beta-cells by decreasing the ATP/ADP ratio or modulating the production of reactive oxygen species. This chapter describes the proposed implications of UCP2 as a modulator of insulin secretion in beta-cells. The contribution of UCP2 in glucose metabolism and sensing in other cell types is also discussed.

Mitochondria Participate in the Control of Insulin Secretion

In the pancreatic beta-cell, mitochondria oxidize in a high proportion of carbons derived from glucose. In these organelles, pyruvate is a substrate for both pyruvate dehydrogenase and pyruvate carboxylase. The former enzyme provides the tricarboxylic acid with acetyl-CoA. The latter enzyme forms oxaloacetate, providing anaplerotic input to the tricarboxylic acid cycle. Reducing equivalents generated by the Krebs cycle are substrates of respiratory complexes, which activate the electron transport

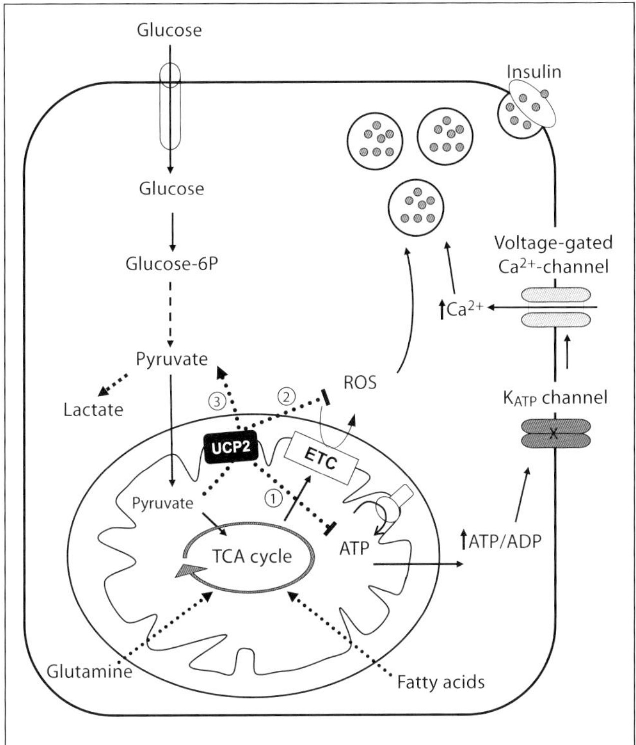

Fig. 1. Simplification of the critical steps leading to insulin secretion in pancreatic beta-cells and putative roles of UCP2 controlling glucose metabolism. Degradation of glucose by glycolysis produces pyruvate that enters the mitochondria and feeds the TCA cycle, producing reducing equivalents that are oxidized by the electron transport chain (ETC). The increase in the ATP/ADP ratio leads to closure of the K_{ATP} channel, depolarization of the plasma membrane, opening of voltage-gated Ca^{2+} channel, influx of calcium, and finally insulin exocytosis. Moreover, ROS produced during mitochondrial electron transport are required metabolic signals for insulin secretion, although the exact mechanism is uncertain. The gray dotted lines represent the proposed roles of UCP2 as a negative regulator of insulin secretion: (1) as a consequence of an uncoupling activity, UCP2 would decrease mitochondrial membrane potential and lower the ATP/ADP ratio; (2) UCP2 could attenuate insulin secretion by decreasing mitochondria-produced ROS levels; and (3) UCP2 as a carrier exporting pyruvate would act as a metabolic sensor for the choice of substrates supplying the TCA cycle.

chain resulting in hyperpolarization of the mitochondrial membrane, generation of a proton gradient and ATP formation by mitochondria, ADP phosphorylation being coupled to reoxidation of reduced coenzymes, and respiration. Consequently, mitochondrial metabolism increases the ATP/ADP ratio. The increase in cytosolic ATP and/or the decrease in free ADP promotes the closure of ATP-sensitive potassium (K_{ATP}) channels and depolarization of the plasma membrane [1]. As a consequence, cytosolic Ca^{2+} is raised by the opening of voltage-gated Ca^{2+} channels. The increase in cytosolic Ca^{2+} is the main trigger for exocytosis, the process by which the insulin-containing secretory granules fuse with the plasma membrane (fig. 1). In addition,

ATP also exerts a permissive action on insulin exocytosis [1]. Therefore, respiration, ATP synthesis, the ATP levels itself, and the ATP/ADP ratio directly control insulin release. Consequently, any factor or change impairing mitochondrial metabolism, decreasing the [ATP]/[ADP] ratio, prevents depolarization-driven Ca^{2+} influx, and thereby suppresses insulin release. Accordingly, it is known that mutations in both the *ABCC8* and *KCNJ11* genes encoding K_{ATP} channel subunits SUR1 (sulfonylurea receptor 1) and Kir6.2 provoke the most severe congenital hyperinsulinism (CHI) [2]. Other metabolites linked to mitochondria metabolism and affecting insulin secretion are calcium, glutamate, certain amino acids, alpha-ketoglutarate, and reactive oxygen species (ROS; particularly mitochondrial ROS) [1, 2].

Mitochondrial Carriers Are Essential Regulators of Metabolism and Cell Bioenergetics

Whereas the outer mitochondrial membrane is permeable to small metabolites, the permeability of the inner mitochondrial membrane is tightly controlled in order to maintain the 180- to 190-mV electrochemical gradient generated by the respiratory chain necessary for ATP synthesis by the mitochondrial ATP-synthase. The transport of metabolites and other solutes across the mitochondrial inner membrane is critical for both the supply of substrates for oxidation, such as organic acids and amino acids, and for the release of products such as ATP and organic acids to the cytosol. The inner membrane actually links the biochemical pathways in the cytosol, such as glycolysis, with those in the mitochondrial matrix, such as the citric acid cycle (also referred to as the tricarboxylic acid or Krebs cycle), respiratory chain/OXPHOS system, fatty acid oxidation helix, urea cycle, and gluconeogenesis.

To ensure this crosstalk between cytosolic and mitochondrial metabolic pathways, the inner membrane has to transport anion substrates such as ADP, ATP, phosphate, oxoglutarate, citrate, glutamate, malate, acylcarnitines, and others. These transport steps are important for the generation of ATP from the oxidation of sugars and fat, breakdown of amino acids, synthesis of heme and iron sulfur clusters, heat production, and macromolecular synthesis. These transport steps are catalyzed by a series of specific substrate carrier proteins that operate as exchangers/cotransporters and span the inner membrane of mitochondria. Such proteins are present over the inner mitochondrial membrane and include ADP, ATP carrier protein (also referred to as ADP/ATP translocase or adenine nucleotide translocator), 2-oxoglutarate/malate carrier protein, phosphate carrier protein, tricarboxylate transport protein (or citrate transport protein), acylcarnitine transporter, uncoupling proteins, Graves disease carrier protein, and many others. These transporters are not entirely characterized yet and the functions of only half of the members of mitochondrial carrier family are known [3].

All members of the mitochondrial carrier family are 300–340 amino acids long and are encoded by nuclear genes. Most of them contain a primary structure exhibiting three more or less repeated regions of roughly 100 amino acids, with some variation in one or two signature sequences. These mitochondrial carriers consist of a basket-shaped structure with six transmembrane helices according to predicted structure and to the resolved structure of the adenine nucleotide translocator [3]. These carriers are generally referred to as the SLC25 family [3]. Dysfunctional carriers are associated with rare but severe human diseases, such as metabolic disorders (carnitine/acylcarnitine carrier deficiency), triple H syndrome (hyperammonemia, hyperornithinemia, and homocitrullinemia), aspartate/glutamate isoform 2 deficiency, sideroblastic anemia, neurodegenerative diseases (Amish microcephaly, neonatal myoclonic epilepsy), and muscular dystrophy [3].

The Mitochondrial Uncoupling Proteins

The observation of an obligatory and tight coupling between respiration (nucleotide reoxidation, oxygen consumption, and H_2O synthesis) and ATP synthesis (ADP phosphorylation) culminated around 1970 with the demonstration of Mitchell's theory based on the generation of a mitochondrial proton gradient through the mitochondrial inner membrane by complexes I, III, and IV of the respiratory chain, followed by the consumption of this gradient during the simultaneous activation of the mitochondrial ATP-synthase. Mitchell's theory predicted that any proton leak through the inner membrane not coupled to ATP synthesis would represent an uncoupling of respiration and result in thermogenesis [4]. Such an uncoupling can be artificially obtained using chemical uncouplers such as 2,4-dinitrophenol or FCCP that promotes proton reentry in the mitochondrial matrix. Interestingly, such a natural uncoupling of respiration to ADP phosphorylation was discovered. It is represented by uncoupling protein UCP, presently referred to as UCP1, a unique component present in the inner membrane of brown adipocyte mitochondria where it dissipates energy of fatty acid oxidation as heat upon physiological demand [4, 5].

Brown adipocytes are specialized mesenchymal cells containing many mitochondria and lipid droplets, and form depots of brown adipose tissue. These cells are activated by sympathetic nerves when heat production is required by the brain to maintain body temperature during exposure to the cold or at birth, or to rapidly increase body temperature upon arousal from hibernation. The noradrenergic stimulation of brown adipocytes implicates immediate activation of UCP1 acting as an uncoupler of respiration from ATP synthesis and provoking a marked loss of energy oxidation as heat. UCP1 has a triplicated structure and is a characteristic member of the mitochondrial transporter family. It is unique to brown adipocytes, but can uncouple respiration of any type of cells expressing it recombinantly. It works as a proton carrier activated by fatty acids, bypassing the mitochondrial ATP-synthase without coupling to any other energy-consuming process and activating a futile proton current through the membrane. The downregulation of the proton gradient and of the mitochondrial membrane potential strongly activates the respiratory chain which greatly enhances heat production since ATP synthesis is nonactive in a situation when coenzyme reoxidation is greatly stimulated by the low membrane potential [4, 5].

In 1997, UCP2, a protein homologous to the initial UCP then renamed UCP1, was identified [5, 6]. Other related mitochondrial transporters were also identified in animals as wells as plants; based on their high level of identity towards UCP1 and 2, they were named UCP3, stUCP, UCP4, or BMCP1/UCP5 (reviewed in [5–8]). Clearly, among the family of mitochondrial anion transporters, a subfamily of uncoupling proteins was identified. However, the exact biochemical and physiological functions of these UCPs is still a matter of debate and the question of their true uncoupling activity has not been solved yet.

UCP2

UCP2 was identified as a membranous mitochondrial carrier having 57% amino acid identity to UCP1 [6]. Unlike UCP1, UCP2 was shown to be expressed in many cell types and tissues, such as macrophages, lymphocytes, brown and white adipocytes, skeletal muscles, lung, gut, heart, thymus, spleen, bone marrow, brain, and pancreatic islets [5–8]. Initial functional experiments in transformed yeast revealed that UCP2 was able to decrease the mitochondrial membrane potential and to partially uncouple respiration [6].

However, the exact physiological role of UCP2 is poorly understood, mainly since the precise catalytic activity of this mitochondrial transporter remains unclear. We believe that UCP2 transport activity is related to the anaplerotic control of the Krebs cycle in such a way that it promotes fatty acid oxidation and limits glycolysis-derived pyruvate utilization [9] (fig. 1).

Interestingly, studies of mice null for the *Ucp2* gene revealed two distinct phenotypes: (1) a stimulation of macrophage activity linked to a role of UCP2 as a negative regulator of ROS level in immune cells [10], and (2) a moderate hypoglycemia due to a role of UCP2 as a negative regulator of insulin release [11]. This latter point is discussed in more detail below. The ability of UCP2 to downregulate macrophage response and control ROS production in cells agrees with its observed role in protection against atherosclerosis, neuron degeneration, and cancer development [5, 12]. Functional and genetic studies confirmed the potential role of UCP2 in cell proliferation [9] and several autoimmune diseases such as encephalomyelitis, type 1 diabetes, rheumatoid arthritis, systemic lupus erythematosus, Wegener's granulomatosis, Crohn's disease, and ulcerative colitis [13, 14].

UCP2 Is an Inhibitor of Insulin Secretion in Animal Experiments and a Putative Regulator of Insulin Secretion in Humans

As explained above, any protein affecting mitochondrial activity and ATP levels or the ATP/ADP ratio is a potential regulator of insulin secretion. More precisely, any protein such as a UCP or a mitochondrial carrier putatively able to modulate the efficiency of oxidative phosphorylation may potentially control insulin secretion. A positional candidate approach and QTL analysis were in favor of a possible role of UCP2 in obesity and diabetes and led us to initially propose *Ucp2* as a gene linked to hyperinsulinemia [6]. Importantly, in agreement with this hypothesis, Zhang et al. [11] described a moderate hyperinsulinemia and hypoglycemia in *Ucp2*$^{-/-}$ mice, establishing UCP2 as a negative regulator of insulin secretion in response to glucose. This proposal was confirmed by several reports of overexpression of UCP2 in rat pancreatic islets or insulinoma cells [15, 16] describing a severe blunting of glucose-stimulated insulin secretion. In other respects, inhibition of *Ucp2* expression using either RNAi in pancreatic beta-cells or whole-body attenuation of UCP2 expression by antisense oligonucleotide enhanced glucose-stimulated insulin secretion and reversed hyperglycemia in models of diabetes and insulin resistance [15–17]. Finally and in agreement with this, inhibition of UCP2 activity by genipin, a natural compound from *Gardenia*, reversed high glucose- and obesity-induced beta-cell dysfunction [18].

In addition to stimulation of beta-cells by glucose, other mechanisms affecting insulin secretion are mediated by UCP2. Wang et al. [19] reported that ghrelin inhibits insulin secretion though the AMPK-UCP2 pathway in beta-cells, and Bordone et al. [20] identified Sirt1 as a repressor of UCP2 and consequently as a positive regulator of insulin secretion. Recently, Sun et al. [21] suggested that microRNA-15a promoted insulin biosynthesis by inhibiting UCP2 expression. In addition, there is also evidence in humans that a functional polymorphism in the *Ucp2* promoter correlated with lower levels of insulin secretion and reduced insulin sensitivity and a higher risk for the development of type 2 diabetes [22, 23].

Search for *UCP2* Mutations in Congenital Hyperinsulinism Patients Reveals Loss of Function of *UCP2* and May Explain Congenital Hyperinsulinism in Two Infants

Description of the Patients

All of these data highlighting the marked ability of UCP2 to inhibit insulin secretion, at least in rodents, prompted us to investigate whether UCP2 could have a role in humans, especially in newborns presenting disorders of insulin secretion such as CHI. Severe CHI is frequently due to mutations in *ABCC8* and *KCNJ11* encoding K_{ATP} channel subunits SUR1 and Kir6.2 [2], but it is accepted that the responsible gene is unknown in 40% of CHI cases. Therefore, we searched for *UCP2* mutations in 10

```
Patient 1             160       170   DV  180      D190       200       210
UCP2_HS         GGRRYQSTVNAYKTIAREEGFRGLWKGTSPNVARNAIVNCAELVTYDLIKDALLKANLMTDD
UCP2_RN         GGRRYQSTVEAYKTIAREEGIRGLWKGTSPNVARNAIVNCTELVTYDLIKDTLLKANLMTDD
UCP2_PS         GGRRYQSTVEAYKTIAREEGIRGLWKGTSPNVARNAIVNCAELVTYDLIKDTLLKANLMTDD
UCP2_MM         GGRRYQSTVEAYKTIAREEGIRGLWKGTSPNVARNAIVNCAELVTYDLIKDTLLKANLMTDD

Patient 2           220       230       240       250       260       G
UCP2_HS         LPCHFTSAFGAGFCTTVIASPVDVVKTRYMNSALGQYSSAGHCALTMLQKEGPRAFYKGFMP
UCP2_RN         LPCHFTSAFGAGFCTTVIASPVDVVKTRYMNSALGQYHSAGHCALTMLRKEGPRAFYKGFMP
UCP2_PS         LPCHFTSAFGAGFCTTVIASPVDVVKTRYMNSALGQYHSAGHCALTMLRKEGPRAFYKGFMP
UCP2_MM         LPCHFTSAFGAGFCTTVIASPVDVVKTRYMNSALGQYHSAGHCALTMLRKEGPRAFYKGFMP
```

Fig. 2. Amino acid changes in patients 1 and 2. Comparison of the amino acid sequences of the second moiety of UCP2 from *Homo sapiens* (HS), *Rattus norvegicus* (RN), *Phodopus sungorus* (PS), and *Mus musculus* (MM). Bold black letters in the upper line represent the amino acids found in patients 1 and 2. Light gray letters correspond to amino acids present in all species.

CHI hyperinsulinemic patients with no detectable mutations by DNA direct sequencing in the *ABCC8*, *KCNJ11*, *GCK*, or *GLUD1* genes. Parentally inherited heterozygous *UCP2* variants encoding amino acid changes were found in 2 unrelated children out of these 10 CHI patients [24] (see 'Molecular studies'). Both patients responded to diazoxide. Patient 1, a girl, was born at a gestational age of 38 weeks from 2 unrelated healthy Caucasian parents. She developed neonatal hypoglycemia and was successfully treated by diazoxide over 1 year. Then, diazoxide was stopped without hypoglycemia recurrence. Patient 2, also a girl, was born at a gestational age of 37 weeks from 2 unrelated Caucasian parents. She presented with seizures at 8 months of age which revealed hypoglycemia. Clinical and biological investigations confirmed the diagnosis of hyperinsulinism. Pancreatic venous sampling revealed a diffuse insulin secretion suggesting a diffuse form of CHI that was successfully treated by diazoxide. Hypoglycemia in patient 2 also resolved after 2 years of age. Her mother was found to be occasionally hypoglycemic in adulthood and had been treated by an antiepileptic drug for seizures during infancy.

Molecular Studies and Prediction of Structural Changes in UCP2 Mutants

PCR analysis of UCP2 exons from peripheral blood leukocytes was carried out. An abnormal DHPLC pattern was detected for 2 unrelated patients. DNA sequence analysis identified three and one heterozygous single nucleotide changes in patients 1 and 2, respectively, all of them leading to an amino acid change (fig. 2). Mutations of patient 1 were a G to A transition changing a conserved glycine into an aspartic acid (G174D), a C to G transversion changing a conserved leucine into a valine (L175V), and a C to A transition changing a conserved alanine into an aspartic acid (A187D). All mutations were inherited from the father. The mutation of patient 2 was inherited from her mother and was a C to G transversion that changed a conserved alanine into a glycine. The amino acid changes identified in these 2 patients were not found in 100 control subjects. All these residues are highly conserved in UCP2 protein from different species (fig. 2). The amino acids G174 and L175, mutated in patient 1, are localized at the end of the second matrix loop, just before nucleation of the predicted fourth transmembrane alpha-helix. The residue A187, involved also in the first patient, is in the predicted fourth transmembrane alpha-helix. The A268, which is mutated in patient 2, is located at the end of the third matrix hydrophilic loop, before the sixth transmembrane domain of UCP2.

Functional Studies of Human UCP2 Mutants in Yeast

To measure respiratory uncoupling, we assessed the proton conductance of spheroplasts from yeast overexpressing wild-type and the mutated UCP2 proteins carrying the amino acid changes found in patients 1 and 2 (in the case of patient 1, the three amino acid substitutions were included in the construct). As we had shown previously, overexpression of wild-type UCP2 in yeast mitochondria increased the proton leak and thus partially uncoupled mitochondrial respiration, compared to control spheroplasts [24, 25]. The activity of the mutated forms of UCP2 (patient 1 or patient 2) was also measured in yeast spheroplasts. Interestingly, yeasts expressing patient 1 and patient 2 UCP2 proteins showed lower proton permeability compared to the ones expressing wild-type UCP2, suggesting that both mutated proteins were less active than wild-type UCP2 (data not shown here, see [24]). In the case of patient 1, the three variants were not tested individually.

Functional Studies in Insulin-Secreting Cells

To assess whether the modification of UCP2 activity observed in patients 1 and 2 could affect insulin secretion by beta-cells, we subjected an insulin-secreting pancreatic insulinoma cell line (INS-1E) to adenoviral expression of wild-type and mutated UCP2 in mitochondria. Insulin secretion by INS-1E cells expressing wild-type and mutant UCP2 proteins was determined in the presence of 15 mM glucose. As expected, adenoviral UCP2 infection significantly reduced insulin release by INS-1E cells (nearly 40% compared to infection with control adenovirus). In contrast, infection of INS-1E cells with AdhUCP2Patient 1 or AdhUCP2Patient 2 did not modify the insulin secretion levels from control values (fig. 3) [24]. These data clearly established that the mutations observed in the 2 patients presenting CHI hampered the normal inhibition of insulin secretion due to UCP2 activity and were potentially responsible for hyperinsulinism. These data were the first description of a potential role of UCP2 in the regulation of insulin secretion and glucose metabolism in humans [24]. Up to now, siblings were not tested and we have not replicated the study in other cohorts to see whether UCP2 mutations are a common occurrence in diazoxide-responsive neonatal hypoglycemia. In other respects, no distinguishing features of the phenotype in the two affected cases were noticed (e.g. protein-

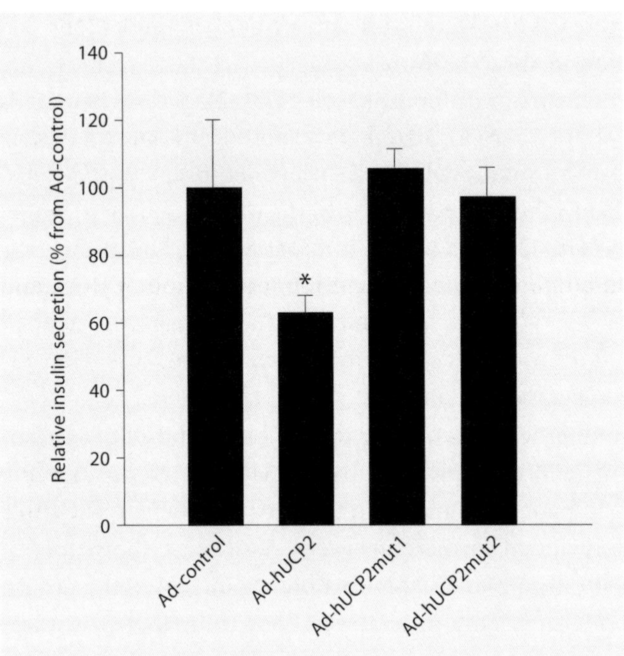

Fig. 3. Effects of mutations in patients 1 and 2 on insulin secretion in response to glucose. Insulin release by INS-1E cells expressing adenoviral wild-type human UCP2 (Ad-hUCP2), mutated UCP2 from patient 1 (Ad-hUCP2mut1), and mutated UCP2 from patient 2 (Ad-hUCP2Patient2) compared with control (Ad-control, containing the GFP gene and the inverted sequence of human UCP2 cDNA). In the case of patient 1, the three amino acid substitutions were included in the construct. Values represent insulin secreted into the medium as a percentage of the insulin secreted by cells infected with control adenovirus (Ad-control) in the presence of 15 mM glucose. The level of statistical significance of the differences between cells infected with control adenovirus and with hUCP2adenovirus is indicated: * $p < 0.001$ (t test). These experiments were described in Gonzalez-Barroso et al. [24].

sensitive hypoglycemia or not, abnormalities of temperature regulation, differences in appetite/behavior).

UCP2 and Experimental Type 1 Diabetes in Mice

In addition to a role of UCP2 in insulin secretion in response to glucose, the ability of UCP2 to limit ROS levels in macrophages and immune cells prompted Emre et al. [13] to look for a role of UCP2 in autoimmune type 1 diabetes in an experimental model of mice treated by streptozotocin. In this study, massive infiltration of macrophages in pancreatic islets followed by lymphocytes preceding insulitis, beta-cell destruction and diabetes was stronger and earlier in *Ucp2*$^{-/-}$ mice. Therefore, at the pancreatic level, UCP2 appears to be an important and dual regulator both of insulin secretion and activity of immune cells controlling the immune/autoimmune status of islets.

Activity of UCP2 in Regulation of Glucose Metabolism also Implicates Pancreatic Alpha-Cells, Adipose Cells, and Hypothalamic Neurons

Since UCP2 is widely expressed in cells and tissues, roles for this mitochondrial carrier were investigated in cells other than pancreatic beta-cells. Interestingly, Diao et al. [26] reported that UCP2 was highly expressed in pancreatic alpha-cells and influenced glucagon secretion. Chevillote et al. [27] observed that UCP2 controls adiponectin gene expression in adipose tissue through the modulation of ROS, and Zhou et al. [28] reported that UCP2 inhibition by genipin reduced insulin-stimulated glucose uptake in adipocytes. An important structure controlling glucose metabolism is the hypothalamus. Remarkably, Parton et al. [29] demonstrated that UCP2 controls the sensing of glucose by the hypothalamic POMC neurons and regulates glucose homeostasis. The same team recently demonstrated that the K_{ATP} channel-mediated glucose excitation of MCH-expressing neurons in the lateral hypothalamus was negatively regulated by UCP2 [30]. All of these data reinforce a wide and strong role for UCP2 in glucose metabolism beyond a simple role in the control of insulin secretion.

Understanding UCP2 Activity and Regulation Will Help to Better Understand Hyperinsulinism, Regulation of Insulin Secretion by ROS, and Glucose Metabolism

UCP2 and UCP1 not only differ in their activity, but also in their regulation. Interestingly, whereas fatty acids activate UCP1 artificially expressed in pancreatic beta-cells, they are unable to activate UCP2 in the same cells [31]. Although a number of data highlight the ability of UCP2 to inhibit insulin secretion, contrary to a few groups attributing this effect of UCP2 to its true respiration uncoupling activity, i.e. its ability to reduce ATP synthesis by mitochondria, many studies strongly indicate that the inhibitory effect of UCP2 on insulin secretion is rather due to its main activity as a regulator of ROS production. In particular, preliminary data suggest that human UCP2 mutants described above, contrary to UCP1 tested in INS-1E cells, were not acting through a simple inhibition of ATP synthesis due to a genuine uncoupling activity of UCP2 (Gonzalez-Barroso and Ricquier, unpubl. data). Previously, Affourtit et al. [32] reported that UCP2 attenuates glucose-induced insulin secretion in INS-1E insulinoma cells by lowering mitochondrial ROS. Lee et al. [33] also reported that UCP2 regulates ROS formation in islets and influences susceptibility to diabetogenic action of streptozotocin. Pi et al. [34] documented a persistent oxidative stress in beta-cells due to absence of UCP2 associated with impaired beta-cell function, and, importantly, highlighted the role of genetic background in mice as well as the effect of backcrosses of mutants. Contrary to most other studies, Produit-Zengaffinen et al. [35] observed that increasing UCP2 in pancreatic beta-cells did not alter glucose-induced insulin secretion, but decreased the production of ROS

Table 1. Physiological roles proposed for UCP2 according to the data obtained from *Ucp2* knockout mice

Organ/tissue	Cell type	Role of UCP2
Pancreas	beta-cell	decrease of ROS production; inhibition of insulin secretion; decrease of ATP level
Pancreas	alpha-cell	decrease of ROS production; uncoupling of respiration; reduction of glucagon content
Brain	POMC neurons	decrease of ATP level; glucose sensing
Brain	NPY/AgRP neurons	decrease of ROS production; glucose sensing; mediation of ghrelin-induced food intake
Brain	MCH neurons	inhibition of glucose excitation
Adipose tissue	adipocytes	decrease of ROS production; activation of adiponectin synthesis; decrease of ghrelin-induced lipogenesis; activation of fatty acid oxidation
Immune system	macrophages	decrease of ROS production; inhibition of macrophage activation; activation of fatty acid oxidation; activation of glutamine oxidation
Embryo	fibroblasts	decrease of cellular proliferation; activation of fatty acid oxidation
Aorta	endothelial cells	decrease of ROS production; atherosclerosis protection

nevertheless. Moreover, a role mediating ghrelin's action on hypothalamic neuronal populations has been proposed for UCP2 by lowering free radicals [36]. Interestingly, these data on UCP2 agree with the growing evidence that ROS are not just deleterious by-products of respiratory metabolism in mitochondria, but can be essential elements for many biological responses, including glucose-stimulated insulin secretion by beta-cells [34].

Conclusion

Mitochondria are considered as central players in the coupling between glucose metabolism and insulin secretion. Indeed, mitochondria function as a glucose sensor and trigger a cascade of metabolic signals that lead to the secretion of insulin by pancreatic beta-cells. UCP2 appears to be an important regulator of insulin secretion and represents an excellent example of a mitochondrial protein involved in this control. However, beyond pancreatic beta-cells and insulin secretion, UCP2 appears to be an important regulator of glucose metabolism in many types of cells that are also implicated in glucose sensing (table 1). UCP2 activity has a negative impact on insulin secretion and, on the contrary, the absence or loss of function mutations in *UCP2* leads to enhanced insulin secretion. Although the primary function of UCP2 remains controversial, there are three main proposals that could explain the impact of UCP2 in insulin secretion (fig. 1): (1) UCP2 is an uncoupling protein that lowers mitochondrial membrane potential and ATP production, (2) UCP2 is a negative regulator of ROS production, and (3) UCP2 modulates glucose oxidation promoting fatty acid oxidation and limiting glycolysis-derived pyruvate utilization. Understanding the real physiological activity of UCP2 is an important challenge to clarify whether UCP2 could be a therapeutic target for diseases in which insulin secretion is altered.

Acknowledgements

The research of the authors was funded by the Centre National de la Recherche Scientifique and European Union-funded Concerted Action Grant (QLG1-2000-00513, PdL), an European Union sixth framework program (Diabesity contract LSHM-CT-2003-503041, DR), and by the GIS-Institut des Maladies Rares (P.d.L.).

References

1 Wolheim C, Maechler P: Beta-cell mitochondria and insulin secretion: messenger role of nucleotides and metabolites. Diabetes 2007;51:S37.
2 Palladino AA, Stanley CA: The hyperinsulinism/hyperammonemia syndrome. Rev Endocr Metab Disord 2010;11:171.
3 Palmieri F: Diseases caused by defects of mitochondrial carriers: a review. Biochim Biophys Acta 2008;1777:564.
4 Nicholls DG: The physiological regulation of uncoupling proteins. Biochim Biophys Acta 2006;1757:459.
5 Rousset S, Alves-Guerra MC, Mozo J, Miroux B, Cassard-Doulcier AM, Bouillaud F, Ricquier D: The biology of mitochondrial uncoupling proteins. Diabetes 2004;53:S130.
6 Fleury C, Neverova M, Collins S, Raimbault S, Champigny O, Levi-Meyrueis C, Bouillaud F, Seldin MF, Surwit RS, Ricquier D, Warden CH: Uncoupling protein-2: a novel gene linked to obesity and hyperinsulinemia. Nat Genet 1997;15:269.
7 Boss O, Hagen T, Lowell BB: Uncoupling proteins 2 and 3: potential regulators of mitochondrial energy metabolism. Diabetes 2000;49:143.
8 Affourtit C, Crichton PG, Parker N, Brand MD: Novel uncoupling proteins. Novartis Found Symp 2007;287:70.
9 Pecqueur C, Bui T, Gelly C, Hauchard J, Barbot C, Bouillaud F, Ricquier D, Miroux B, Thompson CB: Uncoupling protein-2 controls proliferation by promoting fatty acid oxidation and limiting glycolysis-derived pyruvate utilization. FASEB J 2008;22:9.
10 Arsenijevic D, Onuma H, Pecqueur C, Raimbault S, Manning BS, Miroux B, Couplan E, Alves-Guerra MC, Goubern M, Surwit R, Bouillaud F, Richard D, Collins S, Ricquier D: Disruption of the uncoupling protein-2 gene in mice reveals a role in immunity and reactive oxygen species production. Nat Genet 2000;26:435.
11 Zhang CY, Baffy G, Perret P, Krauss S, Peroni O, Grujic D, Hagen T, Vidal-Puig AJ, Boss O, Kim YB, Zheng XX, Wheeler MB, Shulman GI, Chan CB, Lowell BB: Uncoupling protein 2 negatively regulates insulin secretion and is a major link between obesity, beta cell dysfunction, and type 2 diabetes. Cell 2001;105:745.

12 Paradis E, Clavel S, Bouillaud F, Ricquier D, Richard D: Uncoupling protein 2: a novel player in neuroprotection. Trends Mol Med 2003;9:522.

13 Emre Y, Hurtaud C, Karaca M, Nubel T, Zavala F, Ricquier D: Role of uncoupling protein UCP2 in cell-mediated immunity: how macrophage-mediated insulitis is accelerated in a model of autoimmune diabetes. Proc Natl Acad Sci USA 2007;104: 19085.

14 Yu X, Wieczorek S, Franke A, Yin H, Pierer M, Sina C, Karlsen TH, Boberg KM, Bergquist A, Kunz M, Witte T, Gross WL, Epplen JT, Alarcón-Riquelme ME, Schreiber S, Ibrahim SM: Association of UCP2 -866 G/A polymorphism with chronic inflammatory diseases. Genes Immun 2009;10:601.

15 Chan CB, Harper ME: Uncoupling proteins: role in insulin resistance and insulin insufficiency. Curr Diabetes Rev 2006;2:271.

16 Affourtit C, Brand MD: Uncoupling protein-2 contributes significantly to high mitochondrial proton leak in INS-1E insulinoma cells and attenuates glucose-stimulated insulin secretion. Biochem J 2008;409:199.

17 De Souza CT, Araújo EP, Stoppiglia LF, Pauli JR, Ropelle E, Rocco SA, Marin RM, Franchini KG, Carvalheira JB, Saad MJ, Boschero AC, Carneiro EM, Velloso LA: Inhibition of UCP2 expression reverses diet-induced diabetes mellitus by effects on both insulin secretion and action. FASEB J 2007;21: 1153.

18 Zhang CY, Parton LE, Ye CP, Krauss S, Shen R, Lin CT, Porco JA, Lowell BB: Genipin inhibits UCP2-mediated proton leak and acutely reverses obesity- and high glucose-induced beta cell dysfunction in isolated pancreatic islets. Cell Metab 2006;3:417.

19 Wang Y, Nishi M, Doi A, Shono T, Furukawa Y, Shimada T, Furuta H, Sasaki H, Nanjo K: Ghrelin inhibits insulin secretion through the AMPK-UCP2 pathway in beta cells. FEBS Lett 2010;584:1503.

20 Bordone L, Motta MC, Picard F, Robinson A, Jhala US, Apfeld J, McDonagh T, Lemieux M, McBurney M, Szilvasi A, Easlon EJ, Lin SJ, Guarente L: Sirt1 regulates insulin secretion by repressing UCP2 in pancreatic beta cells. PLoS Biol 2006;4:e31.

21 Sun LL, Jiang BG, Li WT, Zou JJ, Shi YQ, Liu ZM: MicroRNA-15a positively regulates insulin synthesis by inhibiting uncoupling protein-2 expression. Diabetes Res Clin Pract 2011;91:94.

22 D'Adamo M, Perego L, Cardellini M, Marini MA, Frontoni S, Andreozzi F, Sciacqua A, Lauro P, Sbraccia P, Federici M, Paganelli M, Pontiroli AE, Lauro R, Perticone F, Folli F, Sesti G: The -886A/A genotype in the promoter in the human uncoupling protein 2 gene is associated with insulin resistance and increased risk of type 2 diabetes. Diabetes 2004; 53:1905.

23 Wang H, Chu WS, Lu T, Hasstedt SJ, Kern PA, Elbein SC: Uncoupling protein-2 polymorphisms in the type 2 diabetes, obesity, and insulin secretion. Am J Physiol 2004;286:E1.

24 Gonzalez-Barroso MM, Giurgea I, Bouillaud F, Anedda A, Bellanné-Chantelot C, Hubert L, de Keyzer Y, de Lonlay P, Ricquier D: Mutations in UCP2 in congenital hyperinsulinism reveal a role for regulation of insulin secretion. Plos One 2008;3: e3850.

25 Rial E, Gonzalez-Barroso MdM, Fleury C, Iturrizaga S, Sanchis D, Jiménez-Jiménez J, Ricquier D, Goubern M, Bouillaud F: Retinoids activate proton transport by the uncoupling proteins UCP1 and UCP2. EMBO J 1999;18:5827.

26 Diao J, Allister EM, Koshkin V, Lee SC, Bhattacharjee A, Tang C, Giacca A, Chan CB, Wheeler MB : UCP2 is highly expressed in pancreatic alpha-cells and influences secretion and survival. Proc Natl Acad Sci USA 2008;105:12057.

27 Chevillotte E, Giralt M, Miroux B, Ricquier D, Villarroya F: Uncoupling protein-2 controls adiponectin gene expression in adipose tissue through the modulation of reactive oxygen species production. Diabetes 2007;56:1042.

28 Zhou H, Zhao J, Zhang X: Inhibition of uncoupling protein 2 by genipin reduces insulin-stimulated glucose uptake in 3T3-L1 adipocytes. Arch Biochem Biophys 2009;486:88.

29 Parton LE, Ye CP, Coppari R, Enriori PJ, Choi B, Zhang CY, Xu C, Vianna CR, Balthasar N, Lee CE, Elmquist JK, Cowley MA, Lowell BB: Glucose sensing by POMC neurons regulates glucose homeostasis and is impaired in obesity. Nature 2007;449:228.

30 Kong D, Vong L, Parton LE, Ye C, Tong Q, Hu X, Choi B, Brüning JC, Lowell BB: Glucose stimulation of hypothalamic MCH neurons involves K(ATP) channels, is modulated by UCP2, and regulates peripheral glucose homeostasis. Cell Metab 2010; 12: 545.

31 Galetti S, Sarre A, Perreten H, Produit-Zengaffinen N, Muzzin P, Assimacopoulos-Jeannet F: Fatty acids do not activate UCP2 in pancreatic beta cells: comparison with UCP1. Pflugers Arch 2009;457:931.

32 Affourtit C, Jastroch M, Brand MD: Uncoupling protein-2 attenuates glucose-stimulated insulin secretion in INS-1E insulinoma cells by lowering mitochondrial reactive oxygen species. Free Radic Biol Med 2011;50:609.
33 Lee SC, Robson-Doucette CA, Wheeler MB: Uncoupling protein 2 regulates reactive oxygen species formation in islets and influences susceptibility to diabetogenic action of streptozotocin. J Endocrinol 2009;203:33.
34 Pi J, Bai Y, Daniel KW, Liu D, Lyght O, Edelstein D, Brownlee M, Corkey BE, Collins S: Persistent oxidative stress due to absence of uncoupling protein 2 associated with impaired pancreatic beta-cell function. Endocrinology 2009;150:3040.
35 Produit-Zengaffinen N, Davis-Lameloise N, Perreten H, Bécard D, Gjinovci A, Keller P, Wolheim CB, Herrera P, Muzzin P, Assimacopoulos-Jeannet F: Increasing uncoupling protein-2 in pancreatic beta cells does not alter glucose-induced insulin secretion but decreases production of reactive oxygen species. Diabetologia 2007;50:84.
36 Andrews ZB, Liu ZW, Walllingford N, Erion DM, Borok E, Friedman JM, Tschöp MH, Shanabrough M, Cline G, Shulman GI, Coppola A, Gao XB, Horvath TL, Diano S: UCP2 mediates ghrelin's action on NPY/AgRP neurons by lowering free radicals. Nature 2008;454:846.

Dr. Daniel Ricquier
Service de Biochimie Métabolique
Hôpital Necker-Enfants Malades
Assistance Publique Hôpitaux de Paris
149 rue de Sèvres
FR–75743 Paris Cedex 15 (France)
Tel. +33 1 44 49 58 09, daniel.ricquier@nck.aphp.fr

Stanley CA, De León DD (eds): Monogenic Hyperinsulinemic Hypoglycemia Disorders.
Front Diabetes. Basel, Karger, 2012, vol 21, pp 172–181

Exercise-Induced Hyperinsulinism: A Failure of Monocarboxylate Transporter 1 Expression Silencing

Timo Otonkoski[a,b] · Thomas Meissner[c]

[a]Children's Hospital, University of Helsinki and Helsinki University Central Hospital, and [b]Research Programs Unit, Molecular Neurology, Biomedicum Stem Cell Centre, University of Helsinki, Helsinki, Finland; [c]Department of General Pediatrics, University Children's Hospital Düsseldorf, Düsseldorf, Germany

Abstract

Exercise-induced hyperinsulinism (EIHI) is a rare disorder, which has so far only been described in two families as a dominantly inherited trait and in one isolated individual. It is characterized by hypoglycemia which is triggered most prominently by anaerobic exercise. Blood glucose levels fall as blood pyruvate and lactate levels increase and, typically, hypoglycemia develops immediately following exhaustive exercise. The insulin secretion of these individuals is responsive to intravenous pyruvate unlike in healthy controls. In all patients, mutations have been found in the regulatory regions of the *SLC16A1* gene, which encodes the monocarboxylate transporter 1 (MCT-1) protein. MCT-1 transports lactate and pyruvate into the cell and is expressed in practically all cell types, except the pancreatic beta-cell where it is transcriptionally silenced. The pathogenesis of EIHI is based on the failure of MCT-1 silencing, leading to inappropriate insulin secretion triggered by anaerobic exercise. Although the patients are responsive to diazoxide in terms of a general increase of blood glucose, diazoxide does not completely prevent exercise-induced hypoglycemia. Most patients do not need specific treatment because they do not have significant symptoms if they avoid strenuous exercise.

Insulin Secretion during Exercise

In healthy humans, moderate as well as excessive exercise is not associated with severe hypoglycemia. Several factors contribute to a tight control of glucose levels. Increased hepatic glucose production, which occurs in response to moderate-intensity exercise, compensates for increased glucose demand of the muscles. An exercise-induced fall in insulin and the increase in glucagon are thought to be the primary stimuli for the increment in hepatic glucose production. During exercise, insulin secretion is in part inhibited by beta-cell alpha-adrenergic receptor activation [1–3].

During intense exercise, there is a rapid increase in the need for glucose. In this situation, glucose mobilized from muscle and liver glycogen is the exclusive muscle fuel. Intense exercise is characterized by marked increments of glucose production rising seven- to eightfold. After intense exercise, rising glycemia requires a substantial increase in insulin secretion for 40–60 min to restore pre-exercise levels [4–6], but without decreasing glucose levels into the range of hypoglycemia.

Although mild hypoglycemic symptoms during prolonged moderate exercise are common, the acute development of severe hypoglycemia during intense exercise is a rare feature. We describe otherwise healthy individuals in whom heavy exercise is associated with massive insulin secretion resulting in symptomatic hypoglycemia.

Clinical Picture and Treatment

The main clinical characteristics of the patients are listed in table 1. The index patient for this disorder was a 16-year-old German boy of Caucasian origin who presented with a 2-year history of recurrent syncope. These episodes usually occurred a few minutes after vigorous exercise. Hypoglycemia was found during one of these episodes (blood glucose <1.6 mmol/l; normal range: 3.0–5.5), which responded rapidly to intravenous glucose with relief of symptoms. During a fasting test, he developed symptomatic hypoglycemia after 12 h (blood glucose 2.2 mmol/l; insulin 20 mU/l). Ketone bodies and free fatty acids were very low during hypoglycemia, and hyperinsulinism was confirmed. First an insulinoma was suspected, but diagnostic laparotomy with manual exploration of the pancreas, intraoperative ultrasonography, and pancreatic biopsies failed to show any abnormalities. Family history was unremarkable in this patient. When the patient reported that he always suffered from hypoglycemia (home measurements of glucose and symptoms of hypoglycemia) after exercising with dumbbells at home, we tested his blood glucose and insulin levels after 5 min of intense dumbbell exercise and found a dramatic rise of insulin (49 mU/l) resulting in hypoglycemia in the recovery phase (glucose 1.9 mmol/l) [7].

The second indentified individual was a Finnish girl who presented at the age of 11 months, when she was admitted with convulsions. She had suffered from a concussion on the previous day and had been eating poorly. Blood glucose was low at 0.9 mmol/l. Subsequently, she had several hospital admissions for hypoglycemic episodes and syncope. Spontaneous blood glucose values in the range of 0.9–2.0 mmol/l were measured several times during early childhood. Extended fasting did not provoke hypoglycemia, but prolonged exercise, particularly swimming, seemed to cause hypoglycemic symptoms that were different from exhaustion and fatigue, although biochemical hypoglycemia was never documented. At the age of 15 years, a bicycle exercise test was performed with monitoring of plasma glucose and insulin. The test was stopped after 10 min and blood glucose concentration measurements 20 min later revealed hyperinsulinemic hypoglycemia (insulin 50 mU/l, glucose 1.8 mmol/l)

Table 1. EIHI individuals and their main symptoms

Case no.	Family history	Symptoms	Treatment
1	index patient, no family history	severe episodes of hypoglycemia with syncopes after soccer (at 14 years of age) or dumbbell exercise	diazoxide had a partial effect, but did not prevent hypoglycemia after anaerobic exercise
2	index patient, family 1	hyperinsulinemic hypoglycemia at the age of 1.2 years; epilepsy	diazoxide for 18 years, partial response
3	closely related to case 2	no symptoms; obesity	–
4	closely related to case 2	symptoms associated with physical exercise	–
5	mother of case 2	symptoms of hypoglycemia related to physical exercise; avoidance of physical exercise	–
6	closely related to case 2	symptoms of hypoglycemia related to physical exercise	–
7	brother of case 2	hypoglycemic symptoms since childhood	–
8	niece of case 2	symptoms of hypoglycemia related to physical exercise	–
9	niece of case 2	no symptoms	–
10	index patient family 2	hypoglycemic episodes since infancy; after puberty associated with physical exercise	intermittent use of diazoxide, partially effective
11	father of case 10	impaired exercise tolerance	frequent snacks
12	aunt of case 10	mild symptoms of hypoglycemia related to physical exercise	–
13	cousin of case 10	prolonged mild neonatal hypoglycemia	–

[7]. Since these 2 cases appeared to represent a new form of hypoglycemia in which exercise was associated with inappropriate insulin secretion, we named the condition exercise-induced hyperinsulinism (EIHI).

Subsequently, another Finnish patient was identified and exercise testing of family members revealed 10 additional EIHI patients for the 2 Finnish cases [8]. The age at diagnosis of these individuals varied widely between 1.5 and 60 years (median: 27). The clinical symptoms varied remarkably. Two of 9 adult patients had never recognized episodes of hypoglycemia; however, one of them was at the time of evaluation severely overweight (BMI: 36). Most of the 9 adult patients reported recurrent hypoglycemic symptoms associated with strenuous exercise. For many, swimming had often been linked with hypoglycemia-like symptoms since childhood. Aerobic mild exercise was usually well tolerated, and most subjects learned to adjust their activities so that they did not develop episodes of serious hypoglycemia. Only the 2 Finnish index cases suffered from recurrent severe episodes of hypoglycemia starting in early childhood. Prolonged neonatal hypoglycemia was reported for the patient who was 1.5-years-old at the time of diagnosis. One index patient suffered from epilepsy.

The 3 index cases had benefited from medical treatment with diazoxide, a potassium channel opener which acts by inhibiting insulin release. Diazoxide relieved their symptoms only to some extent. It was helpful to enable a longer fasting period; however, it did not totally prevent hypoglycemic episodes after exercise. Therefore, none of the patients have found it necessary to continue with the medication. Avoidance of anaerobic exercise is the most effective way to prevent severe post-exercise hypoglycemia. In addition, carbohydrates after physical exercise might be helpful, but have to be tested individually.

Clinical Physiological Studies

Different studies with changing intensity of exercise were performed. Reactions of blood glucose with and without treatment with diazoxide were investigated. After identification of the first 2 cases of EIHI, a protocol to diagnose this condition was established. Exercise testing was found necessary to clearly identify affected individuals.

Physical Exercise Testing

Most EIHI-individuals were diagnosed based on a 10-min bicycle exercise. The aim was to increase the pulse rate to an age-adjusted target of 220 minus age in years. Blood tests for glucose, insulin, pyruvate, and lactate were taken at –10, 0, 5, 10, 15, 20, 25, 30, 35, 40, 50, and 60 min.

All individuals were normoglycemic after the overnight fast and before the test (blood glucose: 3.5–5.2 mmol/l). During exercise, and particularly immediately after it, blood glucose levels decreased in the patients, whereas a slight increase was observed in the control subjects (fig. 1). A clearly hypoglycemic level (<3.0 mmol/l) still remained in 5 of 11 patients at 60 min after the onset of exercise. The patients reported mild hypoglycemic symptoms during and after the test [8]. The increases in blood pyruvate (fourfold from basal level) and lactate (tenfold) were similar in patients and control subjects up to the 15-min sample. Serum insulin levels increased during and immediately after exercise in the patients and were significantly higher at 20 min after exercise in patients compared to control subjects (39 vs. 11 mU/l, $p < 0.05$; fig. 1).

Anaerobic exercise testing to exhaustion seems to be even more diagnostic for EIHI. Exercise with an intensity corresponding to 130% VO_2 max, which means that exercise leads to exhaustion, within 2–3 min elicited comparable maximal lactate levels in an EIHI patient and controls (10–11 mmol/l). The German index patient for EIHI was further tested at an institute of sports medicine. He, but not the controls,

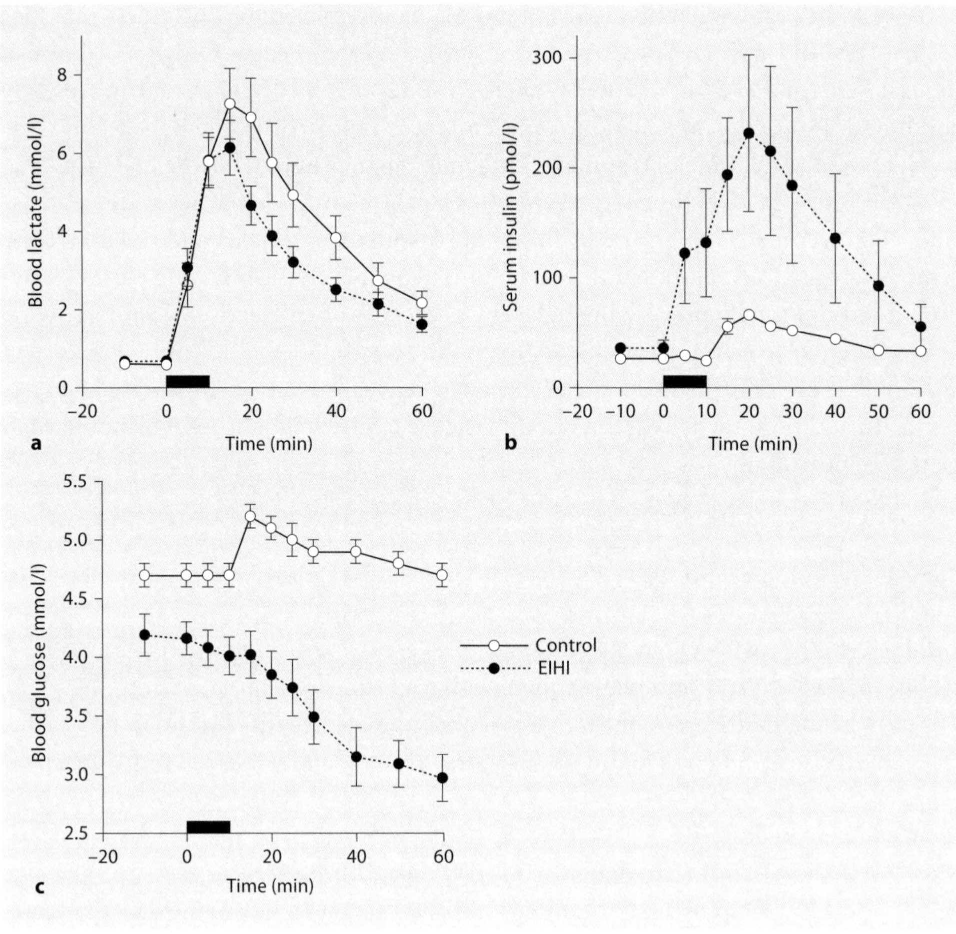

Fig. 1. Physical exercise test. Blood lactate (**a**), serum insulin (**b**), and blood glucose (**c**) concentrations before, during, and after a 10-min bicycle exercise (black bar) in healthy controls (white circles, n = 7) and EIHI patients (black circles, n = 11). Modified from Otonkoski et al. [8].

experienced a massive increase in insulin from 34 to 649 mU/l after the intense anaerobic test (fig. 2) [9]. The increase in insulin was much more pronounced with this protocol compared to milder exercise tests done earlier (insulin increase to 50–90 mU/l) in the same individual.

Suggested Exercise Protocol

Since the data for affected individuals are still sparse, we recommend the following extended protocol for exercise testing in adults after exclusion of cardiac risk factors. The increase in lactate is a particularly important aspect for the diagnosis. The protocol has to be individually adapted for children.

The bicycle exercise test should start after an 8- to 12-hour overnight fast without any significant exercise in the preceding 24 h. If this is not possible, a 4-hour fast

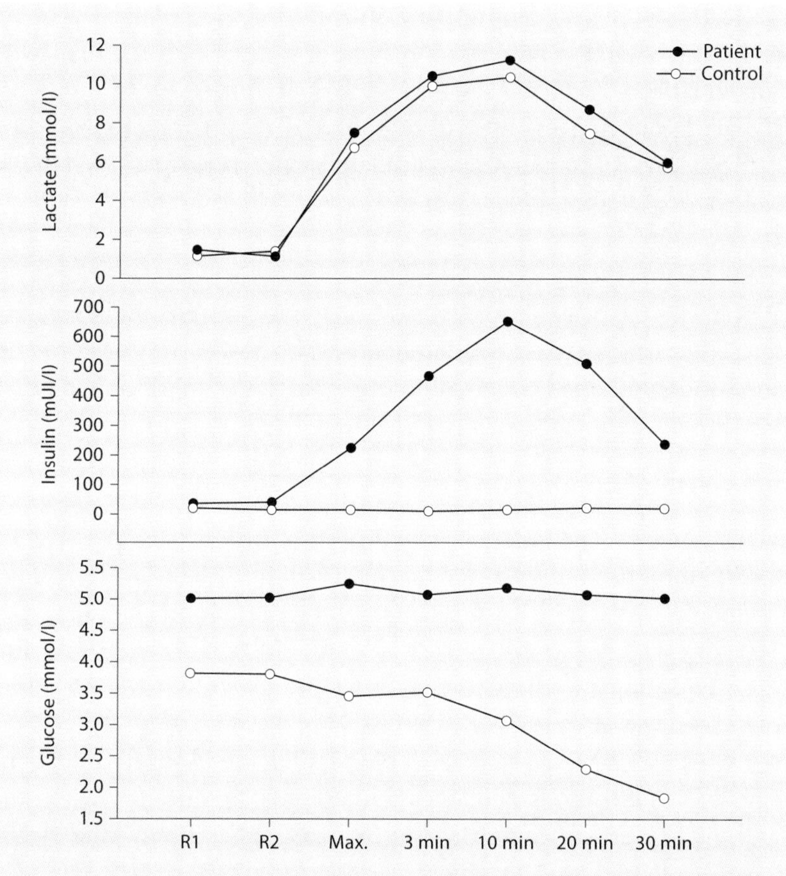

Fig. 2. Anaerobic exercise testing in an EIHI patient and a control on an electrically braked cycle ergometer with intense exercise leading to exhaustion within 2–4 min. Data are shown for lactate, insulin, glucose measured at rest (R1, R2) at maximal exercise (max.), and during recovery (3, 10, 20, 30 min). In the patient, the increase of lactate is accompanied by a rise of insulin resulting in hypoglycemia during the recovery phase. Lactate increased similarly in the control, but insulin did not rise and glucose remained stable.

will also be suitable. An intravenous cannula is inserted into a large (e.g. antecubital) vein for blood sampling. Blood is sampled at two 10-min intervals before the beginning of exercise to ensure a steady state. Blood samples are drawn on a total of about 10 occasions (including at –20, –10, and 0 min before the test; 2-min intervals during the exercise period and early recovery; and 5, 15, 30, 45, and 60 min during later recovery). Glucose, insulin, and lactate are measured. After a 5-min warm-up phase with low intensity, the workload is increased every minute until the patient is exhausted within 5–7 min (to make the total exercise test 8–12 min). Exhaustion is defined by the subject at the time at which he or she is unable to continue cycling due to leg muscle fatigue. The increase of the workload has to be fast to ensure that the total duration of the test is not more than 8–12 min, including the warm-up phase. Typical for EIHI is a marked increase of insulin in parallel with the change in lactate. This results in a drop of glucose during the recovery phase 20–45 min after exercise. It is essential that during and after testing there is awareness for symptoms of hypoglycemia and necessary preparations (availability of i.v. glucose) have been taken to treat severe hypoglycemia.

Intravenous Pyruvate Loading
The intravenous pyruvate test was performed to test the hypothesis that exercise-associated hypoglycemia is associated with an abnormal beta-cell response to circulating pyruvate. This hypothesis was based on experimental studies showing that in vitro overexpression of monocarboxylate transporter 1 (MCT-1) in the beta-cell conferred sensitivity of insulin release to exogenous pyruvate, but not lactate. To achieve lactate-induced insulin release, lactate dehydrogenase also had to be overexpressed [10]. Therefore, the patients received an intravenous bolus injection of sodium pyruvate (300 mmol/l; duration of 1 min) after an overnight fast. The dose was 46.3 ml (13.9 mmol)/1.7 m^2 body surface area. Samples for blood glucose, pyruvate, and serum insulin were taken at 0, 1, 3, 5, 10, and 30 min. As expected, the blood pyruvate concentration increased rapidly after the injection to levels comparable with those measured after physical exercise [8]. There was no response on circulating insulin whatsoever in the control subjects after the pyruvate injection. However, the patients' insulin levels had already increased significantly at 1 min after injection, and the highest concentrations were measured at 3 min. The 3-min peak response was 5.4 ± 0.9-fold in the patients, as compared with 0.94 ± 0.08-fold in control subjects ($p < 0.001$).

Pyruvate is an excellent substrate for mitochondrial ATP production, yet it does not stimulate insulin release when added to beta-cells. This phenomenon has been named the pyruvate paradox [11]. Experimental studies in rodents have shown that MCTs are not expressed in beta-cells, and that overexpression of MCT-1 in islets could induce pyruvate-induced insulin secretion [10]. As found for pyruvate in the controls, lactate infusion during low-intensity exercise (4-hour cycle exercise at 33–34% maximal O_2 uptake) in untrained fasting humans also revealed no major insulin increase despite a substantial rise of lactate concentration [12]. Against this background, it appeared likely that the basic pathogenetic mechanism in EIHI was an abnormal transport of pyruvate and lactate into the beta-cells, perhaps due to failed silencing of the MCTs. Because of the very low expression of lactate dehydrogenase in the beta-cell, pyruvate is more likely to be the direct stimulus for insulin secretion in the EIHI patients, as clearly shown by the pyruvate loading test.

The intravenous pyruvate test is a rapid, specific, and apparently safe test for EIHI associated with inappropriate pyruvate sensitivity of the beta-cells. This should be used as a secondary diagnostic test in individuals who demonstrate inappropriate exercise-induced insulin secretion.

Mutations in the Regulatory Regions of *SLC16A1*

The coding regions of all eight MCT genes (MCT-1 to MCT-8) were sequenced and revealed no disease-associated variants [8]. We then proceeded by performing a genome-wide linkage analysis with DNA samples of 10 EIHI patients from two families, using 430 microsatellite markers. A dominant analysis model revealed linkage to chromosome 1. Several genes of potential relevance were present within the linkage peak. However, the most obvious of them was *SLC16A1*, which encodes the MCT-1 protein. Since the coding region had already been shown to be normal, sequencing was targeted to the 5′ UTR and promoter regions. This time, disease-associated variants were found in both of the Finnish families. In one family, this was a single nucleotide polymorphism (a G → A change in exon 1). In the other family a 25-bp duplication immediately upstream of the transcription start site was found. In the German index patient, several candidate sequence variants were present. However, their association with the disease has not been definitively proven [13].

All of the identified mutations lie within the binding sites of several transcription factors, consistent with the idea that they could affect the regulation of the *SLC16A1* gene. This was supported by electrophoretic mobility shift analysis, which showed differential protein-binding activity of nuclear extracts from various cell types to the variant sequence containing the disease-associated single nucleotide polymorphism. Interestingly, one distinct band was lost specifically in the nuclear extract of the murine beta-cell line MIN6, suggestive of the disruption of a binding site in the beta-cell [13].

Experimental Studies of Pathogenetic Mechanisms

At this point it appeared very likely that the pathogenetic mechanism of EIHI involved failure of the transcriptional silencing of MCT-1 in the pancreatic beta-cells. However, it was impossible to obtain direct evidence of this because patient beta-cells could not be studied. Strong indirect evidence suggests that this is indeed the case. The evidence is based on three lines. First, in skin fibroblasts derived from EIHI patients, the transcriptional level of MCT-1 mRNA was twice as high as that in healthy controls, while the levels of MCT-4 mRNA were similar. Second, quantification of MCT-1 mRNA levels in a broad panel of mouse tissues showed broad variation, with a >100-fold difference between the highest (heart) and lowest tissue (thymus and pancreas). Remarkably, when pancreatic islets and acini were studied separately, practically all of the MCT-1 mRNA was found in the acinar fraction [13]. This further confirmed that MCT-1 is present in practically all other cell types, except the beta-cell, where it is transcriptionally silenced [14]. Finally, using a MCT-1 promoter reporter assay in MIN6 beta-cells, the variants found in the EIHI families were associated with four- to tenfold higher transcriptional activity as compared with the wild-type promoter.

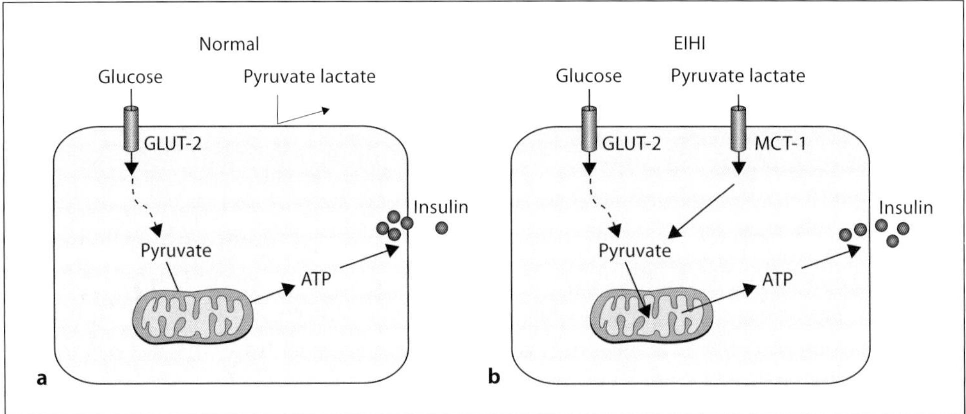

Fig. 3. Schematic presentation of the essential components of the presumed EIHI pathogenesis. During anaerobic exercise, the circulating levels of lactate and pyruvate increase sharply. In a healthy individual, these metabolites cannot enter into the beta-cell due to the lack of MCT-1 (**a**). In EIHI, MCT-1 is present and allows exogenous pyruvate to contribute to glycolytic ATP generation in the mitochondria, resulting in increased insulin secretion (**b**).

A mouse model conditionally overexpressing MCT-1 in the beta-cells was created by Pullen and Rutter [15]. Preliminary results from this model suggest that beta-cell-specific MCT-1 overexpression leads to pyruvate-induced insulin secretion, just as in the patients. Interestingly, the mice are also marginally glucose intolerant, consistent with the idea that the absence of MCT-1 in the beta-cell serves a dual function: (1) it prevents inappropriate insulin secretion due to exogenous pyruvate; and (2) it prevents the loss of pyruvate generated by glycolysis, ensuring that glucose is efficiently oxidized by mitochondria, allowing maximal ATP generation to trigger insulin release. Following this notion, the EIHI patients should be susceptible to type 2 diabetes. However, in our small clinical sample, there is no evidence for this.

Based on these studies, the molecular pathogenesis of EIHI can be summarized as outlined in figure 3.

Conclusion

The phenotype of EIHI is quite clear in our 3 index patients as well as in some of their affected family members. However, since the initial description of these individuals, no other clearly diagnosed cases have been found, even though we have tested a number of candidates who have had hypoglycemic symptoms associated with exercise. If the condition is so rare, it is remarkable that we identified the 3 cases in a very short time. Based on the experience from the less affected family members of our index cases, who would probably not have been diagnosed without the specific hypothesis-driven testing, it seems to us that mild forms of EIHI may be much more common than has been realized. The suspicion of EIHI should be kept in mind whenever the patient has symptoms suggestive of hypoglycemia triggered by anaerobic exercise. In these cases, specific testing should be considered using the exhaustive exercise and intravenous pyruvate tests as we propose.

References

1 Berger CM, Sharis PJ, Bracy DP, Lacy DB, Wasserman DH: Sensitivity of exercise-induced increase in hepatic glucose production to glucose supply and demand. Am J Physiol 1994;267:E411–E421.

2 Jenkins AB, Furler SM, Chisholm DJ, Kraegen EW: Regulation of hepatic glucose output during exercise by circulating glucose and insulin in humans. Am J Physiol 1986;250:R411–R417.

3 Shih ZQ, Wasserman DH, Vranic M: Metabolic implications of exercise and physical fitness in physiology and diabetes; in Porte D, Sherwin R (eds): Ellenberg and Rifkin's Diabetes Mellitus: Theory and Practice, ed 5. New York, Appleton and Lange, 1997, pp 653–687.

4 Marliss EB, Simantirakis E, Miles PD, Purdon C, Gougeon R, Field CJ, et al: Glucoregulatory and hormonal responses to repeated bouts of intense exercise in normal male subjects. J Appl Physiol 1991;71:924–933.

5 Marliss EB, Simantirakis E, Miles PD, Hunt R, Gougeon R, Purdon C, et al: Glucose turnover and its regulation during intense exercise and recovery in normal male subjects. Clin Invest Med 1992;15: 406–419.

6 Sigal RJ, Fisher S, Halter JB, Vranic M, Marliss EB: The roles of catecholamines in glucoregulation in intense exercise as defined by the islet cell clamp technique. Diabetes 1996;45:148–156.

7 Meissner T, Otonkoski T, Feneberg R, Beinbrech B, Apostolidou S, Sipila I, et al: Exercise induced hypoglycaemic hyperinsulinism. Arch Dis Child 2001;84: 254–257.

8 Otonkoski T, Kaminen N, Ustinov J, Lapatto R, Meissner T, Mayatepek E, et al: Physical exercise-induced hyperinsulinemic hypoglycemia is an autosomal-dominant trait characterized by abnormal pyruvate-induced insulin release. Diabetes 2003;52:199–204.

9 Meissner T, Friedmann B, Okun JG, Schwab MA, Otonkoski T, Bauer T, et al: Massive insulin secretion in response to anaerobic exercise in exercise-induced hyperinsulinism. Horm Metab Res 2005;37: 690–694.

10 Ishihara H, Wang H, Drewes LR, Wollheim CB: Overexpression of monocarboxylate transporter and lactate dehydrogenase alters insulin secretory responses to pyruvate and lactate in beta cells. J Clin Invest 1999;104:1621–1629.

11 Sener A, Kawazu S, Hutton JC, Boschero AC, Devis G, Somers G, et al: The stimulus-secretion coupling of glucose-induced insulin release. Effect of exogenous pyruvate on islet function. Biochem J 1978;176: 217–232.

12 Roef MJ, de Meer K, Kalhan SC, Straver H, Berger R, Reijngoud DJ: Gluconeogenesis in humans with induced hyperlactatemia during low-intensity exercise. Am J Physiol Endocrinol Metab 2003;284: E1162–E1171.

13 Otonkoski T, Jiao H, Kaminen-Ahola N, Tapia-Paez I, Ullah MS, Parton LE, et al: Physical exercise-induced hypoglycemia caused by failed silencing of monocarboxylate transporter 1 in pancreatic beta cells. Am J Hum Genet 2007;81:467–474.

14 Zhao C, Wilson MC, Schuit F, Halestrap AP, Rutter GA: Expression and distribution of lactate/monocarboxylate transporter isoforms in pancreatic islets and the exocrine pancreas. Diabetes 2001;50:361–366.

15 Pullen TJ, Rutter GA: Inducible expression of monocarboxylate transporter 1 (Mct1/Slc16a1) in the beta cell of transgenic mice: a model of exercise induced hyperinsulinism (abstract). Diabetologia 2010;53(Suppl 1):S36.

Timo Otonkoski, MD, PhD
Biomedicum Helsinki, Room C507b
PO Box 63
University of Helsinki
FI–00014 Helsinki (Finland)
Tel. +358 9 191 25692, E-Mail timo.otonkoski@helsinki.fi

Stanley CA, De León DD (eds): Monogenic Hyperinsulinemic Hypoglycemia Disorders.
Front Diabetes. Basel, Karger, 2012, vol 21, pp 182–190

HNF4A and Hyperinsulinemic Hypoglycemia

Ritika R. Kapoor · Chela T. James · Khalid Hussain

Clinical and Molecular Genetics Unit, The Developmental Endocrinology Research Group, Institute of Child Health, University College London and Great Ormond Street Hospital for Children NHS Trust London, London, UK

Abstract

Hepatocyte nuclear factor 4-alpha (HNF-4alpha encoded by the *HNF4A* gene) is a transcription factor that plays a key role in pancreatic development, maintenance of beta-cell mass, and regulation of insulin secretion. Mutations in the *HNF4A* gene cause young onset autosomal dominant diabetes mellitus (known as maturity-onset diabetes of the young type 1 or MODY1). Paradoxically, *HNF4A* gene mutations also can cause hyperinsulinemic hypoglycemia (HH) and macrosomia in the neonatal period. The HH due to *HNF4A* mutations typically presents in the first few days of life, and can be mild and transient or severe and persistent, requiring prolonged medical treatment. The hypoglycemia in this condition responds to treatment with the ATP-sensitive potassium channel agonist, diazoxide. These observations suggest that HNF-4alpha might have different roles in regulating pancreatic development, maintenance of beta-cell mass, and insulin secretion during the fetal, neonatal, and adult periods. The exact mechanism/s of HH due to mutations in *HNF4A* has not been elucidated yet.

Hepatocyte nuclear factor 4 alpha (HNF-4alpha) is a transcription factor encoded by the *HNF4A* gene. HNF-4alpha is known to play an important role in pancreatic development, maintenance of beta-cell mass, and regulating insulin secretion. Heterozygous mutations in the human *HNF4A* gene classically lead to maturity onset diabetes of the young subtype 1 (MODY1), a progressive type of early onset diabetes mellitus characterized by autosomal dominant inheritance and impaired glucose-stimulated insulin secretion from pancreatic beta-cells [1]. In addition, variations in the beta-cell-specific promoter (P2) elements of the *HNF4A* gene in humans are associated with increased risk of type 2 diabetes [2].

Recently, it has been demonstrated that heterozygous mutations in the *HNF4A* gene not only cause reduced insulin secretion in childhood/adult life, but also lead to increased insulin secretion during the in utero, neonatal, and childhood periods [3–

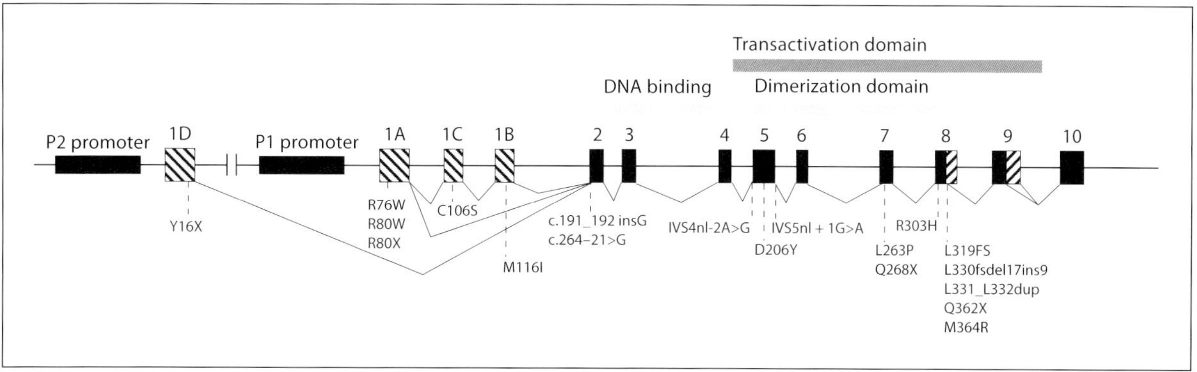

Fig. 1. Location of mutations in *HNF4A* known to cause hypoglycemia. *HNF4A* has 10 exons with up to 8 splice variants and 2 promoter regions.

7]. The consequences of this increased insulin secretion are fetal macrosomia (with the associated morbidity) and either transient or persistent hyperinsulinemic hypoglycemia (HH) [3–7]. The purpose of this chapter is to (1) provide a background to HNF-4alpha, and (2) review the recent literature describing the role of HNF-4alpha in relation to macrosomia and neonatal HH.

Background on *HNF4A*

HNF-4alpha is a transcription factor of the nuclear hormone superfamily with two zinc fingers as DNA-binding domains (fig. 1). The functional domains of HNF-4alpha are made up of an N-terminal activation function (AF-1, also known as A/B domain), two zinc fingers responsible for DNA binding (called the C domain), a potential ligand-binding domain (E domain), and the F domain [8]. The C-terminal domain has a region which is required for homodimerization, activation, and suppression. HNF-4alpha seems to play an important role in early embryonic development as homozygous *HNF4A* knockout mice die in utero [9]. During mouse embryogenesis, the *HNF4A* gene is first expressed in primary endoderm at E4.5, but is restricted to the visceral endoderm from E5.5 to 8.5 days [9]. Thereafter, expression of *HNF4A* becomes confined to the liver diverticulum; hindgut; mesonephric tubules of the kidney; and developing stomach, intestine, and pancreas [10]. In the adult mouse, *HNF4A* expression has been reported in liver, kidney, intestine, stomach, and pancreas [10].

The *HNF4A* gene is located on human chromosome 20q13.1–13.2. The gene has two promoters, P1 and P2, with P2 being upstream to P1. Nine isoforms (*HNF4A1–9*) are known to be produced by the gene by means of alternate splicing, polyadenylation [addition of poly(A) tail to the RNA molecule] and production of different transcripts by the two promoters [11]. The P1-derived isoforms are most abundant in the hepatic tissues, while the P2 promoter represents the major transcription site in beta-cells [11]. Isomers HNF4A1 to HNF4A6 are coded from the hepatic promoter (P1), whereas isoforms HNF4A7 to HNF4A9 are transcribed from the pancreatic P2 promoter. The *HNF4A* P2 promoter has functional binding sites for the transcription factors HNF-1alpha, HNF-1beta, and PDX1 [12]. *HNF4A* isoforms demonstrate both temporal and spatial variation in expression as well as a developmental switch in relative expression [11]. Fetal pancreas contains transcripts derived from the P1 promoter from 9 weeks to 19–26 weeks, whereas adult pancreas has no transcripts derived from the P1 promoter [11].

In the adult pancreatic beta-cell, HNF-4alpha has a key role in regulating the multiple transcriptional factor networks, and in combination with other hepatocyte nuclear factors (such as HNF-1alpha) has been proposed to form a functional regulatory loop [13, 14]. HNF-4alpha seems to be an abundant transcription factor in the islet and regulates a significant fraction of the pancreatic islet transcriptomes by binding directly to a large number of actively transcribed genes [13]. HNF-4alpha and HNF-1alpha occupy one another's promoters in the islets, thus establishing a hierarchical regulatory relationship between these two genes. In the pancreatic islet, HNF-4alpha expression depends on HNF-1alpha, and this effect is mediated through the direct occupation by HNF-1alpha of an alternate promoter in the *HNF4A* gene [13].

The expression of several genes which encode components of the glucose-dependent insulin secretion pathway are dependent upon HNF-4alpha [15]. These include glucose transporter 2, the glycolytic enzymes aldolase B and glyceraldehyde-3-phosphate dehydrogenase, and liver pyruvate kinase [15]. HNF-4alpa is critical for normal mitochondrial function and glucose-induced ATP generation with subsequent insulin secretion. The loss of HNF-4alpha function also leads to multiple defects in mitochondrial metabolism (including defective mitochondrial metabolism, impaired mitochondrial tricarboxylic acid cycle enzyme activity, and partial uncoupling of the mitochondrial respiratory chain), which further impairs glucose-stimulated insulin secretion [15]. Using the INS-1 cell line, it has been demonstrated that HNF-4alpha alters the mRNA expression of the mitochondrial E1 subunit and UCP2 (uncoupling protein 2) [15]. Defects in both of these contribute to impaired metabolism-secretion coupling. Hence, HNF-4alpha is critical for regulating glucose transport, glycolysis, and mitochondrial metabolism; and in doing so is crucial for glucose-stimulated insulin secretion.

HNF-4alpha also plays an important role in regulating beta-cell mass. The proliferative response (and activation of the Ras/ERK signaling cascade) of beta-cells seems to be dependent on HNF-4alpha. A significant number of genes and metabolic pathways involved in the regulation of beta-cell proliferation are dependent on HNF-4alpha [16].

Table 1. Table summarizing the duration of hypoglycemia due to *HNF4A* mutations in patients reported to date

Total number of cases identified	26
Duration of disease <1 month	12 (46.15%)
Duration of disease 3–6 months	2 (7.7%)
Duration of disease >6 months	12 (46.15%)

Hyperinsulinemic Hypoglycemia Due to Mutations in *HNF4A*

Mutations in the *HNF4A* gene typically lead to MODY 1, which is associated with impaired insulin secretion from the beta-cell. Recently, however, newborns with mutations in the *HNF4A* gene have been reported to have HH. In the first study describing the association of HH with mutations in the *HNF4A* gene, Pearson et al. [3] retrospectively examined birth weight and hypoglycemia in 108 patients from families with maturity onset diabetes mellitus due to *HNF4A* mutations. They found that *HNF4A* mutation carriers were born macrosomic, with a birth weight increased by a median of 790 g compared to family members that did not carry the mutation ($p < 0.001$). In addition to macrosomia, transient hypoglycemia was reported in 8 of 54 of these infants with heterozygous *HNF4A* mutations, with documented HH in 3 of the 8 cases. Of these 8 infants with hypoglycemia, 4 inherited the *HNF4A* mutation from their mother and 4 from their father, suggesting that hypoglycemia is independent of maternal glycemia. Subsequently, two further reports have described macrosomia and transient neonatal HH in MODY1 pedigrees with mutations in the *HNF4A* gene [4, 6].

However, the phenotype of HH due to *HNF4A* mutations is not limited to the mild transient hypoglycemia as reported in the first few studies. In 2008, we described a severe and persistent phenotype of HH coexisting with MODY1 in three families with novel *HNF4A* mutations [5]. The children with HH in these families were markedly macrosomic and developed severe HH requiring high concentrations of intravenous dextrose and subcutaneous glucagon infusions to maintain normoglycemia. Contrary to previous reports, the HH in the three infants did not resolve in the neonatal period and persisted well into childhood. Despite the severity of the initial presentation, the hypoglycemia was well controlled on diazoxide in all the patients. Recently, another family with neonatal macrosomia, MODY1, and persistent HH (up to 3 years) was described [17]. The duration of hypoglycemia in the patients reported so far has been summarized in table 1. Twelve of 26 patients (46%) have been reported to have persistence of hypoglycemia >6 months, of which 5 are known to have hypoglycemia for >2 years, with the longest duration being >8 years.

The prevalence of *HNF4A* mutations in a large cohort of patients with diazoxide-responsive HH (n = 220) was recently investigated and reported to be 5% [7]. In this large series, the distinctive features of *HNF4A* mutations were confirmed to be high birth weight (birth weight +2.4 SDS) and early age of presentation (median of 1 day). This series also confirmed that *HNF4A* mutations can cause persistent HH, and reported the oldest patient as being 8 years of age with ongoing hypoglycemia. Interestingly, a family history of diabetes was not a consistent feature of HH due to an *HNF4A* mutation in this study (4 of the 11 mutations had arisen de novo). The locations of the mutations described so far are summarized in figure 1. Due to the small number of patients reported so far, there is no clear genotype and phenotype correlation.

Mechanism/s of Hyperinsulinemic Hypoglycemia Due to *HNF4A* Mutations

Given that *HNF4A* plays a key role in regulation of pancreatic development, maintenance of beta-cell mass, and regulation of insulin secretion, it is not surprising that *HNF4A* mutations are associated with disorders of glucose homeostasis. The mechanism(s) by which mutations in *HNF4A* lead to MODY 1 includes defects in glucose-stimulated insulin secretion, mitochondrial dysfunction, and increased apoptosis. However, the mechanism(s) of HH due to *HNF4A* mutations is currently not known. It is possible that beta-cell exhaustion follows the early hypersecretion of insulin [3] or that the different phenotypes are a consequence of abnormal expression of different target islet genes. It is also possible that *HNF4A* might have a different role in the fetal period compared to adulthood in regulating pancreatic beta-cell mass, and there may be differences in temporal and spatial expression during development of the beta-cell.

Another possible mechanism of HH in patients with *HNF4A* mutations might involve the loss of interaction between HNF-4alpha and other nuclear receptors. Peroxisome proliferator-activated receptor-alpha (PPAR-alpha) is a member of the family of nuclear receptors that are activated by fatty acid ligands. Activated PPAR-alpha induces the transcription of genes involved in peroxisomal and mitochondrial beta-oxidation. PPAR-alpha plays an important role in regulating insulin secretion by controlling fatty acid oxidation in the beta-cell. Fasting upregulates PPAR-alpha which in turn activates fatty acid oxidation and prevents the accumulation of lipid signaling molecules required for insulin exocytosis. Gupta et al. [18] have shown that in HNF-4alpha-deficient beta-cells, the expression of PPAR-alpha is reduced. The reduction in the expression of PPAR-alpha could lead to the accumulation of lipids such as malonyl-CoA which are important in triggering insulin section [19]. In support of this hypothesis, PPAR-alpha null mice develop fasting HH [20].

As homozygous *HNF4A* knockout mice die early due to defective gastrulation [9], other attempts have been made to understand the role of HNF-4alpha using a beta-cell-specific knockout model. Using a Cre-*loxP* system, Gupta et al. [18] generated beta-cell-specific HNF-4alpha knockout mice and assessed glucose homeostasis in adult mice. As expected, deletion of HNF-4alpha in these mice led to glucose intolerance, but paradoxically also fasting and fed hyperinsulinism. Further studies in these mice showed there was no alteration of islet architecture or beta-cell mass. However, the beta-cell-specific HNF-4alpha knockout mice had a significant reduction in the mRNA levels of the Kir6.2 subunit of the pancreatic ATP-sensitive potassium channel subunit. In cotransfection assays, it was shown that HNF-4alpha binds and activates the promoter region of the Kir6.2 gene (*KCNJ11*). Thus, the reduction in the mRNA levels of the Kir6.2 subunit might explain the hyperinsulinism in these mice.

In another study, Pearson et al. [3] also used the Cre-*loxP* system to generate beta-cell-specific HNF-4alpha knockout mice and assessed glucose homeostasis during late gestation (E18.5 to E20). They found that these mice had increased insulin concentrations during the in utero period and HH in the newborn period. However, in contrast to the study by Gupta et al. [18], these mice showed no change in the expression of the *KCNJ11* gene. The findings of Pearson et al. [3] with regard to the expression of *KCNJ11* gene are supported by another study of beta-cell-specific HNF-4alpha knockout which also confirms normal expression of *KCNJ11* [21].

Thus, the precise mechanism by which mutations in HNF-4alpha lead to HH is currently unknown, but it is likely that defects in HNF-4alpha alter different gene expression patterns during early and later life (fig. 2).

Clinical Implications of *HNF4A* Mutations

The observations that *HNF4A* mutations can lead to macrosomia and HH in the neonatal period have several important clinical implications. In a pregnancy where the family is known to carry a mutation of the *HNF4A* gene, close surveillance for macrosomia and neonatal hypoglycemia is required regardless of whether the mother or the father carries the mutation or whether the affected parent has developed diabetes. Macrosomic infants are at an increased risk of developing shoulder dystocia with Erb's brachial palsy (increasing the risk of perinatal asphyxia), facial nerve palsy, and clavicular and humeral bone fractures, and will thus require close monitoring. Neonates with a family history of *HNF4A* mutations must have their blood glucose levels checked and monitored. Any newborn with unexplained macrosomia and HH should be tested for mutations in the *HNF4A* gene. The presence of a *HNF4A* mutation indicates that this patient is at risk of developing diabetes mellitus later in life and will require annual surveillance. The early detection of diabetes mellitus in these patients will allow early intervention and possibly reduce the impact of long-term diabetic complications.

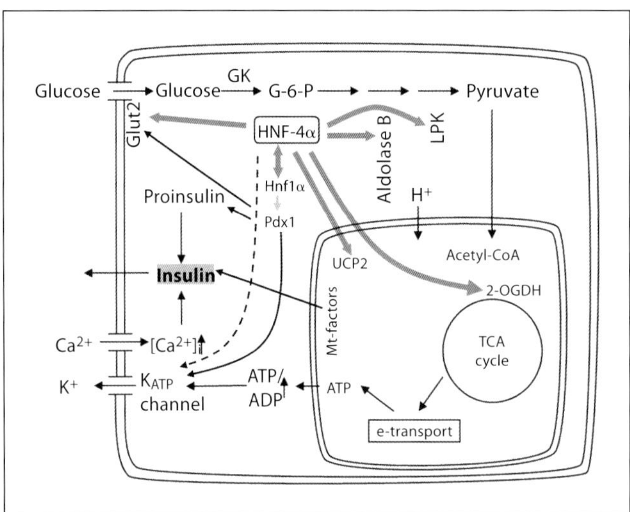

Fig. 2. Role of HNF-4alpha in the pancreatic beta-cell. HNF-4alpha regulates the expression of several genes involved in controlling glucose-induced insulin secretion. These include aldolase B, L-pyruvate kinase (LPK), glucose transporter 2 (Glut-2), UCP2 (uncoupling protein 2), 2-oxologlutarate dehydrogenase (2-OGDH) and transcription factor HNF-1alpha. HNF-1alpha in turn regulates PDX1 (pancreatic and duodenal homeobox 1) [22], which itself plays an important role in processing of proinsulin [23]. HNF-4alpha might also have a role in the regulation of the pancreatic beta-cell ATP-specific potassium (K_{ATP}) channel.

Conclusion

HNF-4alpha is a key transcription factor involved in regulation of pancreatic development, maintenance of beta-cell mass, and insulin secretion. Mutations in the *HNF4A* lead to a dual phenotype of MODY1 and neonatal HH with macrosomia. The HH can vary in severity and duration, and all cases reported so far have responded to treatment with diazoxide. The precise mechanism of HH is unclear, but could involve HNF-4alpha altering different gene expression patterns during early and later life. Neonates with a family history of *HNF4A* mutations must have their blood glucose levels checked and monitored. Any newborn with unexplained macrosomia and HH should be tested for mutations in the *HNF4A* gene. The presence of a *HNF4A* mutation indicates that this patient is at risk of developing diabetes mellitus later in life and will require annual surveillance.

References

1 Yamagata K, Furuta H, Oda N, Kaisaki P, Menzel S, Cox NJ, Fajans SS, Signorini S, Stoffel M, Bell GI: Mutations in the hepatocyte nuclear factor-4alpha gene in maturity-onset diabetes of the young (MODY1). Nature 1996;384:458–460.

2 Silander K, Mohlke KL, Scott LJ, Peck EC, Hollstein P, Skol AD, Jackson AU, Deloukas P, Hunt S, Stavrides G, Chines PS, Erdos MR, Narisu N, Conneely KN, Li C, Fingerlin TE, Dhanjal SK, Valle TT, Bergman RN, Tuomilehto J, Watanabe RM, Boehnke M, Collins FS: Genetic variation near the hepatocyte nuclear factor-4 alpha gene predicts susceptibility to type 2 diabetes. Diabetes 2004;53:1141–1149.

3 Pearson ER, Boj SF, Steele AM, Barrett T, Stals K, Shield JP, Ellard S, Ferrer J, Hattersley AT: Macrosomia and hyperinsulinaemic hypoglycaemia in patients with heterozygous mutations in the HNF4A gene. PLoS Med 2007;4:e118.

4 Fajans SS, Bell GI: Macrosomia and neonatal hypoglycaemia in RW pedigree subjects with a mutation (Q268X) in the gene encoding hepatocyte nuclear factor 4alpha (HNF4A). Diabetologia 2007;50:2600–2601.

5 Kapoor RR, Colclough K, Flanagan S, Wales J, Conn J, Ellard S, Hussain K: Persistent hyperinsulinaemic hypoglycaemia and maturity onset diabetes of the young (MODY1) due to heterozygous mutations in the HNF4A gene. Diabetes 2008;57:1659–1663.

6 Conn JJ, Simm PJ, Oats JJ, Nankervis AJ, Jacobs SE, Ellard S, Hattersley AT: Neonatal hyperinsulinaemic hypoglycaemia and monogenic diabetes due to a heterozygous mutation of the HNF4A gene. Aust NZ J Obstet Gynaecol 2009;49:328–330.

7 Flanagan SE, Kapoor RR, Mali G, Cody D, Murphy N, Schwahn B, Siahanidou T, Banerjee I, Akcay T, Rubio-Cabezas O, Shield J, Hussain K, Ellard S: Diazoxide-responsive hyperinsulinemic hypoglycemia caused by HNF4A gene mutations. Eur J Endocrinol 2010;162:987–992.

8 Ryffel GU: Mutations in the human genes encoding the transcription factors of the hepatocyte nuclear factor (HNF)1 and HNF4 families: functional and pathological consequences. J Mol Endocrinol 2001;27:11–29.

9 Chen WS, Manova K, Weinstein DC, Duncan SA, Plump AS, Prezioso VR, Bachvarova RF, Darnell JE Jr: Disruption of the HNF-4 gene, expressed in visceral endoderm, leads to cell death in embryonic ectoderm and impaired gastrulation of mouse embryos. Genes Dev 1994;8:2466–2477.

10 Taraviras S, Monaghan AP, Schültz G, Kelsey G: Characterization of the mouse HNF-4 gene and its expression during mouse embryogenesis. Mech Dev 1994;48:67–79.

11 Harries LW, Locke JM, Shields B, Hanley NA, Hanley KP, Steele A, Njølstad PR, Ellard S, Hattersley AT: The diabetic phenotype in HNF4A mutation carriers is moderated by the expression of HNF4A isoforms from the P1 promoter during fetal development. Diabetes 2008;57:1745–1752.

12 Thomas H, Jaschkowitz K, Bulman M, Frayling TM, Mitchell SM, Roosen S, Lingott-Frieg A, Tack CJ, Ellard S, Ryffel GU, Hattersley AT: A distant upstream promoter of the HNF-4alpha gene connects the transcription factors involved in maturity-onset diabetes of the young. Hum Mol Genet 2001;10:2089–2097.

13 Odom DT, Zizlsperger N, Gordon DB, Bell GW, Rinaldi NJ, Murray HL, Volkert TL, Schreiber J, Rolfe PA, Gifford DK, Fraenkel E, Bell GI, Young RA: Control of pancreas and liver gene expression by HNF transcription factors. Science 2004;303:1378–1381.

14 Boj SF, Parrizas M, Maestro MA, Ferrer J: A transcription factor regulatory circuit in differentiated pancreatic cells. Proc Natl Acad Sci USA 2001;98:14481–14486.

15 Wang H, Maechler P, Antinozzi PA, Hagenfeldt KA, Wollheim CB: Hepatocyte nuclear factor 4alpha regulates the expression of pancreatic beta-cell genes implicated in glucose metabolism and nutrient-induced insulin secretion. J Biol Chem 2000;275:35953–35959.

16 Gupta RK, Gao N, Gorski RK, White P, Hardy OT, Rafiq K, Brestelli JE, Chen G, Stoeckert CJ Jr, Kaestner KH: Expansion of adult beta-cell mass in response to increased metabolic demand is dependent on HNF-4alpha. Genes Dev 2007;21:756–769.

17 Pingul MM, Hughes N, Wu A, Stanley CA, Gruppuso PA. Hepatocyte nuclear factor 4α gene mutation associated with familial neonatal hyperinsulinism and maturity-onset diabetes of the young. J Pediatr 2011;158:852–854.

18 Gupta RK, Vatamaniuk MZ, Lee CS, Flaschen RC, Fulmer JT, Matschinsky FM, Duncan SA, Kaestner KH: The MODY1 gene HNF-4alpha regulates selected genes involved in insulin secretion. J Clin Invest 2005;115:1006–1015.

19 Prentki M, Joly E, El-Assaad W, Roduit R: Malonyl-CoA signaling, lipid partitioning, and glucolipotoxicity: role in beta-cell adaptation and failure in the etiology of diabetes. Diabetes 2002;51:S405–S413.

20 Gremlich S, Nolan C, Roduit R, Burcelin R, Peyot ML, Delghingaro-Augusto V, Desvergne B, Michalik L, Prentki M, Wahli W: Pancreatic islet adaptation to fasting is dependent on peroxisome proliferator-activated receptor alpha transcriptional up-regulation of fatty acid oxidation. Endocrinology 2005;146:375–382.

21 Miura A, Yamagata K, Kakei M, Hatakeyama H, Takahashi N, Fukui K, Nammo T, Yoneda K, Inoue Y, Sladek FM, Magnuson MA, Kasai H, Miyagawa J, Gonzalez FJ, Shimomura I: Hepatocyte nuclear factor-4alpha is essential for glucose-stimulated insulin secretion by pancreatic beta-cells. J Biol Chem 2006;281:5246–5257.

22 Gerrish K, Cissell MA, Stein R: The role of hepatic nuclear factor 1 alpha and PDX-1 in transcriptional regulation of the pdx-1 gene. J Biol Chem 2001;276:47775–47784.

23 Wang H, Iezzi M, Theander S, Antinozzi PA, Gauthier BR, Halban PA, Wollheim CB: Suppression of Pdx-1 perturbs proinsulin processing, insulin secretion and GLP-1 signalling in INS-1 cells. Diabetologia 2005;48:720–731.

Dr. Khalid Hussain
Clinical and Molecular Genetics Unit
The Developmental Endocrinology Research Group
Institute of Child Health
University College London
30 Guilford Street
London WC1N 1EH (UK)
Tel. +44 20 7 905 2128, E-Mail K.Hussain@ich.ucl.ac.uk

Author Index

Subject Index